SEX, DRUGS
AND SCRUBS
MORE THAN A LOVE STORY
BY J.A. Alexander

This is a work of fiction. Names, characters, businesses, places, events, locales, and incidents are either the products of the author's imagination or used in a fictitious manner. Any resemblance to actual persons, living or dead, or actual events is purely coincidental.

All rights reserved
Copyright © 2021
This book is copyright under the Berne Convention.
No part of this book may be used or reproduced in any manner whatsoever without written permission from the author.

ISBN: 978-1-7367599-0-5

Printed in the United States of America

To the doctors, the real physicians; the nurses, the angels of mercy; and the health care workers, the unsung heroes, who are called upon daily to struggle to relieve suffering, prevent disability, and prolong life. Thank you for your dedication, your sacrifice, and your selflessness.
And to Claire, thank you for the future.

"All you have to do is write one true sentence. Write the truest sentence you know."

—Ernest Hemingway

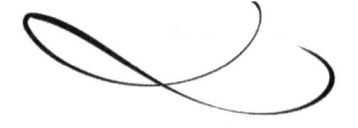

Introduction

The United States is ranked 11th in the world among industrialized nations in health care, yet the cost of health care in this country is the highest in the world and double the cost in France, the country with the best-ranking in health care. There are multiple reasons why Americans pay more and get less, but one major factor is physician quality.

Health care quality is tied to physician quality. This country once had the best health care in the world because it had the best physicians in the world. Those physicians were trained in a system that went back to Dr. William Osler, the Father of Modern Medicine.

However, the original methods damaged doctors during their training period and left many of them with a type of post-traumatic stress syndrome. Reforms were instituted to protect them while doing their internships and residencies, but those reforms left deficits in their training experience.

The medical profession needs to find a way to replicate the previous training experience without compromising the physician in the process. To do that, the scope of the training in a given field could be narrowed or the time spent in training increased. The scope of the different fields of medicine could be decreased and the number of fields increased so less time would be necessary to become proficient in a narrower field. The basic sciences could be moved to college and made prerequisites for medical school entrance, thus opening up most of medical school for clinical training. But to solve the problem, physicians need to take their profession back. Turning health care over to the private sector and giving corporations control has resulted in an escalation in cost coupled with a decrease in quality. Physicians should be controlling health care, not those driven by profit or political gain.

Since life is the most precious thing anyone possesses, health care should be a priority, and relieving suffering, preventing disability, and prolonging life should be a fundamental sociological premise. In order to fulfill that mandate, well-trained, dedicated, intelligent physicians are needed. The practice of medicine can only attract the best and brightest if physicians are respected members of society, adequately compensated, and given the opportunity to live productive lives.

Health care becoming a business changed all that and diminished the profession's ability to attract the type of individuals who make good physicians.

    This work of fiction is a story about what it took to make a doctor when doctors were physicians, not providers. It is about a young doctor doing his internship in a city/county hospital in the early seventies and what it took for him to become a competent, well-trained physician. It is about his struggle to have a normal life, to find love, and to maintain hope in the face of the daunting challenges he faced. It is one year in the life of a young doctor going through hell, but finding heaven in the love of a beautiful, exceptional, young woman.

> "The few own the many because they possess the means of livelihood of all ... The country is governed for the richest, for the corporations, the bankers, the land speculators, and for the exploiters of labor. The majority of mankind are working people. So long as their fair demands—the ownership and control of their livelihoods—are set at naught, we can have neither men's rights nor women's rights. The majority of mankind is ground down by industrial oppression in order that the small remnant may live in ease."
>
> —Helen Keller, *Rebel Lives: Helen Keller*

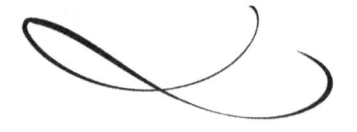

Table of Contents

Part 1: Orientation
- Chapter 1: Sharon 1
- Chapter 2: Lysergic Acid Diethylamide 52
- Chapter 3: The Concert 64
- Chapter 4: Falling in Love 87
- Chapter 5: Dr. Sheffield 101

Part 2: Internal Medicine
- Chapter 6: The Wards 115
- Chapter 7: The ED 176

Part 3: Surgery
- Chapter 8: The Wards 213
- Chapter 9: The Halloween Party 235
- Chapter 10: The ED 250
- Chapter 11: The Trauma Service 263

Part 4: OB/GYN
- Chapter 12: New Year's Eve 274
- Chapter 13: The ED 293
- Chapter 14: Labor and Delivery 311
- Chapter 15: The Wards 319

Part 5: Pediatrics
- Chapter 16: The Wards and the Match Game 325
- Chapter 17: The Nursery and the California Trip 354
- Chapter 18: Sharon's Fight for Life 378
- Chapter 19: The ED 395
- Chapter 20: It's Over 401

Epilogue 427

Essay on Health Care in the U.S. 430

About the Author 437

"And therefore, never send to know for whom the bell tolls; it tolls for thee."

—John Donne

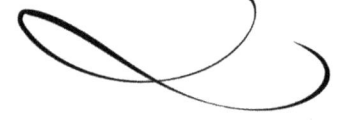

Part 1: Orientation

"I have written a wicked book, and feel spotless as a lamb."

—Herman Melville

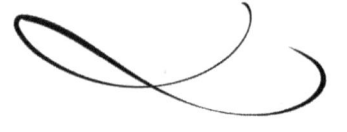

1
Sharon

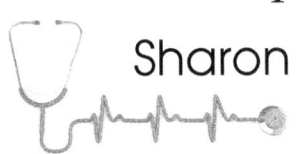

Dave walked out of the white-hot heat of the Southern summer sun and into the buzz and hum of the muggy humid atmosphere of the administrative offices of the hospital. The place had the smell and shabby well-worn appearance of every other city/county teaching hospital in the country. He was going to complete his registration, sign his contract, and officially begin his internship at University Hospital, a teaching hospital associated with a top medical school in the South. Like the Grady in Atlanta, Charity in New Orleans, or Parkland in Dallas, University Hospital served the indigent population of a large metropolis and its surrounding area.

There were still a number of new interns milling around in the reception area when he entered, and about a dozen were standing in a line at the front desk. Dave recognized two of his friends in the line: Henry, a fraternity brother and college roommate, and Mike, one of his roommates from medical school. Dave introduced his two former roommates and joined them on the front steps of the administration building after he completed his registration.

Henry greeted him. "When did you get in, Dave? Do you have a place to live yet? I am living in a house on the Park, and one of my roommates left today to do his internship at Harvard. It's a big house with four bedrooms—well, five, but we turned the one downstairs into a zoom room."

"Zoom room?" Dave asked and laughed.

"One of my roommates is an audiophile. He came up with the idea of putting a killer sound system in the room, taking all the furniture out, covering the floor with cushions and pillows, putting black-out paper over the window, and replacing all the light bulbs with black lights. The results: zoom room," Henry explained.

"Or opium den. How much herb are you smoking these days, Henry?" Dave asked.

"I am just a social smoker, but my roommates indulge fairly frequently. I prefer an expensive scotch with a splash of water. There are four flight attendants who live next door, the park is right there, and the area is considered the coolest and hippest place in the city to live. What do you say? I was going to pick up the rent on the other bedroom and turn it into a study, but for you, I will continue to share a bathroom." Henry was enthusiastic about Dave moving in and the two of them living together again.

Henry's family was wealthy. He had a trust fund that gave him a significant income, plus he got revenue from his family's holdings. He had never attended public school.

"Sounds great, but I already have a place. I rented a one-bedroom apartment on the north side in a singles complex that has a great pool. But what about Mike?"

Mike had been following the conversation closely just waiting to be asked. "I am staying in a Motel 6 trying to find a place. How much is the rent?"

Mike was from a blue-collar, working-class background. His grandparents were immigrants, and he was the first one in his family to attend college.

"It is a hundred a month." Henry thought maybe it was better to have the extra room than to share a bathroom with someone he didn't know, even if there were two sinks. "There is a party tonight. You can come by, meet the other two guys, and we can talk about it. Dave, you need to make the party tonight. Like I said, there are four stewardesses who live next door. One is really something, I mean she is drop-dead gorgeous with a great body. She dated Bar for a while but dumped him when she found out he was doing his internship in Boston. The house on the other side is owned by a gay couple, and they are the ones giving the party. It's to celebrate Bar moving out because he was a little less than tolerant of gays."

"You know I would never miss a party. Who is this Bar guy? Why don't you date this flight attendant if she's so hot?" Dave asked.

"Bar was something else. He was the number one guy in our class and had the highest score in the country on the National Boards. Bar is not his name; he uses his initials as a nickname. He is a narcissistic sociopathic asshole." Henry frowned, then brightened. "I have a girlfriend I have been seeing for about a year. She is an account manager for a PR firm with clients all over the South, so she travels a lot. I have to pick her up at the airport later this afternoon. She makes enough money to keep me in the style I am accustomed to," Henry joked.

"Since when do you need someone else's money? Wait, her family is wealthy too? Is this a family merger, rather than a romance?" Dave ribbed Henry.

Mike was more than a little envious. He had the view that things came way too easily for guys like Henry, but Dave appreciated Henry and the way he "got" life. Henry saw things clearly. To Henry, life was short, and in the overall scheme of things, the individual was insignificant. He was too educated, too smart, and too well read to think otherwise. His understanding of the pathos of the human condition and the state of mankind was why he had become a doctor.

Mike was the exact opposite of Henry in every way.

Henry laughed off Dave's comment. "My girlfriend and I come from similar backgrounds. I like her a lot; I could move in with her, but I am staying at the Park house for now. I have to admit she seems perfect for me but—one more but—I know this year is going to be tough, and I don't want any distractions," Henry explained.

Henry was aware people pursued him for his wealth. He knew that women targeted him, and men wanted to benefit from knowing him. He had never dated a girl who didn't have money, and he was very particular about whom he associated with, always carefully evaluating them to make sure they were genuine. Dave Cameron was as genuine, honest, and open as anyone could be; he was trusting, idealistic, and truthful to a fault. Henry's relationship with him was based on Dave's solid character and integrity; Henry felt Dave was his best friend.

"You can meet Sherry tonight, and I want to introduce you to Sharon, the flight attendant I was telling you about. I think the two of you will connect." Henry smiled at Dave.

"This is not like you, Henry, getting involved and setting someone up," Dave responded.

"I'm not; I'm simply facilitating a meeting between two people I like. Besides, I want her to be with someone decent. Wait until you meet her. I am not kidding; she is beautiful and smart with the best body I have seen." Henry added, "She's had a lot of men after her since she dumped Bar, hitting on her and asking her out, but she turns most of them down. I think she will like you though because you two are a lot alike." As Henry continued to tell Dave about Sharon in glowing terms, Dave started to get excited about meeting her.

The heat and humidity got to them after a while. Henry and Dave exchanged addresses and phone numbers, Henry gave Mike his address for the party that night, and Mike left. Henry continued to talk to Dave after Mike left. "He seems OK, but I am not sure. He is pretty rough around the edges."

"I was rough around the edges when we met," Dave countered.

"You weren't rough around the edges. You were a diamond in the rough. All you needed was a little polishing. I am not sure this guy is even a gem stone, much less a diamond. Well, we will see." They said goodbye with Dave promising to be at the party.

Dave smiled to himself as he thought about the way Henry had "polished" him. Henry had taught Dave how to dress and about wine, food, art, and culture. He pointed Dave to the great writings that were the foundation of Western civilization. Dave read the classics, along with the points and counterpoints of religion, politics, and philosophy. Henry had indeed polished him, expanding his knowledge and understanding of almost everything. Thanks to Henry, he became better read, better educated, and more sophisticated.

Dave drove to his apartment on the north side. The apartment was perfect for him, and it was also a hundred and fifty a month. His salary was four hundred and fifty, with a hundred for his car note, about fifty for gas, phone, and withholding, that left him around two hundred a month to live on. He would take most of his meals at the hospital, his dry cleaning was free, and the apartment had a washer and dryer in his section of the complex, so all he had to do for laundry was buy was detergent. His benefits covered everything else. His one luxury was his car. Dave was a car guy, so he figured the hundred a month was worth it to enjoy his car.

Dave hadn't had a date for three months. When the student nurse he had been dating found out he was moving to take an internship in another city and he didn't ask her to go with him, they parted. Thinking of her caused Dave to remember his other relationships.

During his junior year in high school, he starting dating a sophomore cheerleader. They were the American fairy tale, a real piece of true Americana—the star football player and the cheerleader. She was blond, cheerleader cute with dimples, big blue eyes, great legs, and well-developed breasts. They went through a period of making out in his car then later that year, when it came down to it, she said yes.

She was fifteen and he was sixteen. They had unprotected sex in the back seat of his Chevy. Fortunately, her eighteen-year-old sister went to a different doctor from the one she usually saw, got a prescription for BCPs, and gave the pills to her younger sister.

They went out every weekend, ending up in the back seat of the Chevy getting it done. Dave had a key to his grandfather's beach house, and when he was sure no one was going to be there, they would drive for over an hour to spend time there. They were innocent, open, and crazy about each other, so they learned about sex with no inhibitions or restraints. She told him what she liked, he told her what he liked, they tried new things and experimented until they got it right. They would shower together before they had to go back, and they explored each other's bodies as they soaped and washed one another.

In the summer, she would get her girlfriends to cover for her so they could spend the night together at the beach house. They would go to the beach and swim in the morning, then go sailing in the afternoon, and have sex at night. They went skinny dipping some nights and had sex on the beach. Of course, there were always the showers.

When he started college, he drove home every weekend to see her. Then he pledged a fraternity and there were parties on the weekends he wanted to go to and was expected to attend as a pledge. He stopped going home and started dating college girls. She started dating a basketball player, and the next summer, he heard they got married after they graduated. He did not know it at the time, but it would be a long time before he had a relationship that even came close to what he had with her.

He dated a number of sorority girls in college with a lot of making out but nothing that got serious enough for sex on a regular basis. He spent the summer between college and med school at the beach house, sailing and reading. Occasionally, some friends would drive down. They would hang out on the beach during the day then spend the nights playing table shuffle board and drinking beer at the dive beach bar down the road. But it was strictly a stag affair. On the weekends his parents were at the beach house, he would go home to water ski with friends who had stayed home or returned after college. But almost everyone he knew from high school was married.

The summer ended, and he went back to start medical school in the same city where he attended college. Tommy was dating the girl he dated in college. She was in graduate school at the university and when she finished grad school, they got married. Tommy stayed at the hospital associated with the med school they attended to do a straight Surgery internship, but he and Dave drifted apart after he married.

High school had been the early 60s, college was the mid-60s, but medical school was the late 60s. The sexual revolution was in full swing. Dave smiled to himself as he remembered the women, and they were women, not high school or college girls, he had been with before he met the student nurse. They were independent women who had not married their high school or college boyfriends but instead had joined the work force. They were strong, confident, hedonistic, and not necessarily looking for love. They were looking for Mr. Goodbar; if they found love, that was fine, but it would be with Mr. Goodbar.

Two of them were just fuck buddies; not even friends with benefits, but straight up fuck buddies. He met both of them at the pool, and their bikinis did little to hide their assets or their intent. He never knew what they did or where they worked. In fact, he never went out with them and everything took place in the afternoons at their apartments. In the summer, he would find one at the pool and when it wasn't pool weather, he would simply go to one's apartment and knock on the door.

He knew they went out with other guys and may have even been seeing someone regularly, but that didn't bother him. The sex was too good. They never talked much; they just fucked, and that was what it was—fucking and nothing else. One had red hair and very pale skin that showed sexy tan lines in the summer. The other was blond, but it was bottle blond, and she was tan all over. They were both hot, uninhibited, and had no restraint on their libidos.

He dated a NASCAR hostess. She posed in revealing bikinis for the calendars you see in auto repair shops advertising motor products or in skimpy outfits in magazines and catalogs promoting the same motor additives. She presented the Champagne to the winner at NASCAR races. She also did regional TV commercials for NASCAR and a national spot for one the motor products. She was like Dave's own personal centerfold. Even though there was a lot of sex, there was also companionship and conversation, but she was divorced and wanted no part of a meaningful relationship. She had an itch, and Dave scratched it for her, that was all.

During the school year, Dave and Tommy stuck to their routine during the week and didn't go out. Classes and labs went from eight in the morning until five in the afternoon. After class, they got something to eat, studied until ten or eleven then had a beer or two and went to bed. If they knocked off at ten, they would go to a college bar they had frequented as undergrads, drink a couple of beers and play pool. If they stopped at eleven, they would have a beer in the apartment, talk, and watch a little late-night TV.

Dave was a good athlete and excelled at sports, so he excelled at "sport fucking." In truth, Dave was practicing and perfecting his craft those two years just as he did with all the other sports he played. It didn't occur to him at the time that he was using sex and the women he was seeing to help him deal with the stress of medical school.

He met the student nurse his first day on the Medicine wards his junior year. She was petite, cute, and even under the starched formless student nurse's uniform, he could tell she had curves. The medical students and nursing students were getting tours of the hospital when the two groups intermingled. She flirted with him, and he asked her out on the spot. She reminded him a lot of the cheerleader except she had dark brown eyes and soft brown hair; after they went out that night, his "sport fucking" days were over.

They had the same kind of relationship he had with the cheerleader. Their time together taught him that sex just for the physical pleasure of it was great, but it was hollow. There had to be an emotional connection and that intangible spark between two people for it to be good. The pornographic, raw, anything-goes stuff brought him immense pleasure, but there was something missing. She showed him what it was. As he lay there, he wondered if he would ever find it again, and he fell asleep thinking about her and the cheerleader with a sense of loss.

He slept for a few hours and woke up with a slight ache in his heart. He lay for a while thinking about the woman he was going to meet tonight, then he thought what a pitiful loser he was, obsessing about someone he had never met.

Dave had a country cousin he grew up with, and they had remained close. At the height of his womanizing, she had told him, "I hope you don't fly over all the flowers in the garden and land on a pile of manure in the barn yard." He had surely flitted over two flowers, and he knew he had landed on a few piles of manure in his "sport fucking" days.

But no matter how good those two relationships had been, they had not been great love affairs. He knew that even though he feared he would never find anyone like the cheerleader or the student nurse again, they were not what he wanted. Maybe he had thrown away as good as it gets for something that didn't exist; that worried him, yet he knew what he wanted. He wanted someone he could not live without, someone to experience life with until they grew old together and died in each other's arms. He wanted a love so strong they could not be parted even in death. He wanted passion, desire, and uncontrollable lust coupled with a deep everlasting love. Maybe he was just too idealistic and naive, but that was who he was and that was what he wanted. He started to sing "Tonight" from *West Side Story* in the shower but stopped thinking how lame and pathetic he seemed he was who he was, and that was a naïve romantic guy looking forward to tonight and the girl he was going to meet.

He doused himself with incense oil, put on his favorite T-shirt, jeans, and his tire tread sandals. The T-shirt was grey with Gandalf's image and Lord of the Rings printed on the back. Dave loved Tolkien. On his bookshelf were bound versions of *The Hobbit* and *The Lord of the Rings*. Tolkien understood there was evil in the world and good had to unite to confront evil, but when good combated evil, it was often consumed in the process, like matter and anti-matter.

As a doctor, Dave wanted to facilitate the fight against pain, suffering, disability, and the greatest evil of all—death. But there was more to it than that. The senseless, never-ending Vietnam War, bigotry and hate, the racism of the Jim Crow South that was the legacy of slavery, the unbridled greed of unregulated capitalism, and man's never-ending inhumanity to man were other issues Dave wanted to see eradicated. Among his books were the works of Charles Dickens. He felt the lines in *A Christmas Carol* regarding the two children of mankind, Ignorance and Want, were among the most important in literature. "Beware of these two children, Ignorance and Want, but beware of this boy, Ignorance, most of all."

The concentration of wealth, and the power it brought, led to ignorance and want. The cycle of dictator or king; versus oligarchy or rule by the aristocracy, the few; versus a representative government had been present throughout the history of Western civilization. Plato explored the subject extensively. Like Pericles, Dave believed it took an educated, informed, and engaged populous to sustain a representative government. He thought the ancient Greeks had established the correct path for humanity to follow thousands of years ago, yet humans continued to make the same mistakes that allowed ignorance and want to plague mankind. Occupying a place of prominence with his other books was a leather-bound version of *The Iliad*.

Dave hoped his generation would end the vicious cycles of history, and through the revolution of the 60s counter-culture, set humanity on the right path. There had to be a better way, and he believed it was the Greek way of science, reason, and representative government coupled with humanism. That book was on his shelf too, *The Greek Way*.

He knew that every generation before his hoped for an end to war, poverty, and injustice. His grandfather had served on a destroyer in the North Atlantic fighting German submarines in the First World War, the war to end all wars. It didn't end all wars. His father had driven a tank across Europe with the Third Army in World War Two—a war that almost destroyed the entire world. His father wrote a letter to his mother telling her that the reason he was fighting was so his son, whom he had never seen, would not have to fight a war. But the sons of the men of his father's generation were currently fighting a war they could not win, for no valid reason, in Vietnam.

His grandfather had hoped his generation would end war, and his father had hoped his generation would set things right. Now, Dave hoped his generation would demand a better future, but deep in his heart, Dave knew what Tolkien and Dickens knew—there is evil in the world.

Hemingway's books were on his shelf, *A Farewell to Arms*, *The Old Man and The Sea*, and *For Whom the Bell Tolls*. Like the characters in Hemingway's books, Dave would try to make things better even in the face of insurmountable odds, and maybe in the process, he could improve the human condition just a little.

One of the problems was the struggle individuals faced in holding on to the benefits of their efforts. The crux of that struggle lay in the basic concept of government. Did government exist to benefit the governed, or did the governed exist to benefit those who govern? Did government exist to benefit everyone, or did government exist only to benefit those in power or those who had wealth? Did wealth and power rule, or did everyone have a voice? He had read Marx, but rejected collectivism and the communist utopia because he knew it could never work. But Steinbeck was another story. Dave loved Steinbeck like he loved Dickens. Organizing to protect the many from exploitation by the few, laws to protect the worker, and helping those in need—these were things that did work. Dave believed in Eleanor Roosevelt's concept that had been proven over and over: we do well when we all do well. Things were always better when everyone had something, no one had nothing, and no one had everything. He had *The Grapes of Wrath* on his shelf, but he also had the other works by Steinbeck, like *Sweet Thursday*. In his LPs was an album of Woody Guthrie's songs.

Regardless of all that, tonight Dave was full of hope, not hope for mankind, but for himself. Hope this girl was everything Henry said she was and that they would connect.

It was easy to find the house. There was an expressway that led from downtown out to the north side where Dave's apartment was. The expressway went past the Park, and there was a street that circled the Park Area following its contours with other streets coming into it like the spokes of a wheel. He took the exit on the expressway for one of those streets, then followed Park Street around until he found the right number on the house.

The grassy park was large with a lake at one end, trees and landscaping, a soccer field, football field, baseball field, basketball court, and tennis court. At the far end was an open area with a raised stage with a high wooden wall behind it. The lake had a jogging trail around it, and there were picnic tables everywhere scattered throughout the park.

On the park side, the street was lined with a gravel border for parking, and on the other side, there was a curb, gutter, and sidewalk. The house was a large old Victorian with a similar house on the left, and it looked as if they had been built by the same builder. On the right was a smaller, more elegant, well-kept house in a slightly more modern style with a yard and landscaping. He parked on the grassy side, crossed the street, and walked to the house.

The door was open, and he could hear people talking, so he walked in. The house had high ceilings with wainscoting, hardwood floors, and plaster walls. The entry was a long hall leading to a staircase with a landing at the top. There was an opening on the left into the dining room where a pony keg with the accompanying red plastic cups was on one end of a large table and wine bottles with disposable plastic wine glasses were on the other end. Various food trays were in the middle of the table along with paper plates and plastic flatware. The chairs for the table had been pushed against the walls. Behind the opening to the dining room was a smaller opening into the kitchen and a door further down on the other side of the hall that Dave assumed was the zoom room.

There was a larger opening on the right into a big living room that was furnished with second-hand, worn, mismatched couches and chairs, plus the ever-present card table found in all male-dominated communal living quarters.

Henry was sitting on one of the couches between two women. The one on the right was turned from Dave listening to Henry talk. She was a small woman dressed in an expensive work casual outfit, and everything about her was prim, trim, neat, and proper, from her hair to her shoes. That was Sherry, Dave knew, because she was like every girl Henry had ever dated. But the one on the left literally stopped Dave in his tracks, and all he could do was stand and stare at her. She had her head turned slightly toward Henry, so Dave saw only her partial profile at first; she was a classic beauty with fine, even features and an alluring mouth. She was the most beautiful woman Dave had ever seen.

Her long hair was light auburn with golden highlights, and her skin flawless. She had on a close-fitting white blouse that was tied above her waist with long tails. The blouse had buttons, but they were left buttoned exposing just the right amount of the swell of her breast. She was wearing a short black skirt, which accentuated and drew attention to her long, slim, perfectly shaped legs that ended in black come-fuck-me heels. Her style was distinctly European. European women knew how to dress in a way that accentuated their best features, and if she had worn a scarf tied around her neck, he would have been certain she was French. She had that flair.

She must have sensed he was staring at her because she turned her head to look at him, and that is when he saw her eyes. They were large, sensual, and almost colorless. He had never seen eyes like that before. They made her look like some ethereal being. Those eyes met his in an unwavering gaze. He knew his mouth was hanging open, so he tried to smile to cover his astonishment. She returned his smile with the slightest hint of mirth in her eyes and only the very corners of her mouth. Then she looked him up and down. He heard women talk about guys undressing them with their eyes, and now he knew what they meant. She was evaluating him from head to toe, and he felt completely exposed, not just physically but as if she could see into his very essence with those remarkable eyes.

He regained his composure and broadened his smile into a grin. *Don't just stand here grinning like an idiot*, he told himself. He started walking toward her and Henry saw him.

"Dave," Henry said as he stood up. The other woman turned to look at him. Dave had seen that look before, and he could read her thoughts. *Henry, this is your college roommate you told me so much about? My God, he is a hippie!* She did not stand up.

The ethereal creature stood up and Dave saw just how striking she was. She was tall, lithe, and graceful with long legs, a small waist, a firm posterior, and high, full, firm breasts. It occurred to him that was why she stood up, not to be introduced to him, but so he could see just how stunning she was. He was stunned. All he could think was, *she is not human, she must be an elf, a beautiful elf.*

Henry turned to the woman on his left. "Sherry, this is Dave, my roommate from college." Sherry extended a limp hand to Dave as if she were afraid to touch him. He took her hand gently and acknowledged her.

"This is Sharon Kelly, a flight attendant who lives next door. Sharon, this is David Cameron. We are both doing internships at University Hospital." She did not extend her hand but just stood there and let him take her in.

"Sherry, move over a little so Dave can squeeze in beside Sharon." Henry sat back down and moved to his left. As Dave and Sharon sat down, Dave had to put his arm on the back of the couch for them to fit; when he did, she turned to face him. Her makeup drew attention to her translucent eyes. They were large with dark emerald green rings around irises that were so pale, they were almost white. They were so unusual, Dave was transfixed by them. When she turned back, she had a satisfied smile on her face because she knew he was hooked. All she had to do was reel him in and decide if she wanted to keep him or throw him back. Dave was completely aware where things stood after that look.

A love story and social commentary

"Dave, you need a drink. There is beer and wine in the dining room." Henry pointed to the opening across the hall.

Sharon stood up. "I need something too. I'll show him."

She extended her hand. Dave stood up, took her hand, and they walked to the dining room. Dave glanced back at Henry and saw a raised eyebrow, followed by a satisfied smile. When Dave and Sharon reached the table, he asked what she wanted.

"A beer is fine," she answered.

"I didn't take you for a beer girl." Dave was sure she was going to ask for a glass of wine.

"Normally you would be right, but if I had a glass of wine and it was good, I would want another, and then maybe another, and I am not looking to get hammered tonight. I can sip and nurse a beer a lot longer than a glass of good wine." Their eyes met, she smiled at him, and her smile literally made him weak in the knees.

Dave was not looking to get hammered either; he was looking to not blow it with the most remarkable woman he had ever met. He took two red cups, pulled two beers from the keg, and handed one to her. Their eyes met again, and he almost blurted out, *You have the most beautiful eyes I have ever seen.* Her eyes demanded and compelled him to say it, but how many other guys before him had told her how beautiful her eyes were? It was a line she had definitely heard before, so it would sound trite.

This was an intelligent, sophisticated, educated, confident woman. She was all too knowing and aware to fall for a line or his smooth Southern charm. He had to go straight at her with truth and honesty, exposing himself for who he was. If she liked who he was, then she would keep him; if not, she would throw him back. Dave had never wanted anything more in his life than not to be thrown back and rejected by the most desirable woman he had ever met.

"Do you want to go back and talk to Henry and Sherry?" Sharon asked after Dave handed her the beer.

"No. I have heard everything Henry has to say, and he has heard everything I have to say. Besides, Sherry doesn't like me. I can tell by the way she looked at me," Dave answered.

She laughed. "I picked up on that too, but what about your other friend? Isn't he coming tonight? He may already be here. Don't you want to go check?"

"No, I have heard everything he has to say too. I would much rather stay here and talk to you, unless you want to go back?" He knew it was a critical moment. If she said she wanted to go back, then she was throwing him back. If she wanted to stay and talk to him, he still had a chance with her.

She looked at him, and he knew she was making the decision, so he added, "Henry introduced us because he thought we had a lot in common and would like each other. He told me about you, and I know he told you about me. I know Henry, and he doesn't normally get involved. He just doesn't do that, so he must have had a good reason for introducing us. I think we should trust him, give it a chance, and see what happens. I want to stay here, talk to you, and get to know you. I only hope you feel the same way about me." He made his move being as honest and open as he could.

Their meeting was why she came, why she had spent a lot of time getting ready, and why she had stood in front of him to let him see just how incredible she was. She gazed directly into his eyes. Her eyes no longer made him uncomfortable because they were soft, vulnerable, and had a slight touch of fear in them. He wanted to say more. He knew both of them were wounded and looking for a way to heal their wounds. They were coming off relationships they had ended, but the pain was still there, even though the wounds were self-inflicted. She had been with Bar for almost six months, and he had been with the student nurse for nearly two years. You don't spend that much time with someone on the most intimate of terms and just walk away unscathed. To heal their wounds, they had to take a chance. He was willing, but was she?

They stood there looking into each other's eyes until she broke the spell. "So, you are a frat rat, who went to Woodstock, smoked pot, joined the revolution, and became a hippie." She was going to give him a chance. The vulnerability and fear left her eyes as they danced with mischief showing she was ready to play the timeless game men and women play.

"I was in a fraternity with Henry, but I am not a frat rat. I can tell you exactly what Henry told you about me. He told you I was a naive idealist out to save the world," Dave answered.

"That is pretty much right on, except you left out all the accolades. He believes you are special, one of the few people he trusts, and his best friend. He thinks quite lot of you," Sharon countered.

"Wow, he really built me up. Are you impressed? I am," Dave said and laughed.

"What did he tell you about me?" Sharon asked, smiling at him with her eyes twinkling.

"He said you are smart, sophisticated, and together. He likes you a lot and thinks you are special too. I think that is why he wanted to introduce us. I am going to leave out all the accolades because they are too numerous to mention," Dave answered, then he added with his most charming smile, "He told me you were beautiful, but not that you had lovely elfin eyes."

"Henry told me about that too or he warned me about it—the smooth Southern charm. I wondered when it would come out. I can tell you, if it had come out sooner, I would have dropped you for the seducer you probably are, in your Gandalf T-shirt talking about elfin eyes," Sharon countered without a smile.

"You are too beautiful to be human—you have to be an elf, *and* you know who Gandalf is," Dave persisted.

"I read Tolkien; I am not an elf. So, dial-down the charm," Sharon answered coolly. "Tell me about Woodstock. What changed you so much? I bet you were a preppy dresser like Henry and now look at you. Is the way you dress the only thing Woodstock changed? I want to hear about it from someone who was there," she continued.

"No, but it's a long story. Can I give you the cliff notes version now, then tell you the whole story another time over a glass of good wine at my apartment?" Dave answered.

"I will take the cliff notes version now," Sharon responded.

"You are right. I dressed like Henry because he taught me how to dress. Woodstock changed that and everything else about my life. Cliff notes version: I went to Woodstock, smoked pot for the first time, had a life-changing experience, heard the most incredible music you can imagine, and came home a different person," Dave continued. "Now, can we talk elves?"

"No, the elves were involved in the wars; I skipped over those parts. Those books are really about Hobbits. They had things in perspective and knew what was important in life. Sam was the real hero. Frodo tried to save the world, but it was Sam who saved it. Sam showed what was possible if you embrace contentment and happiness." Sharon loved Hobbits. "It is obvious you identify with Gandalf, but I don't identify with any of the elves. I identify with Sam. If I am anything, I am a Hobbit."

"You certainly don't look like a hobbit, you look like...." Sharon glared at him. "OK, I get it." Dave put his hands up, then added, "I guess my whole philosophy of life has been shaped by writers like Tolkien."

"Who else? I am curious. I think we have read some of the same authors," Sharon asked.

"Shakespeare of course, or whoever really wrote Shakespeare, Bacon or his contemporaries, Melville, Dickens, Steinbeck, Michener, Hemingway—"

Sharon interrupted him. "Hemingway! He was a chauvinistic misogynist who glorified war." Her eyes flashed and Dave realized they could be weaponized.

"Hold on, and let me explain. *The Old Man and the Sea* for one thing, *A Farewell to Arms* and *For Whom the Bell Tolls* are both antiwar and glorify love. Hemingway understood we are all flawed, and we can never win in the struggle, but we continue to fight regardless. The Hemingway hero, or flawed antihero, is a typical Hemingway man. He is damaged and knows he can't win, but he continues to fight for what is right even in the face of impossible odds." Dave tried to justify his love for Hemingway.

"That is a male thing. It is how you justify yourselves and your actions. Hemingway did not portray women well in his books, and he did not treat them well in his personal life. The same goes for Dickens. His social commentary is second to none, except maybe Steinbeck's, but like Hemingway, he did not handle women well in his writing or in his real life." Sharon made her point.

"I adore women, especially an elfin creature like you." Dave tried to redeem himself.

She was not having it. "Knock off the elfin stuff and drop the Southern charm. We are having a serious discussion here. If you can't get your dick out of the way long enough to have a serious conversation with a woman, then I guess you are a Hemingway man." Her eyes were still flashing.

He was on dangerous ground; the Hemingway reference had put him there, but he was who he was, and if this was going to work, she had to like him for who he was, not some fabrication of himself concocted to draw her in. He didn't want to just seduce her. He wanted much more than that from her.

"I am sorry, but I knew I had offended you. I was trying to lighten things up. I promise I will not do it again. My dick is not in the way anymore. I am just not used to having this kind of dialog with a beautiful woman." Dave was scrambling for footing and traction.

"Do you mean if a woman is attractive, she is not smart enough, educated or well-read enough to have this kind of discussion with you?" He was on even shakier ground. She had him on the run; he had to recover and recover fast, or it would be all over.

"Again, I am sorry, and this is not Southern charm or a line, but I have never met anyone like you. Maybe my dick is in the way. Like referring to you as an elf and trying to charm you. I will not let that happen again, I promise. I will put my dick away. There see, my dick is put away. No dick. See, my dick is gone. No more dick. I am totally dickless. Can we continue?" Dave was desperate.

Her eyes softened. "You are cute, but I think you are dangerous too, and I doubt you are dickless. I didn't mean to snap at you, but don't disappoint me by being just another guy on the make. After what Henry told me about you, I expected more than that from you. I can tell you this, speaking of dicks, it is what is above your shoulders, not what is below your waist, that interest me. OK, who else?"

Dave knew she had dated the smartest guy in the room, not some pretty boy or muscle-bound Neanderthal. "I think Huxley had the most influence on me. He was a genius. *Brave New World, Point Counter Point*, and *The Doors of Perception*. I felt like it was OK to take mescaline because of him. Not only did it enhance everything, but I was able to see the world, the cosmos, the whole universe in perfect perspective." He was still in the game.

"Yet despite *Doors of Perception*, Huxley rejected hallucinogens in the end. Chemicals, in one form or another, have been used to enhance thinking, art, literature, and music long before Huxley, Kesey, or Leary. Their use has produced positive results, but the effects on the users have been negative in many instances. Look at the twenty-seven club—Janis Joplin, Jim Morrison, and Jimi Hendrix. I have never taken anything, but I would like to try it sometime and see for myself." She was back with him in spite of the Hemingway thing.

He wanted to reach out and take her in his arms. She had read Huxley. She was his fantasy, his dream, his perfect woman. He moved toward her, causing her to step back.

"I am sorry," Dave recovered and stopped very close to her.

"That's OK," she said, then she leaned into him.

She leaned against him and looked into his eyes. "Are we trying too hard? Are we two people on the rebound trying to connect because someone we respect told us we would? All that discussion seemed a little strained. I broke up with a guy a few months ago, and I know you left a girl behind when you moved here. Did Henry push us together, not for the reasons he told us, but because he likes us and felt sorry for us?" Once again, he saw sadness, venerability, and a little fear in her eyes. How did she do that? Her eyes were so expressive, she could use them to communicate like a form of telepathy. He put his arm around her.

"Like I told you, that is not like Henry, but even if you are right, I still want to give us a chance. And this is not a line: you are the most amazing, remarkable woman I have ever met, and I want to get to know you."

She touched the beads at his throat. "Are these real?" Her face was turned to his, she was leaning into his chest with his arm around her, and now her eyes were smoky and soft. She was not frightened anymore, and he was not worried about her rejecting him. They had let their guard down, opened up to one another, and connected.

They stood there looking into each other's eyes totally unaware the dining room was full of people getting beer, wine, and food. Most of the people in the room knew her or at least who she was, but none of them knew who he was, yet it was obvious to everyone the two of them weren't interested in greetings or introductions, so everyone just walked around them.

"I think they are real African trader beads. I bought them from an Arab street vendor in front of the Paradiso in Amsterdam. He was selling a lot of stuff from North Africa, including Moroccan hash. I bought the beads and some hash. They put the hash in wooden match boxes—you just slide the bottom out, scrape some off into a pipe and light it. It is righteous stuff, and it gets you really high," Dave answered.

"I love Amsterdam! The Paradiso, was that in the Red-Light District?" She pulled away, and he saw she was excited.

"No, it was a sort of club or whatever. It used to be a church. It was full of a lot of fucked-up people jumping up and down dancing to that European techno music. You could buy anything you wanted on the street out front. There were guys standing on the sidewalk shouting, 'Hashish! Mescaline! LSD! Psilocybin!' like they were vendors at a ballpark shouting, 'Hot dogs, popcorn, cold beer!'" Dave laughed. "The locals would buy something, take it, then head into the Paradiso to dance the night away all fucked-up."

"Is that where you got the mescaline you took?" Sharon was interested in the mescaline.

"No, I got the mescaline from a friend in medical school who made it. Where else have you been in Europe besides Amsterdam?" Dave asked.

"Only Paris. I became a flight attendant because I wanted to travel." She looked a little sad. "Or maybe I just wanted to get away. I was set to go to grad school, but I just flew away instead." She brightened. "We fly to Mexico and Canada from almost everywhere in the US. From the West Coast, we fly to Hawaii, Australia, and New Zealand. From here, I can bid trips to Amsterdam, London, Paris, and Rome. I have only been flying for four years, so I am too junior to hold any of those trips, but if I am on-call and a girl gets sick or has some kind of emergency, I get to fill in for her. I would love to go to Rome, but I feel bad about wanting someone to get sick so I can go. Is it bad for me to want someone to get sick so I can go to Rome?" Sharon looked at him mischievously under her brows.

"No comment. I guess you went to the Rijksmuseum in Amsterdam and the Louvre in Paris." Dave wanted her back leaning against him with his arm around her.

"Yes, but I also took a night canal trip in Amsterdam, and I went to Notre Dame in Paris. The flight to Europe is an all-nighter, but you know that. It is a hard service and a long trip with no sleep; you get there in the morning and have to fly back the next morning, so you have only a day and a night to do things. I went as hard as I could, for as long as I could, until I fell in bed exhausted. You have to get a good night's sleep because the trip back is even harder. How long were you in Europe, and where did you go?" Sharon leaned into him, he put his arm around her waist again, and he could feel the physical tension building between them.

"I was there for a month with a backpack and a Eurail pass. We traveled at night, slept on the train to save on hotel bills and to leave the days open to do things. We landed in Luxembourg, went to Paris, London, Amsterdam, Zurich, Salzburg, Vienna, Athens, Rome, the Riviera, Barcelona, Madrid, and back to Luxenberg to fly home. We only stayed two or three days in each place, but that trip was more of a life-changing experience for me than Woodstock or the mescaline. I love Europe."

Dave tried to pull her tighter against him, but she jumped away again. "I hate you. I want to do something like that. I assume the 'we' referred to the girl you left behind when you moved here."

"She was a student nurse at the time. We were together from my junior year of med school until three months ago. She wanted to come with me, but I knew the only reason she wanted to come with me was to get married, so it ended. After she graduated, she took a job at the hospital where we went to school, and I heard she is dating a GI fellow now." Dave was a little sad as he spoke, and Sharon picked up on it.

"Déjà vu all over again. Only I didn't want to marry Bar or go to Boston with him." Sharon sounded more angry than sad. "What should I do with one day in Rome if I ever get there."

"The usual: the coliseum, the forum, and the Pantheon. You can do all that in one day if you hustle. But there is so much more." Dave wanted to hold her again.

"Not the coliseum. That is an evil place. I can't stand violence, even if it happened thousands of years ago or is in a book. Let's talk about Paris. It's my favorite." She moved closer to him.

"Me too. I love the Louvre, but I also like the National Gallery. Renoir is my favorite Impressionist. Everything he did was so light and happy. I thought the light in his pictures was Impressionistic, then I went to the Luxenberg Gardens and realized he was painting exactly what he saw. The light there is amazing. I thought the same thing about the trees in Italian paintings until I was in Italy and saw the trees really look like that. In the Louvre, you are overwhelmed by so much, and I love it all, but I am drawn to the neoclassical painters, David and Delacroix. Liberty Leading the People gives me chills. There is so much to see and learn in Europe, not only in the great cities like Paris and the ancient ruins of Rome and Athens, but the history of Western civilization is everywhere." Dave put his arm around her waist again.

A love story and social commentary

They continued to talk, letting the sexual tension build between them as Dave kept his arm around her waist, and she put her hand on his chest occasionally. They laughed and debated, agreeing or disagreeing on a variety of subjects. They began to understand why Henry had brought them together. They were both bright, inquisitive, innocent, open, trusting, full of a desire for life and what it had to offer. They had read the same books, they had the same core belief system, they liked and enjoyed the same things. They stood there talking with their warm beers abandoned on the table, enjoying each other's company, letting the physical chemistry between them develop until they were interrupted.

She was standing in front of him talking enthusiastically about what a beautiful writer Fitzgerald was, when Dave saw a man come up behind her. "Hello, Gorgeous." He put his arms around her from behind. Dave was instantly jealous. Of course, what was he thinking, a woman like her? Did he really think she had been sitting around just waiting to meet him? Henry told him there were guys lined up trying to fuck her, and this jerk was one of them. In fact, he acted like he was already fucking her. He had his hands all over her. Dave was crushed.

She pulled away laughing. "Phillip!" He looked like he was in his early forties, moderately handsome, slender, and dressed like he was on his way to Studio 54 with shiny square-toed shoes, flared designer slacks, and a silk disco shirt partially unbuttoned. There was another guy behind him dressed the same way, only he was about ten years younger, not in the least bit handsome, short and heavy set with thinning hair.

"Phil and Bob, this is Dr. David Cameron. He was Henry's roommate in college and has just moved here to do his internship at University Hospital. Dave, this is Phil and his partner Bob. They own the house next door and the most exclusive clothing store in the city. This is their party."

Partners who own the house next door—they were the gay guys! Dave almost burst out laughing at himself. Boy he was hooked, landed, in the boat, stored in the ice chest, and the boat was on the way back to the dock. He was insanely jealous over a woman he had just met.

"He's pretty. Is he straight?" Phil asked as he looked at Dave.

"Yes, he is straight," Sharon answered smiling.

"Pity. How do you know?" Phil went on.

"I can tell by the way he looks at me." Her eyes were warm as she looked directly into Dave's eyes.

"Are you sure? Look at that hair," Phil continued, teasing her.

"Yes, I am sure. I have gaydar, and I can tell you he definitely does not set it off." Sharon laughed.

"I am right here. Why are you two acting like I am not here? I am right here. I am not gay. I can answer for myself," Dave interjected.

"Too bad, with those shoulders and that cute butt," Phil responded.

"Is my butt really cute?" Dave looked at his backside then back at her.

"Yes, it is." Sharon said, looking at his rear.

"I think the female is in heat, and the male is aroused. He is definitely not gay," Bob said, speaking for the first time.

She turned on them. "OK, that is enough. What has gotten into you two?"

"What has gotten to us is some outrageous dope. We are very stoned," Phil responded.

"The question is what has gotten into you, or more to the point, what is going to get into you? This guy has you all hot and bothered," Bob said looking at Dave.

"Stop it!" Sharon pouted.

"I have never seen you as happy as you are with … what's his name?" Phil added.

"That's no excuse for being crude. I know you thought you were being funny, but I just met Dave, and I don't want him to get the wrong impression of me." Sharon was upset with them.

"I could never get the wrong impression of you. I think you are perfect. Nothing anyone could say would ever change that impression of you." Dave looked at her as he spoke.

"See, he gets you, Gorgeous. He would never mistake our fun for anything other than that—just fun. Right, Dave, is it?" Bob added.

"God, one of them spoke to me. They do know I am here." They all laughed as Sharon leaned into Dave, and he put his arm around her waist again. "Do gay men not talk to straight guys?" Dave asked.

For the first time since they walked up, Bob and Philip actually paid attention to Dave. Philip looked at Dave, not Sharon, as he spoke. "Looks, brains, manly build, straight-forward honesty, and I think he believes every word he just said about you. God, he is Dudley Do Right.

His front tooth probably sparkles when he smiles. You deserve it after that homophobic, controlling, cold asshole Bar. Let him compliment you and tell you how great you are. Let yourself bask in his attention and know that you deserve it. I have never seen you as happy as you are tonight. Let yourself go. Don't be afraid. Embrace that happiness. " Then Phil rolled his eyes. "I know *he* wants to embrace more than your happiness."

Dave interrupted. "My name is Dave. It is obvious you guys are Sharon's friends, and I hope we can be friends too, because I want to see more of her." Dave stuck out his hand.

Phil took his hand then looked at Sharon as he shook it. "I told you, Dudley Fucking Do Right, and he wants to see more of you." Phil looked her up and down smiling as he shook Dave's hand.

Sharon leaned against Dave. "Thanks."

"For what?" Dave asked.

"For not being homophobic," Sharon answered.

"Yeah, the jerk she was seeing before was a real piece of work," Bob said as he took Dave's hand.

"Bob and Phil don't like Bar, as you may have ascertained, because he is a tad homophobic." Sharon put her hand on Dave's chest, and he put his arm around her waist.

"It's not that he is homophobic; we deal with that all the time. It's the way he treated you. That's why we don't like him, Dave. He treated her like she was a hood ornament. She was there only for show. He is the great Bar, smarter than you and superior to you in every way—just look at the really gorgeous woman he is fucking. He only used her to enhance his image." Bob explained his disdain for Bar in no uncertain terms. Dave really didn't like thinking about Sharon being fucked by Bar or anyone else.

"Dave, you two have been talking for some time. What were you talking about? Please tell me you were wooing her with tasteful eroticisms. No, I'll bet not. What were you talking about?" Phil asked.

"We were talking about writers, books, art, travel," Dave answered.

"You are obviously a smart guy, Dave. You are an educated man and a doctor. Did she hold her own with you on those topics?" Bob added.

"She more than held her own," Dave replied.

"Bar totally controlled her. He belittled anything she said and humiliated her by disproving any point she made. He never let her express her opinion or demonstrate her intelligence. He just wanted to display her. She demonstrated to everyone what a man he was because he was fucking a woman like her." Phil was worked up.

Dave had heard enough about Bar fucking Sharon. He could not control his jealousy; he felt so possessive he took her in his arms and pulled her to him. "Why did you stay with him?"

"They tend to be a little dramatic because they hate him so much. It's complicated. He wasn't into physical fucking; he was into mind fucking. Physically, he was almost asexual, and I certainly wasn't in it for the sex. He looked like Ichabod Crane. He got off on doing things to people to see how they reacted, not by having sex. Now, the last thing I want to talk about or think about tonight is Bar. He is gone and forgotten as far as I am concerned. I don't want anything negative to spoil tonight." She put her arms around Dave's neck as he held her.

"Don't try to paint us as two drama queens, Sharon. You know we are telling the truth. Jesus, can you two stop it for a minute? We came over here to ask you if you wanted to smoke some herb. We have some stuff from Jamaica, real Bob Marley—one hit and the world turns round shit, or do you want to stay here and entertain the dining room with your foreplay?" Phil asked.

Sharon turned in Dave's arms and hit Phil lightly in the chest with her fist. "That's enough. Do you want to smoke some weed?" She looked back at Dave.

"Sure, if you want to," Dave responded.

"Leave us adjourn to the zoom room then." Phil walked away with Bob.

"I heard about this zoom room from Henry. I want to check it out." Dave started to follow them, but Sharon held him back.

"How do you really feel about gay men?" Sharon asked.

"I thought it was obvious," Dave answered.

"You are very smooth and that could have been an act for my benefit. Those two guys are my friends. They have always been there for me. There is not a mean or devious bone in their bodies; they are kind and caring. Straight guys can be very conflicted about gay men. I need to know the truth." Sharon was serious.

"Cliff notes version now, and a real discussion later?" Dave tried to joke about it.

"Honesty and enough meat in the cliff notes so I know where you stand." Her eyes were flat, and he sensed this was not a deal breaker but an important informational item that required an answer.

"I believe in freedom. I believe that if you don't harm anyone else, you should be free to do whatever you want. I may not agree with what you say, but I will defend your right to say it. I may not agree with what you do, but I will defend your right to do it. People have been doing what they do since we climbed down from the trees—in fact, probably before we climbed down. What's more, I oppose hatred and bigotry in any form for any reason. Your friends have nothing to worry about where I'm concerned." Dave answered as honestly as he could.

She put her arms back around his neck and kissed him softly. When the kiss was over, she looked straight into his eyes, and he could feel the warmth in her eyes turn to heat.

They caught up with Phil and Bob at the zoom room door. "What took you so long?"

"We walk slow," Sharon answered.

"I thought you might be administering a gay tolerance test to Dave." Phil looked at Dave.

"That too," Sharon added.

"Did he pass?" Phil asked.

"He is an A student." She patted Dave's chest.

"Only one problem," Dave said. Sharon looked at him with a worried expression. "I have impure thoughts about my teacher."

"I don't blame you. I have impure thoughts about her, and I am gay. I can only imagine how she must affect a straight guy." Bob leered at Sharon.

The unmistakable, pungent odor of pot wafted over them as Phil opened the door to the zoom room. "Smells like we are not the first ones to arrive." They closed the door and waited for their eyes to adjust to the black lights then sat down in a circle near the back wall. Sharon's white blouse glowed like it was electrified.

There was a couple lying in each other's arms in the corner listening to the music. Pink Floyd was playing softly; two other couples were sitting in a circle near the front wall passing a joint around. All six of the other people ignored them.

Phil took a partially smoked joint out of his shirt pocket. "We will finish this. We know our tolerance level. One joint between us is about all we can handle for a night." He reached in his pants pocket and pulled out a baggy full of large buds. "I suggest you use a pipe." He walked over to the shelf beside the door where the stereo components were to get a pipe and lighter from a basket on the shelf.

"Fill a pipe and share it. If you take one hit at a time, you can titrate your high. Let me warn you, more than three hits and you are going to have to remind yourself to breathe." Phil handed Sharon the baggy and pipe, used the lighter on the joint, passed it to Bob, then handed the lighter to Sharon. Sharon followed Phil's instructions. They shared two full pipes, rotating who took the first hit, then Sharon asked Dave if he wanted to do a third pipe.

"I can't believe you would even ask," Dave mumbled.

"Thank God," Sharon said.

They fell back into the cushions and pillows in each other's arms and didn't move for quite a while. When the record finished, Phil got up to change the music. Bob was passed out, the couple in the corner were still there, the other two couples were drinking beer after finishing their joint, and a few more people had wandered in to share a joint. Phil put Crosby, Stills, Nash, and Young on, adjusted the volume up so the four-part harmony filled the room, then he came back and sat down beside Dave and Sharon.

Sharon rolled on top of Dave as he ran his hands down her back then brushed her hair back from her face to kiss her. It was a passionate hungry kiss that continued as she clung to him. Her blouse came untied and she raised up so he could bury his face in the softness of her breasts. Her skirt rode up to her hips as she sat up straddling him and went after his belt.

"You two need to get a room," Phil said as he watched them.

Sharon whispered, "My room is right next door."

"Are you sure. Are you sure you are ready for that?" Dave whispered back.

"I am ready, and I think you are too." She was sitting on him.

"If I get any more ready, I won't be able to walk out of here without attracting attention." Dave breathed.

"I think we are going to get a lot of attention when we walk out of here regardless," Sharon responded softly in his ear.

She retied her top. "I am so high, I forgot we weren't alone." She stood up and adjusted her skirt. "Wow. Wait till you try to stand up."

"I am having trouble sitting up. Some gay guy drugged the hell out of me," Dave said as he struggled to his feet. "Are you positive we can find your room?" Dave asked.

"It's right next door," Sharon said as she adjusted her top and pulled her skirt down.

"Like I said, are you positive we can find your room?" Dave asked again.

"If you two stay here, you are going to put on a live sex show for a dozen people," Phil told them and laughed.

"I can't believe I am so high, I forgot where I was," Sharon said to no one in particular.

"Here. Enjoy." Phil handed the baggy to Sharon.

"That's all I need, to smoke more weed." Sharon didn't take the baggy.

"Save it for next time. We have plenty. For some reason, I don't think this is the last time you two are going to get together." Phil pushed the baggy on her.

"Thanks, tell Bob good night for me if he ever comes around." She took the baggy and walked to the door.

Phil stood up and reached out to Dave. "Hold on a minute. I think you are a good guy, but you need to understand that she is a treasure, and you need to value her. She is not just another lay, or a one-night stand; she is something special. She needs to be cherished, not just used."

"You don't have to tell me how special she is—I know," Dave responded then followed Sharon out unaware everyone in the room had watched what had happened and was watching them leave.

She was waiting for him in the hall leaning against the wall. She handed him the baggie, he took it and put it in his pocket, then he took both her hands in his, intertwined their fingers, and held her hands against the wall above her head. He kissed her, and she responded by pushing her body against his.

"Get a room," someone from the landing called down.

"We are trying. We are just way fucked-up." Dave looked up, but the guy who said it was gone, so he looked back at Sharon and kissed her again. Dave's heart was pounding because he was about to have sex with the woman of his dreams, his fantasy woman, and she was real, standing right in front of him, soft, warm, and willing. He had never felt this excited about anything in his life.

They walked down the hall with their arms around each other's waist. When they passed the opening to the living room, someone commented to Henry, "I wondered how long it would be before those two left to get it on."

Henry was still sitting on the couch with Sherry, but now Mike was sitting with them. Henry started to say something as they passed the opening, but as he watched them walking together, intertwined and looking into each other's eyes, he realized there was nothing to say. He smiled and thought, *I guess I was right.* Everyone in the living room watched them leave as Mike blurted out, "Jesus, she's a stone-cold fox," and Sherry commented, "I thought she had more class than that."

Mike got up and followed them out the front door, stopping on the porch to watch them walk down the sidewalk. They stopped midway between the two houses, and Dave said something to Sharon. She threw her head back and laughed, then she said something back to Dave with her face very close to his, laughed again, and they kissed. They stood there with their arms around each other kissing until finally they walked slowly to the other house.

Mike walked back in, went to the couch, and sat down. "She is really hot. I thought he was going to throw her down and fuck her right there on the sidewalk. They made it to the other house, but I'll bet they are already fucking."

Sherry's mouth dropped open, and Henry said, "I guess I was right about them connecting."

"Of course, you gave her to Dave. He connects with a lot of women. She is just one more." Mike leaned back on the couch and conjured up a lewd pornographic image of Sharon in his mind.

"What do you mean? He only dated one woman for the last two years." Henry was starting to dislike Mike.

"Yeah, but he was fucking a bunch of women regularly before he met her." Mike sulked, didn't say any more, and got up to get another beer.

Sherry had listened to the whole conversation with her mouth open. "That guy is crude, lewd, and socially unacceptable."

Sherry liked Sharon even though she was a little jealous of her. After what Mike had said about Dave, she was worried about her. But Sharon was not her problem. Henry was. She had a plan, and Henry was at the center of her plan. They would get married and move to New York City where Henry would become a top internist. His position would open doors for her, and with their money, she could become a New York socialite and join the most elite, exclusive circle in the country. This Dave person could not interfere with that. It was this Dave person she needed to worry about.

Mike walked into the dining room. Dave was off with a hot woman and he was there pulling another beer—how typical. When he moved in with Dave, he tried to connect with the two women Dave was seeing at his old apartment complex, but they wouldn't even talk to him. He called the NASCAR hostess after Dave started dating the student nurse, but she let him know in no uncertain terms that she wasn't interested. It wasn't as if he were a virgin. He had been with a girl in high school and one in college. He had been with a few women in medical school, but not like the two women at the apartment, the NASCAR hostess, or the woman Dave just left with.

On the way to her house, Dave stopped to tell Sharon what Phil had said—she was a treasure he needed to cherish. She responded that she had a very good idea what he was going to do with her treasure tonight. They laughed and kissed, but the exchange slowed them down.

They walked up the stairs to Sharon's room; it was simple, tasteful, tidy, and girly. He sat on the bed and waited as she went to a portable record player, flipped through the LPs in the rack below it, selected a record and put it on. The soft smooth sound of Miles Davis's trumpet drifted through the room. She walked back to face him, untied and tossed her top aside, unzipped the skirt, stepped out of it and kicked it with the blouse, wiggled out of her thong gracefully and tossed it on the floor with her blouse and skirt. She left the come-fuck-me heels on and stood in front of him.

If Dave had looked up, he would have seen her eyes were bright and glistening, but he couldn't stop looking at her perfect body. He kicked off his sandals, pulled his T-shirt over his head, stood up and pulled off his jeans.

"I don't want you to be disappointed. I need to warn you, I am not very experienced at this." He looked up at her face and realized she was unsure of herself, a little frightened, and didn't know what to do next.

A woman's body can be played like a musical instrument to produce cords of ecstasy. Dave had learned to play the female instrument from very hedonistic women who were intent on achieving maximum pleasure, so he learned to play it with skill, attention, and generosity. Sharon's body was the most exquisite instrument he had ever played, and he played it with the care a fine instrument deserves. Good sex is like good jazz. Each player takes a part, composing, arranging, and playing at the same time, then they come together in perfect harmony and blended perfection. They are always listening to each other, tuned to each other, and playing off each other.

Dave took her in his arms; the feel of her body against his was indescribable. He reached back with one hand and pulled the bed covers back, laid her down gently in the bed, and slid in next to her on his side. "We don't have to do this. We can wait if you are not ready."

She turned on her side to face him. "I'm ready. I was ready in the zoom room." She kissed him, then she moved to bring her body against his. Dave kissed her ear, then her neck from behind her ear to the top of her shoulder. When he reached her shoulder, he rolled her on her back, and moved on top of her, being careful to support his weight with his elbows. Once they were settled, he continued down, brushing her skin lightly with his lips until he reached the swell of her breast. He brushed them with his lips, being careful to pay equal attention to each breast as he used his lips and tongue to tease her nipples.

She took his head in her hands as he moved further down, continuing to brush her skin with his lips. Her breathing became rapid and shallow. He took her between his lips and began to brush her lightly with his tongue. She made a soft moaning sound and threw her arms out, digging her fingers into the bedding.

Dave applied all the techniques he knew. She tossed her head back and forth, alternating between digging her fingers into the bedding and holding his head. She made a louder moaning sound as the skin of her chest blushed a vivid salmon color. She began to tremble as the salmon flush turned to deep red blotches, then she started to shake violently. Finally, she held him to her, bucking wildly, and crying out until she sagged into the bed, limp. She lay there as if she were unconscious for a while. Dave raised up on his hands and knees over her. Her eyes were closed, and it looked as if she was barely breathing. Her hair was spread out around her calm expressionless face, and her whole body was totally relaxed. She looked like the rendition of a fantasy goddess he had once seen on a book cover.

A love story and social commentary

She opened her eyes and reached for him, pulled him down, and kissed him. It was a deep, wet, lustful kiss, like nothing they had done before. Then she pushed him over and moved down until her breast were resting on his thighs. What she lacked in experience, she made up for with enthusiasm.

Dave pulled her on top of him, and she put her knees on each side of his hips as he entered her. He gave her complete control, only responding to her, not taking any initiative. She hugged him with her face buried in his neck. She kissed him and sat up on him like she was posting on a horse with her hands on his chest. She pulled his face to her breast with her hands on his head. When she did that, Dave cupped her breast with his hands and brushed her nipples between his lips with his tongue. When she came back down, he put his arms around her and stroked her back as he moved in unison with her.

Dave rolled her onto her back without disengaging and buried himself in her as deeply as he could, as she wrapped her arms and legs around him, kissing him. It was another wet, lustful, passionate kiss. She seemed to be trying to pull him completely into her body with her arms and her legs, then she broke the kiss, convulsing and crying out again.

Dave's face was over her face. "Open your eyes." She opened her eyes, and he looked directly into them. Her eyes were hazy and soft; he felt as if he was literally falling into her through her eyes. If the eyes really are the windows to the soul, their windows were wide open and welcoming. At that moment as he kissed her, he actually lifted her off the bed as he tried to push deeper into her, then he collapsed on top her. Dave started to move but she hugged him tighter with her arms and legs, pulling him back to her, and they lay there locked together until he was no longer in her. He rolled on his back, and she immediately snuggled under his arm with her head on his chest and her leg over his. They did not move or speak for some time.

When she spoke, it was in a small, soft voice. "I have never experienced anything like that."

"Neither have I," Dave said in a whisper.

She raised up to look at him. "Really?"

He looked back at her. "Really."

"Was it the Jamaican weed?" Sharon asked in the same small, soft voice.

"It was us. The weed may have enhanced it, but it was us," Dave whispered back.

She dropped her eyes. "I guess you think I am a slut."

"Why would I think that?" Dave looked at her.

"Oh, I don't know. Maybe because I had your dick in my mouth a few hours after we met. Nice girls don't fuck someone they just met." She leaned on her elbow with her hand on the side of her head looking at him. "I'm not a slut. I know you don't believe me, but I'm not. I've never done anything like this before. I know you don't believe that either, but it's true. I have never had sex like that before. I didn't even know it could be like that."

"I don't think you are a slut. I hate to admit it, but I have been with some sluts in my time, and you aren't one. We're two people who connected, that's all. I just had the most amazing sex I have ever had in my life, and it wasn't with a slut. It was with an amazingly wonderful woman." Dave pulled her to him.

"I don't know if I believe you. You are very smooth with your Southern charm and an easy manner." Sharon looked hard into his eyes. "Don't think I am a slut." She pleaded with her eyes. "Henry called me this afternoon after he picked Sherry up at the airport. He wanted me to meet his college roommate at the party. At the time, I wasn't planning on going to the party, and I told him so. He told me I had to go and meet this guy. He built you up so much, I decided to go to see if anyone could be that great. I haven't had a lot of luck with men. That's why I am not very experienced." She put her head back down on his chest.

She continued, "Henry likes you a lot, so he said he wanted us to meet. I decided to go all out and put what I have on display to see if you were intimidated by my looks. Some men are. I wanted to know if you could get passed my looks and connect with who I am. Most men don't even try. I didn't believe anyone could be as great as Henry said you were. I wanted to test you. Obviously, you passed the test," she said softly.

Sharon became more animated. "Have you looked in the mirror?" She confessed, "You look like a Viking with your vivid blue eyes and shoulder-length hair. But what made me even give you a chance was your confidence—not arrogance or cockiness, but understated confidence."

Sharon sat up in bed. "I felt that connection Henry thought we would have, and I actually started having fun with you!" She looked down. "It has been a long time since I have had fun like that." She looked into his eyes again.

What is it about her? It's not just her beauty. How can I feel so connected to someone so quickly? Dave wondered. He let her keep talking.

"Everything clicked. You didn't talk about sports, your car, or yourself, like most Southern men do. You actually sought out who I was. You seemed to be exactly who Henry said you were." She blushed a bit and said, "Of course, the weed pushed me over the edge; that plus Phil telling me to let go, enjoy being with a man who was into me, and let him indulge me. I was high and hot for you, and you were right there. I just said to myself, what the hell, why deny yourself what you want, let go, so I did. I am glad I did, but I don't want you to think I am a slut or that I act like this all the time." She looked down again.

She was open and vulnerable, so Dave sat up and reached for her. She looked up, putting her hands out to push him away. "I need to convince you I am not a slut."

Dave ignored her hands and pulled her to him. "How foolish are you? After what we just did, how close we were, the whole night, don't you think I know you are not a slut? Stop trying to justify or dissect something as incredible as what just happened. Really. We are sitting here with nothing on, still high, in the afterglow of the best sex I have ever had. I have never experienced anything like it. Do you want to talk more? We could discuss your misconception about men. You think it's what's above a man's shoulders that counts. Let's talk about that."

She smiled. "You are a horrid man. Don't make fun of me. First, you have an exaggerated opinion of yourself and second, you're wrong." She traced his lips with her finger, stopping after she had gone all the way around, then she pushed her fingertip between his lips, and he brushed it with his tongue. "It is definitely what is above the shoulders that counts." They laughed together.

They were sitting facing each other on the bed. "Look at me. I am too exhausted to take a shower. But I can't go to bed like this." She got up and went to the bathroom. When she returned, he asked, "Do you want me to go?"

"Not unless you want to. I want you to stay, but if you feel like you should go, it's OK. I understand." Her voice was small and soft again.

"I want to stay. I was giving you an out." Dave looked at her.

"I don't want an out. I want you here with me." Sharon turned out the light, got in the bed with him and kissed him good night. As Dave lay there holding her in his arms, he was still high on weed, but he was even higher on how the night had gone. He was living his dream, and the reality was even better than the dream. He did not go to sleep immediately but enjoyed holding Sharon close to him and feeling her warm body against his.

He started thinking about what it had taken for him to reach this point. All the hard work, studying, sacrifice, and delayed gratification. He knew guys who had finished college and grad school, had high-paying jobs, and were married with kids.

In high school, his circle of friends would be out during the week, but he would be at home studying. Then in college, he had labs in the afternoon when the other members of his fraternity were busy enjoying all that college had to offer. He was a biology major plus he had to take premed courses. He took sixteen to eighteen hours a semester, and he had to keep his grade point above a three point with biology, physics, calculus, chemistry, comparative anatomy, quantitative analysis, and the main reason many premed students were weeded out: organic chemistry. But that was nothing compared to med school and the rigid routine he had to maintain in the two basic science years with anatomy, neuroanatomy, histology, physiology, parasitology, pharmacology, hematology, and microbiology.

Then came the two clinical years with the stress, sleeplessness, fatigue, and exposure to death, broken bodies, and horrible disease states. He had to get up at five to be at the hospital by six to draw blood, and he was required to stay at the hospital all night when he was on call. In the face of all that, he had to take classes in medicine, surgery, OB/GYN, and pediatrics plus be grilled about his patients every day by his attendings. He had to compete with ninety-nine other very smart dedicated students to maintain a decent rank in class in order to get a good internship. No—Dave had paid a price for his current happiness. Like the song said, "You got to pay your dues if you want to sing the blues, and you know it don't come easy." Dave had paid his dues, and it hadn't come easy. It had taken dedication, discipline, and a single-minded adherence to purpose to achieve his goal and to be where he was tonight.

The heavy weed smoking had begun in the clinical years. He got stoned and lost himself in the beauty and softness of the student nurse's body to blot out the horrors he was exposed to at the hospital. Dave thought nothing of the fact he was using drugs to cope. The untold, dirty secret of higher academics was drug use. It started in college with the use of amphetamines to study. If you had a hard test and needed to stay up to study, you went to the dispensary to get a few pills. It got worse in med school with the massive load of the basic science years coupled with the need to excel and compete. During the clinical years, he saw the use of white crosses, mainly in the thoracic surgery residents. They were doing three to four major cases a day and the five milligram dexamphetamine tabs kept them going.

He was happy, but that happiness had come with a toll. Next week, he would begin the last phase of his training, and he had no allusions; he knew it would be worse than anything he had been through so far. But tonight, as he held Sharon in his arms with her body against his, listening to her quiet breathing, he knew in this moment he had it all.

He had been having an extremely erotic dream about sex with an elfin princess and woke up in an excited state. He looked over at Sharon. She was still sleeping, breathing slowly and evenly. What was he supposed to do—wake her up and ask her if she wanted some dick? He tried to think about something else, but he could feel her beside him, warm and soft, so that was impossible. How did this happen? How did he end up in bed with her?

Dave knew a woman makes the decision about who she lets into her body. Men think they are in control, that they can talk a woman into sex or seduce her, but that's not true. The woman makes the final decision. The decision-making process is only taken away from a woman through rape or the use of alcohol, drugs, violence, harassment, or abuse. If men would just accept that a woman has control over her own body, it would eliminate a lot of problems. But the male gender refused to do so because in reality, it wasn't about sex. It was about power and control.

Dave understood there were physical reasons why a woman picked a man. In homo sapiens, or homo saps as his college biology professor used to say, not without good cause, the female has the secondary sex characteristics that attract the male. The male is visual, looking for those secondary sex characteristics that indicate fertility. He wants to spread his genes and have offspring; that is his drive for the survival of the species. The female needs a male who can protect her and her offspring. That is her drive for the survival of the species—to raise her young. Her evaluation of a male is much more complicated. Natural selection and evolution are always at work. It is not how a species does; it is how it adapts. The modern female adapted her evaluation process to pick a man with money or the brains and education to get money to provide for her and her young. However, the basic instincts are still there—the need for good, manly physical characteristics that can protect the more cerebral female. He had it all figured out; he was in bed with her because she had chosen him, but that didn't help his problem. Her secondary sex characteristics were right up against him, so he remained ready to spread his genes.

Sharon woke up, put her head on his chest, and her leg over his. "My goodness, someone must have had a good dream." But Dave was not the only one who had been dreaming. Sharon had dreamed she was ravished by a Viking warrior. The dream had disturbed her. She had erotic dreams but never about someone like a Viking warrior. As she lay there, she remembered what she felt when she first saw him. He looked like a Viking with his long blond hair and bright blue eyes, plus he looked a little dangerous. Because of the dream, she was just as ready as he was. There was something she felt with him she had never felt with any of the other guys she dated; there was a sense of danger and excitement, yet there was also a feeling of security. She felt a new type of sexual freedom because she felt safe with him. She pulled him on top of her, and they had sweet morning sex. Though it was nothing like the night before, it was just as satisfying in its own way.

She whispered in his ear, "I am starving. I didn't eat before the party."

He whispered back, "Me too."

"Let's go make breakfast." She put on a sheer short silk robe. He put on his jeans, and they padded barefoot down stairs to the kitchen.

"I can make bacon and eggs. You set the table, get us some orange juice, make toast, and start the coffee." Sharon began to put things together to cook breakfast.

When Dave had the table set with the orange juice, toast, and coffee, he came up behind her while she was cooking the eggs, cupped her breasts, then he slid one hand down her front. The short, shear robe didn't cover much.

She rotated in his arms. "Stop that or I will get distracted and burn the eggs. Behave yourself or you won't get any breakfast." She wiggled out of his arms, and turned back to the eggs, but her breathing had changed, and she felt a tingling from his touch. She smiled and thought, *last night showed me I definitely have been missing something. Maybe he is just what I have needed.*

When the eggs were finished, they sat down to eat, and she decided she had to find out more about him. "I like being with you, but you scare me a little too. It's funny—I have never been with anyone who excited me the way you do. I like it, but I don't like it. There is something wild about you that turns me on, but it makes me a little frightened too. The way you woke up, I will bet you dreamed about fucking some elfin princess in a fantasy about adventure, like in *The Lord of the Rings*."

"Only the elfin princess part." Dave looked at her in a way that let her know she was that princess.

Sharon blushed under his gaze. "Well, I dreamed about being fucked by a Viking. I don't like Vikings, but I liked being fucked by this one. That's why I woke up just as ready as you were. I don't understand why. I hate violence and violent people, so why would I get turned on dreaming about being ravished by a Viking? I think you had something to do with my dream." She looked at him and wondered who he really was.

"I hope he had blond hair and blue eyes." Dave continued looking at her in the same way.

"You know he did. I have to ask—are you really a Viking in hippie clothes? I know you played football, and that is a violent game. Is it just my imagination, or are you really a dangerous Viking, not a peace-loving hippie?" Sharon looked back at him with an unwavering gaze.

"How do you know I played football?" Dave asked.

"Because of the way you are built. You are built like a football player. I am not complaining; you have a great body. But you didn't get those shoulders, arms, and that tight butt from playing golf," Sharon answered smiling.

"I did. Does that make a difference?" Dave was starting to worry.

"Oddly enough for some reason it doesn't. But is that all behind you? Are you over it—the violence, I mean? Lastly, please tell me you don't hunt and kill beautiful wild woodland creatures." Sharon finished and looked at him intently.

"I liked playing football, but I have a bad knee to remind me of the damage it did to me. I don't hunt."

She kissed him. "Let's clean up. It is getting late, and I have to fly tomorrow, so I need to wash my hair and do some things."

"Can I see you tonight?" Dave asked.

"Yes, but I have to get to bed early, because I have an early flight." Sharon looked directly into his eyes, arousing him in ways he had never felt before.

"I have no problem with us getting to bed early." Dave held her with their eyes locked.

"Do you ever think of anything else?" Sharon pulled away, feeling a little flushed.

"Don't worry. I will go. Not willingly, but I will go."

Before he left, they exchanged phone numbers, he gave her his address and directions to his apartment, and she said she would pick up some take-out on the way for dinner. They kissed and he left.

He walked back to the other house to talk to Henry. When he walked through the open front door, he saw a nice-looking, thin young man in glasses with a garbage bag; he was picking up plastic wine glasses, beer cups, and paper plates from last night. "Hi, I am Dave Cameron."

"I know who you are. I am Harven Watson, one of Henry's roommates. You know you crushed about a half-dozen guys' hopes last night. I, for one, was very impressed. You just walked in and walked out with her. You really let the air out of their balloons." The young man continued cleaning up.

"Is Henry here? I want to talk to him. Do you need some help?" Dave asked.

"No, he went to Sherry's last night after the party. He was supposed to be here this morning to help me, but as you can see, I'm it. I am almost finished. Plus, you weren't here long enough to add to the mess." Harven smiled.

"Do you have Sherry's phone number?" Dave asked.

A love story and social commentary

"I have it upstairs. Let me dump this last bag, and I will get it for you." Harven tied the bag, took it out back, and threw it on top of a pile of other bags.

"Your friend is upstairs. He moved in this morning. He is a little hung over. I guess he got pretty hammered last night. It turned into a hell of a party after you left, but I guess you aren't sorry you missed it." Harven looked at Dave with a slight smirk. "Let's go up, and I will get you the phone number and show you where Mike's room is."

They went upstairs and Harven got Dave the number. "Take it easy. I am sure I will see you around." Harven smiled and walked away.

Dave took the phone number from Harven and knocked on the door to Mike's room.

"Come on in," Mike called.

"Hey guy, you need any help?" Dave walked in the room.

"No, I'm finished and all moved in. So, how was it, I mean breakfast, not to mention dinner?" Mike leered at Dave.

"God, she is amazing. I have never met anyone like her. She is beautiful, smart, and I am not even sure she is human. I think she may be some kind of ethereal creature from another world," Dave gushed.

"I saw her. She is really hot. So, she fell for your line, took you home, and fucked your brains out. I thought you two were going to fuck right there on the sidewalk before you even got to her house," Mike said.

"What?" Dave was surprised by Mike's lewd comments.

"I followed you out. I wanted to get a better look at her." Mike smiled.

"You followed us?" Dave was more surprised.

"I just went to the front porch. Hey, she wanted to be looked at. Why do you think she was dressed like that? So, again, was it as tasty as it looked?" Mike wasn't going to let it go.

"You have the wrong impression of her. We are going to keep seeing each other, and that means you are going to be around her, so you need to cool it." Dave was not happy with his friend.

"Are you trying to tell me she isn't a slut? If she isn't a slut, she was sure wearing a slut's uniform last night, and from what I've heard, she sure acted like one in the Zoom Room. How long did you know her before you were fucking her? You think your boyish good looks and irresistible charm caused her to lose her head and start giving you head that quickly?" Mike's voice dripped with venom.

"Long enough. Knock it off. I came by to talk to Henry and to see if you were moving in here. Henry is not here, and you are moved in, so I am going to take off. I need to read the stuff we got yesterday and fill out all the forms. Have you done that yet?" Dave asked, changing the subject.

"Yes, I spent yesterday getting it done. Hey, I get it. You like this slut. Don't worry about me. I will treat her like a lady. But you are far from the first one down that road; I will bet there are ruts in it up to your knees. That field has been plowed many times before you plowed it, but that never bothered you before, so why should it bother you now? You want to get a beer later?" Mike lightened up.

"No, I am seeing her again tonight. I want to spend time with her before we are tied up at the hospital. Are you worried about being responsible for patients rather than just watching?" Dave wondered if Mike was as worried as he was about the coming year.

"No, we will be fine. We're ready. Think of me while you are fucking her tonight. I will be sitting in some bar alone. If I know you are thinking of me, I can enjoy it vicariously." Mike laughed.

"The last thing I want to think about is you while I am with her. See you later." Dave left.

If Dave had been aware of why Mike was talking Sharon down, he would have known Mike was more jealous and envious of him than he could have ever imagined. There had been a lot of girls at the party last night, and Mike had met some of them. Not one of them spent any time with him or said more than, "Nice to meet you." He left the party alone and hammered on beer, while Dave left with Sharon.

Dave drove back to his apartment and called Sherry's number.

"Henry?" Dave said when Henry picked up.

"Yes, Dave. What's up?" Henry answered.

"I don't know what to say. I should say thank you, but that's not adequate. In case you can't tell, I am walking on air and my head is in the clouds. Last night was the most magical night of my life," Dave went on.

"Really," Henry said dryly.

"Have you been talking to Mike?" Dave asked.

"No, Mike has been talking to me and anyone else within ear shot at the party last night." Henry was unhappy with Mike.

"I got some of that this morning," Dave admitted.

"I don't think you get it, Dave. This guy is not your friend. He trash-talked you and the woman you were with to anyone willing to listen. Friends don't do that. I don't want anything to do with him, and you should avoid him too, especially if you are with Sharon. He has some kind of sick, perverted thing for her. I let him move in because you asked me to, but I will spend most of my time at Sherry's," Henry added.

"I know he is a little envious. He has had to work his tail off to get to where he is, so naturally he resents those of us who are more fortunate and have had things easier. But he has a good heart. Don't you believe those of us who are more fortunate should help those who are less fortunate? Am I not my brother's keeper?" Dave said, defending Mike.

"The Bible? Come on, Dave. You are not his social worker or his welfare agent. All I am saying is watch your back with him because he will stab you in it the first chance he gets," Henry told Dave.

"I learned that in Sunday school, and you don't have to be religious to know it's true," Dave responded.

"This is not Sunday school in your family church in Our Town, USA, where you grew up. This is the real world. There are people in it who are toxic. When you identify one, you need to get as far from them as possible, as quickly as possible. That is what you need to do with Mike, because he is toxic," Henry pleaded with his friend.

"I didn't call to talk about Mike. I want to talk about Sharon. How did you know we would connect like we did?" Dave changed the subject because he knew Henry was right.

"I didn't know it would go down like that. Wow! You were doing the wu change lang before the party actually got started. But I knew you would like each other. It is pure narcissism. You see yourself in each other. Each of you looks in the pool of the other and sees your own reflection; you like the image because it's you. You have read the same books, you have the same philosophy of life, you are both attractive—well, Sharon is drop-dead gorgeous, and you are simply a nice-looking man. You both like music and art, you both like to travel. I could go on and on. I had this feeling I knew Sharon from somewhere when I first met her, and then as I got to know her, I felt like she reminded me of someone. It hit me yesterday. It was you. She reminds me of you. I thought you two would connect because you would be connecting with yourselves," Henry said, finishing his dissertation.

"So, it wasn't magic but psychology. I don't believe it. I believe it was pure magic. You know, Henry, sometimes it is best not to see the wires and believe in the magic," Dave told Henry.

"There is no magic. The wires are always there, even if you don't see them. Science and math are behind everything. You know that. You are a biologist," Henry scoffed.

"I'll bet you enjoy telling kids there is no Easter Bunny. I want to talk about Sharon, and you make me talk about Mike. I want to thank you for a magical night, and you tell me it's psychology." Dave wanted to believe some things were magical, and he believed last night was one of those things.

"Like I said, you are a biologist. She is the hottest woman you have ever met; therefore, you want to spread your genes with her. She is an evolved woman, so she is looking for a man with brains to provide for her, and then she meets a man with brains and brawn. Your biology and your dynamics made the connection, not magic. It was just the perfect biological and psychological pairing," Henry lectured.

"It was also fueled by the best ganga I have ever smoked, and we were both very high. I think the weed took her inhibitions to the floor; I don't think she would have acted that way without being completely fucked up. But I don't care. I will not let you spoil my joy." Dave was too happy to let Henry bring him back to reality.

"Don't get me wrong. I share your joy. Two people are happy because of me. I take full credit. Only a person as highly intelligent and intuitive as I am could have orchestrated such a perfect pairing," Henry said proudly.

"I choose to think you facilitated a magical night, but you are more than welcome to congratulate yourself on your intuition and intelligence. I also called because I want to get together and talk about this year. Sharon has a trip tomorrow, and I imagine Sherry is doing her nine-to-five jive at work, so can we meet for a beer?" Dave asked.

"I'll meet you for lunch at this Irish pub I know. We can have a pub lunch and drink some good Irish beer." Henry gave Dave the name of the pub and directions before hanging up.

A love story and social commentary

Dave had lunch and spent the rest of the afternoon reading pamphlets and filling out forms while listening to the Allman Brothers Band. After he finished, he cleaned the apartment and washed his sheets, towels, and the dishes. Then he set two places at the bar, remade the bed, put fresh towels in the bathroom, put out scented candles and sandalwood incense sticks in the bedroom, bathroom, and front room. He drove to the supermarket to buy a bottle of decent white wine, a six-pack of beer, and some flowers that he wrapped in tissue. He put the flowers on one of the beanbag chairs. When he was satisfied that everything was perfect, he took a shower, used a lot of incense oil, and got dressed in a T-shirt and jeans. The last thing he did was put "It's a Beautiful Day" on the turn table.

Dave sat down in the other beanbag chair, rolled a small joint from the baggy Sharon got from Phil, and looked around his apartment with a sense of satisfaction. The front room had sliding glass doors that opened onto a balcony with a view of the pool. There was a counter between the front room and kitchen with two bar stools. A Duel turntable, a big Sansui receiver, a TV, and Dave's books were on a large shelf complex next to the door. On the opposite wall were two big beanbag chairs with a wicker table between them. The hall led past the kitchen to the bathroom on the left, the bedroom on the right, and a storage closet at its end. In the bedroom was the bed with a wicker headboard and a wicker bedside table with an alarm clock and lamp on it. Opposite the foot of the bed were sliding mirror doors to the closet. It had shelves, so he didn't need a chest, and next to the bed was a large window. All the rooms had overhead lighting. Above the big Infinity floor speakers on each side of the shelf complex were framed prints of Venus Rising from the Uffizi in Florence and The Picnic from The National Gallery in Paris. Sitting on the shelves were his medical books and the books that had influenced his life, along with a copy of The David from the Academy in Florence. Dave was not sure what the replica was made of, but it looked and felt like real marble.

On the wall next to the kitchen counter was a framed oil painting of Paris seen from the steps of Sacre Coeur. He and the student nurse had sat on the steps one afternoon splitting a bottle of wine, with some cheese, and a baguette watching the artist paint it.

Behind the beanbags was a large poster for the America's Cup with two twelve-meter boats with their spinnakers and bloopers up running down wind. He had spent the last month of the summer between his freshman and sophomore years in med school on Cape Cod living in a big house in the dunes with friends from college who had summer jobs on the Cape.

They all heard about a music festival in upstate New York near the town of Bethel called Woodstock. He and one other guy who was not working that weekend drove to Woodstock and became a part of the legend. For Dave, it was a life-changing experience. He had not cut his hair since that weekend and he no longer dressed like a preppy fraternity guy in button-down shirts, designer pants, and penny loafers.

His tire-tread sandals had come from a trip to Mexico the last month of the summer between his sophomore and junior years in med school. The large carved lava ashtray on the table between the beanbags had come from the same trip along with the pottery jar under the table. The jar contained weed, papers, and a lighter.

The mother of a friend was from a wealthy Mexican family, and they were involved in the development of a resort on the Mexican Riviera. She gave her son an apartment, complete with a maid and a cook for the summer, so he invited Dave and two other friends down that August.

While he was in Mexico, he read *The Electric Kool-Aid Acid Test* by Thomas Wolf about the Merry Pranksters, Ken Kesey, and the San Francisco acid scene. There was a leather shop in town where he got his tire-tread sandals. Dave had them make him a deer skin leather shirt with fringe like Kesey's leather jacket. He wore the leather shirt in the winter and replaced the sandals with climbing boots from Zermatt, Switzerland. If it was really cold, he wore a copy of Billy Kid's Olympic ski sweater and his down ski jacket. But the hip-hugging bell-bottom jeans were a fixture year-round. At medical school, he had to wear a dress shirt, tie, and slacks with his short white doctor's coat on the wards and in the clinics. The same was true for his internship, only the coat was long, but he still had clothes from college for that.

In his bedroom, above his bed, was a poster for Woodstock with the lineup of bands and a picture of the field on the farm where it took place. He had gotten it from a record shop in Providence Town where he got the America's Cup poster. On the opposite wall from the window was a picture poster of Aldous Huxley in a suit standing in the Hollywood Hills and pointing out over LA, stoned on a hallucinogen. It had accompanied the book, *The Doors of Perception*.

He and his friends brought a burlap bag of peyote buds back from Mexico. They bought weed from one of the beach boys on the beach at the resort, and before they left, they asked him about peyote. The next day, an older guy showed up with the burlap bag of peyote buds. Charlie had an undergraduate degree in chemistry, so he knew what to do with them.

When they got back, he spent a week cooking, and the end product was a dozen capsules of mescaline for each of them. Dave went to three concerts on peyote that year: the Moody Blues, the Grateful Dead, and the mother-fucking Rolling Stones. They were nights filled with great music, cosmic sex, and then a complete understanding of the universe and everything in it. The "doors of perception" opened, and Dave walked through them.

Like the books on his shelf, these trips had a tremendous effect on Dave. His medical school had an agreement with the largest private hospital in the city to hire its medical students during the summer. Medical school started on September 1, and ended May 31, so Dave worked the first two months of the summer then travelled during August during those three years. He saved as much money as possible while working to travel and buy things he wanted, like the stereo component set. He had learned early on that if he wanted to be independent and do what he wanted to do, he had to control the purse strings. To control the purse strings, he had to have his own money, so he worked every summer so he could travel and buy what he wanted, and he saved the rest.

He worked as a urology tech doing catherizations, starting IVs, and helping with minor procedures the first summer. After he had pharmacology his sophomore year, he worked as a medication nurse on a medical floor. The last summer, after he had medicine his junior year, he worked as a CCU nurse. He graduated from med school in late May and did not have to report for his internship until late June, so he worked as the charge nurse in the ED on the eleven-to-seven shifts for a month. The ER charge nurse's salary gave him the money for the car, the move, and his apartment with some left over to add to his savings.

The hospital used this partnership to allow its staff to take summer vacations and still have plenty of coverage. The medical school saw the partnership as good experience for its students, plus it gave them a chance to make extra money as an adjunct to financial aid. It was a win-win situation and Dave took full advantage of it.

While he was waiting for Sharon, he thought about what Henry said. He knew Henry was right about the chemistry between two people, the how's and why's it developed, but Henry had left out the human factor—the soul. Dave felt their souls had touched in some way last night. He knew he was a complex biochemical, electrophysiologic organism, and even the thoughts he was currently having were a result of neurotransmitters turning neurons on and off in his brain, but he felt something magical happened last night, and nothing was going to change his mind about that.

The doorbell rang. He got up, started White Bird with the sound low enough to made a perfect background and opened the door. All he could do was stand and stare at her. She had on white shorts, strappy white wedge sandals, and a red tube top just wide enough to cover and accentuate her breasts. Her makeup was perfect, highlighting her eyes and mouth, the way her outfit highlighted her legs and breasts. She was standing with her hip cocked to one side, her elbows resting on her sides, her arms extended palms up, holding a bag with Chinese letters on it in one hand and a shopping bag in the other.

"I come bearing Chinese takeout and a great album I bought today. Well, are you going to invite me in? If not, there were a couple of cute guys checking me out in the parking lot. I bet one of them will let me in if you don't." She smiled and looked down the stairs as two guys walked by looking up. She had completely unsettled him. She knew how powerful her looks were, and she knew just how to use them.

He reached out and pulled her to him. She put her head back and laughed. "What will your neighbors think?"

He kissed her neck and nibbled at her earlobe. Her breathing quickened as she pressed against him.

"Are you taking advantage of my hands being full to molest me?" she asked.

"You bet," Dave answered as he went back to her neck.

"Well, cool your engines. I promised myself I would act like a lady tonight." Sharon tried to wiggle free.

"That doesn't sound like much fun." He ran his hands down her back to her rear while continuing to kiss her neck, causing her breathing to become more pronounced.

"What am I going to do with you?" she said softly.

A love story and social commentary

"I have a few good ideas." Dave nibbled her ear again.

"OK. That's enough," Sharon said pulling away. "You can't have dessert until you have eaten your dinner. Besides, my arms are getting tired of holding your dinner." She wiggled her way out of his embrace, walked to the kitchen, put the food bag's contents in the oven, and set it to warm. "How did you know I like White Bird? That song and your neck work almost pushed me over the edge, but I knew I had to be strong and fight you off, if I was going to maintain my lady-like demeanor."

Dave closed the door. "I am not sure I like Lady. If you are going to have a case of multiple personality disorder, when is Slut coming back out? I like her better." Dave followed her.

"You are impossible. When 'Beautiful Day' finishes, I want to play my new album. I love Linda Ronstadt. Two members of her back-up group got together with a guy from Poco and one from The Flying Burrito Brothers to form their own group, the Eagles, and they just released a new album. The FM rock station played the whole thing a few days ago. I bought it today while I was out shopping." Sharon walked to the shelf and put the shopping bag in front of it.

"If Lady is out and I have to wait for Slut to come out, do you want to smoke a joint while we listen to it?" Dave asked.

"Sure." Sharon walked over to the beanbags and saw the flowers. "Dave!" She smelled the flowers. "Do you have a vase? We need to put them in water. You come on like a molesting Viking, then give me flowers like a Southern gentleman. Who has multiple personality disorder?"

Dave did not have a vase, so he put the flowers in a pitcher and placed it on the counter between the place settings. Then he went back to the beanbags, sat down and started the joint.

"That smells Jamaican. I can't get fucked up like I did last night. I have to fly early tomorrow." Sharon was a little apprehensive.

"Take a hit, and I will get you a glass of wine." Dave walked to the kitchen to pour Sharon a glass of wine and get himself a beer. He came back and handed her the wine as she finished with the joint.

"Just as I was feeling safe with the Southern gentleman, here comes the Viking again. Sure, take a hit of this killer dope and drink some wine. Don't worry, I won't take advantage of you, not much anyway, said the spider to the fly. I guess I will end up in your bed before the night is over, but I want to hear the Eagles first and eat Chinese by candlelight at the perfect place settings you did. Are you going to light the candles?" Sharon asked.

"I was, but you smell too good. I would rather smell you. What are you wearing?" Dave took the joint.

"Ambush," Sharon answered.

"Wearing Ambush, the way you are almost dressed, teasing me with other guys, 'oh please, Mr. Big Bad Viking Wolf, don't molest me. Oh, well maybe just a little molesting. Well, if you insist maybe a lot of molesting.' Who is taking advantage of whom here?" Dave took a second hit of the J.

"I admit it. I want to be molested by a Viking warrior like the one in my dream. I like Vikings now," Sharon said in a husky voice.

Dave was getting very high, so he tried to hand the number back to Sharon. "No. If I don't stop now, I won't hear the Eagles and will go to bed hungry again tonight. 'A Beautiful Day' is finished. I can't take another hit; I am way fucked up. Put the Eagles on and turn the volume up."

Dave put the joint in the ashtray, went to the shelf, opened the album and put it on the turntable. He adjusted the volume and sat back down to listen.

"They are great," Dave said when the album finished.

"I couldn't wait to buy it," Sharon responded.

Dave poured Sharon another glass of wine, got another beer, then went around the apartment lighting the incense and candles. They went to the kitchen and filled their plates with fried rice, vegetable chow mein, and Peking duck. When they finished eating, Dave put the dishes in the dishwasher, and they went back to the beanbags. "What do you want to hear now?"

"Do you have any Linda Ronstadt?" Sharon asked.

"Sure." Dave put a Linda Ronstadt record on. He finished his beer, and Sharon finished her wine while they listened to the album. "Do you want another glass of wine?"

"Yes, but no. I want one, but I have to get up at four and fly at six. I have already smoked and drank too much. Besides, I want to keep the current buzz going." Dave went through his albums, put Sticky Fingers on the turntable, and cranked the volume again.

"I want to dance." Sharon danced to the middle of the room. Dave was a good dancer, but as he danced over to Sharon, he realized he was an amateur compared to her. She did a perfect Tina Turner, dancing backward and forward, throwing her head down so her long hair fell over her face when she danced forward, then throwing her head and hair back as she danced backwards. Dave felt he was completely out of his league trying to dance with her.

He stopped. "You are a professional dancer."

"Twelve years of ballet from the first grade through my senior year in high school." She stopped and curved her arms in front of her chest and did a tight spin, turning her head to spot as she turned. "Now, put your hands lightly on my waist." She lifted her arms above her head, stood on one foot and turned in his hands. She stopped to face him, put her arms around his neck, and put her head back laughing. "We just did a pas de deux."

She was a dancer. That explained everything. Her slender gracefulness, her perfect legs and rear, the way she moved, her confidence, how she presented herself, her style, how lithe she was—everything. It was all clear to Dave now.

"I haven't danced since college, and I haven't done ballet since high school. Who are you, Dave Cameron? How do you have this effect on me? What's your sign? Where did you come from? How did you make it? Why do I see myself so differently and feel so free when I am with you?" Dave thought about his conversation with Henry, but Dave refused to see any wires. It was all magic, pure magic—he was sure of it.

"Why did you stop dancing?" Dave asked as he held her by her waist.

"Dance is an expression of joy. Something happened that took the joy out of my life; besides, I was too tall, there were a lot of other girls much better than I was, and I knew I wasn't going to make a career out of it. But I don't want to talk about that tonight; I am too happy. I'm ready to be ravished by my Viking now. I want him to make me scream like I did in my dream." She jumped into his arms and wrapped her legs around his waist.

Dave carried her to the bedroom, placed her on the bed, unzipped her shorts, pulled them off and tossed them aside. She had on a small thong like the one she had on last night. She raised her hips so he could pull them off, and then she sat up and he pulled the tube top over her head. She lay back down with her hair spread out around her head, one long leg straight, the other one bent at the knee, and her arms over her head. He stood looking at her as he undressed and thought, my God she is perfect in every way. Then he got on the bed next to her, propped himself up on one elbow, and began to trace her body with his fingertips as she closed her eyes.

It was basically a repeat of the night before, but now they were comfortable with each other, so any awkwardness or uncertainty was gone. They took their time, enjoying every aspect of their pas de deux. They were a tight sexual jazz duet now, playing each other and playing off each other to produce harmonic ecstasy. She screamed because he didn't stop; he pushed her until she convulsed so hard it seemed she was having a seizure. For Dave, it was so intense it was almost painful, so he cried out as she clung to him.

Sharon spoke softly in his ear, "I thought I was going to die. I couldn't breathe, and it felt like my heart stopped. After last night, I didn't think it could get any better. But it did."

Dave could barely collect himself to talk. "Some people call it the little death. I don't know what to say. I have never felt anything that intense in my life."

She snuggled under his arm with her head on his chest. They lay quietly for a while. "What time is it? I have to get up at four. If I get to bed by ten, I will only get six hours of sleep, and I have a hard trip tomorrow."

"It is nine. It's finally dark outside. I can't imagine being in this bed without you tonight. Can we spend the weekend together? It is the last weekend before orientation." Dave cuddled her in his arms.

"I will call you when I get back tomorrow night about the weekend. I have to go now." Sharon got up, went to the bathroom, and when she came back, she was dressed.

"Where are my sandals? You rip a girl's clothes off and don't leave them where she can find them." Dave put his jeans on and followed her to the front room.

Before she left, he held her in his arms, reluctant to let her go, until she whispered, "Please. I have to go."

Dave walked her to her car barefoot with nothing on but his jeans, gave her the flowers, and watched as she drove away after cautioning her several times to drive carefully. He already missed her by the time he saw the tail lights of her car disappear.

Dave walked back to his apartment and sat down in a beanbag. The room seemed empty without her glow and vitality. Her album was propped against the bookshelf, so he put it on and smoked the rest of the joint. Phil had said if you smoked too much, it would put you out—with her gone, he wanted to be out. As he listened to the record, he could see her dancing and laughing in the middle of the room. He had only known her for two days, but now he was terribly lonely without her, and his apartment seemed lifeless. He thought about the last two nights as he stretched out in the beanbag and closed his eyes, floating on the music. The weed did not put him to sleep, but it did put him in La La Land. He played the record again.

After the record finished a second time, he got up and went to the bedroom, pulled off his jeans, and got in bed. He could smell her in the bedding. Ambush. He drifted off to sleep with her smell producing images in his head. Ambush.

He woke up late and a little groggy. He had been dreaming about having sex with a beautiful, fantastic dancer, and the dream had been very vivid, but he knew it was only a dream because women like her only existed in dreams.

His mind began to clear, and that's is when he smelled her on the sheets. Ambush. She was real. He got up, walked to the front room, and saw the album on the turntable where he left it. The stereo system was still on. Of course she was real. "Man, did I get fucked up last night. I smoked too much of that shit." He laughed at himself and did a little naked happy dance.

He went back to the bedroom; it was late, and he had to meet Henry for lunch at noon. He continued to smile and dance around. "I am never going to wash my sheets again. I want my bed to always smell like her." He showered, got dressed and drove to the city to meet Henry. He arrived at the pub before noon, but Henry was already there sitting in a booth in the back.

2
Lysergic Acid Diethylamide

Henry greeted Dave and handed him an envelope. "I got a letter today from Cousin Jane in San Francisco. There are twelve little squares in it. Four of the squares are pieces of blotter paper with images of the Do Da Man from the Grateful Dead album cover stamped on them. There are four others that look like brown caramelized sugar and four that are almost transparent. They are LSD from San Francisco. Cousin Jane said I needed to expand my mind. I thought you might want to do a little mind expanding, too. The blotter paper ones are called Mister Natural. The others are Window Pane and Clear Light; they are stronger, and you are only supposed to take half at a time. Have you ever heard of a guy named Owsley? He made the acid. Jane got it from some musician she is fucking."

"Wow! Twelve hits of Owsley acid from California," Dave exclaimed. "We will do the Mister Natural first. Sharon wants to try it, and Sherry needs to do it too." Dave took the envelope.

"Let's do it this weekend. Are you seeing Sharon again tonight?" Henry asked.

"No, she is flying today and won't be back until late." Dave added, "How is Cousin Jane, and what is she doing in San Francisco?"

"She is living there. She is involved with the artsy-fartsy San Francisco crowd—poets, artist, writers, and musicians. I would call her a groupie, but she has too much money to be a groupie, so I guess she is a star fucker. I hear from her from time to time." The waitress came to take their orders. "Two Guinness drafts and two fish and chips." Henry turned to Dave. "So, what did you want to talk about?"

"I want to talk about this year. How were the clinical years for you?" Dave was serious.

"I drank more, but that is not what you are talking about, is it?" Henry understood exactly what Dave was talking about.

"I'm talking about dealing with the broken bodies, the devastating diseases, the poverty and ignorance, I am talking about the blood, vomit, pus, body fluids, and the smells. I can't deal with the smells. I'm talking about being responsible, not just watching someone else make the decisions. I am not sure I can deal with the on-the-job training we have to do." Dave had been carrying around his insecurities and it felt good to open up to Henry.

"Man, I hear you about the smells. I barfed twice in front of my Medicine team. The nurses laughed at me, made jokes at my expense, and gave me a nickname I will never divulge. But I couldn't help it. The smell hit me, and the barf came out of me. What can I say, Dave? It goes with the profession. Focus on the job. Don't think about anything but the patient's diagnosis and treatment. Keep it scientific. Think of the patient as a diagnosis and focus on getting the best outcome," Henry responded.

"You're talking about depersonalizing the patients. They are just gomers and trolls. They are not people with names; they are the CHF patient, the diabetic, the GI bleed. I know you can't do the job if you get emotionally involved, but I haven't learned how to ignore the humanity of it all, so I compensate by getting fucked up and using a woman's body to counter the horror," Dave confessed.

"I don't know what to tell you. You are right—detached, sociopathic people seem to do better at what we do. People like Bar thrive. You have to find a better way to cope. Empathy is good, but it is a two-way sword that cuts both ways," Henry countered.

"I am sorry, I know this is heavy shit, but I needed to talk to someone about it. I have never been as happy as I am since I met Sharon. God, Henry, she is everything I have ever dreamed about in a woman and more, but this stuff keeps pulling me down," Dave lamented.

"Dave, I know you, and I know you will be fine. Just trust yourself. I know that sounds like a cliché to patronize you, but it's true," Henry said reassuringly. "I am sorry I am not more help. Come to Sherry's tonight for dinner. Her apartment complex has gas grills, picnic tables, and a big pool. We will grill some steaks, play a little Frisbee, and take a swim. I want Sherry to get to know you; plus, we need to get her buy-in to do the acid. I will see you around five. Here's the address." Henry wrote out Sherry's address, they finished lunch, and Dave drove back to his apartment.

Dave spent the afternoon thinking about what Henry had said about insulating himself from the emotional onslaught of working in a city/

county hospital. It was easy to talk about it, but the reality of a place like University Hospital was overwhelming. As a student, he had seen some very disturbing things, and no matter how detached he tried to be, he couldn't help but be affected. How could he manage if he weren't just watching, but he was the one responsible? He was also concerned about the hours, the lack of sleep, and the loss of any personal life, especially now, after meeting Sharon. He knew this internship would take an emotional and a physical toll on him. The interns where he went to school were pale, hollow-eyed, and unhealthy looking.

He decided to smoke a joint before changing clothes. Dave was smoking the joint to drive away his fears and insecurities, but he told himself he was getting high to enjoy dinner with Sherry and Henry. He had to charm Sherry so she would go along with all four of them taking acid, so he needed to be loose, confident, and witty. He pushed the idea he was using a drug to self-medicate out of his mind. He put ZZ Top on the turntable, rolled a number, and forgot about his concerns as he listened to the blues of the little old band from Texas.

Dave put on a flowered Hawaiian shirt with his bathing suit and used Chanel Pour Homme. No incense oil or T-shirt to charm Sherry. He checked the clock to make sure he had time to stop for flowers, stuck the remaining half-joint in his breast pocket in a baggy, and got the last four beers from the six-pack he bought yesterday out of the fridge.

Sherry lived in one of the most exclusive apartment complexes in the city. Dave parked on the street, found the right apartment, and rang the bell. No one answered, so he followed the path out to the pool area. The common area was landscaped with paths that led to a large pool with a waterfall. There were lounge chairs around the pool, tables with big umbrellas further back, and a line of gas grills behind the tables. Dave saw Henry and Sherry setting at one of the tables.

"Hey, Cisco."

"Hey, Poncho." Dave walked to Sherry, handed her the flowers, and set the beers on the table. "Thanks for having me over. I know you worked today so the last thing you wanted to do was cook for me, so if you would like, I can grill the steaks and help with anything else you need. I lived with Henry for two years, so I know he is worthless."

"Well, thank you. Of course, grilling the steaks would help. I have everything else under control." She took the flowers. "These are lovely."

"Not as lovely as you are. Henry is a lucky guy." Dave took one of the beers and offered one to Henry.

"No thanks, I have a scotch going." Henry held up a crystal glass almost full of scotch with only one ice cube. "Like I said at lunch, I drink more these days."

"Sherry, are you sure I can't do more than grill the steaks to help?" Dave asked.

"No, everything else is done. We will eat when it is cooler. But you are sweet to offer. You are right: Henry is worthless. He did call to let me know you were coming, so I could get everything ready. There wasn't much to do—get the steaks and potatoes, make a salad, choose a wine, and set the table." Sherry smiled at Dave.

"I am glad Henry asked me over because I didn't get a chance to talk to you at the party." Dave looked down. "I got, ah …. distracted."

Sherry laughed. "I would say so. Sharon is a beautiful girl." Sherry was starting to warm up to Dave. He wasn't a dirty hippie after all; he was well spoken and polite with excellent manners. Of course, Henry's best friend for the last eight years wouldn't be some low-class individual with no breeding or background, but why did he dress the way he did, and what about the beads and hair? Sherry was in her element. She loved to entertain. She saw it as practice for when she was a New York socialite.

"That's a cute bathing suit. It looks new. Did you get it at Bob and Phil's?" Dave took a shot on a hunch and hit the mark. Sherry was wearing a tasteful black one-piece bathing suit.

"Yes, it is new. Bob and Phil's have the best selection; it is the only place to shop. Henry, did you hear? Dave likes my bathing suit—you know, the new one you haven't noticed." Sherry primped a bit.

"Yes, dear. Sorry I didn't say something sooner." Henry smiled behind his glass of scotch. He smiled knowing Dave could charm the paint off a wall. Dave's charm lay in the fact everything he said was true, and he believed what he was saying. Sherry was pretty. The suit was flattering. Dave simply told the truth, and it came across in an innocent boyish manner.

"Dave, I have to ask. Why is Mike your friend? He is nothing like you. You are different than I thought you would be when I saw you at the party, but he isn't. He is just what he appears to be—crude." Sherry frowned.

"We got close in med school and helped each other through some tough times."

Loyalty, Sherry thought, *another checkmark for Dave.*

"Last question. I don't mean to put you on the spot, but you look so different from anyone I have ever known, yet you seem to be like everyone I have ever known. Why the hair, beads, sandals, and hippie attire? You are a nice-looking man, so why do you hide your looks in that hippie garb?" Sherry asked.

"It is a statement. It means I stand for peace and love; I oppose the war and support the civil rights movement. I wear my philosophy and political stance for everyone to see," Dave answered.

"You are not a communist or radical, are you? I mean, you believe in democracy and capitalism, don't you?" Sherry continued to press Dave.

Henry knew this was dangerous territory, because he was aware of Dave's feeling on those subjects, and they were not conducive to winning Sherry over, so he jumped in. "Dave has some socialistic ideas, and I have to admit, I agree with him, but he is not a radical, communist, anarchist, or anti-American. He and I are pretty much in line politically and sociologically. His family, like mine, is responsible for founding this country. They were some of the earliest settlers in the colonies and fought in the Revolutionary War. He is a direct descendant of one of the families of the Republic of Texas, like I am. You are letting the hair fool you. He is an American, and his family has been here even longer than mine."

"I'm sorry, Dave. I had to ask; you hear so many stories these days, and there is so much on TV about demonstrations and the counter culture. You are Henry's best friend, and I want us to be friends. Please don't take offense. I can see now I was overreacting a bit. Henry is too liberal for me, and frankly you scared me, but I am beginning to understand," Sherry said apologetically.

Dave did not say anything. He knew it was best to let Henry handle the situation.

"Now that you know Dave is not going to murder you in your sleep, burn down the city, or start a revolution, can we have some fun and not be so serious? This coming weekend is our last weekend before we start orientation, and we want to plan something to do."

"That would be great." Sherry felt secure and happy; Dave was one of them after all.

"Dave let's play some Frisbee and take a swim before dinner," Henry suggested.

"You can take the boy out of the frat, but you can't take the frat out of the boy." Sherry sipped her glass of wine and picked up a magazine.

Henry and Dave played Frisbee for a while then dove in the pool. "I am moving out of the Park house and moving in with Sherry," Henry told Dave. "I thought about what you said at lunch and decided I needed a more private, sheltered environment. I don't want any extra drama or aberrant personalities complicating my life."

"I am sorry about Mike. So, you are going to tell her you are moving in with her, and oh by the way, do you want to take some acid this weekend to seal the deal." Dave smiled at Henry.

"Something like that. Just follow my lead," Henry replied.

"Henry, this girl does not know who you are. Socialistic ideas, really? How many hours did you and I spend in college discussing political systems, economic systems, and different forms of government? We dissected Plato's *The Republic*, *The Federalist Papers*, *Das Capital*, and a half-dozen others. You are a socialist. You have lived in the social democracies of Europe and know firsthand the advantages. You taught me humanistic science was the road to a successful society. I could go on, but you get my meaning. Sherry doesn't know any of that about you. 'Henry is too liberal for me,' really? You are not being straight with her, and now you plan to extort her into taking acid with you." Dave had a worried look on his face.

"She knows just what I want her to know about me. She is the type of woman I need. The type of woman I have always needed. I am comfortable with her, just like I was with the others. Unfortunately, they all tend to be conservative, and their families are even more conservative. I let them be comfortable with me, that's all. I am not going to marry her; I just want a good relationship with someone with a similar background," Henry explained.

"Don't worry, I am not judging you, and I am the last one to give relationships advice. Look at my track record." Dave told his friend.

"You can be sure her father knows everything about me and my family. He is a developer with extensive holdings in the South, he is a major donor to a certain political party, and he belongs to a certain conservative group. You can bet he is watching out for his little girl; I have no regrets about my actions," Henry added.

"OK. Lead on, Macduff. I will follow you once more into the breach." Dave laughed.

Dave knew very wealthy people were different. Everyone is a product of their environment and experiences, and the wealthy are raised in a privileged protected environment that leads to a different paradigm. Henry treated those of his class as if there was a different set of rules or codes of conduct for them, and in Henry's case that was not a good thing. If you were an ordinary person, Henry was a model of behavior, but the wealthy needed to look out for themselves where Henry was concerned. It bothered Dave at first, but over time, he had come to accept it. Sherry was Henry's girlfriend and a member of his class, so it was up to him to deal with her. Dave prepared himself to go along with Henry as long as it did not get too far out of hand.

Sherry brought the steaks out while they were in the pool. "Henry, can you get the wine? I have water glasses and a pitcher on the table. Dave, you can start the steaks anytime. I will wait to bring the salad out until the last minute." Henry headed back to the apartment with the Frisbee, while Dave fired up the grill and put the steaks on.

"Dave, I thought you might be a bad influence on Henry, but it is just the opposite. He is so much more relaxed and open around you. He is usually so stiff, guarded, and formal. I like the side of him you bring out." Sherry sat sipping her wine.

"We got close during Hell Week. Henry, Tommy a guy from my hometown, and I pulled each other through. Believe me, we know each other inside out, literally. When you go through something like that, you get close. I guess that's why Henry is relaxed when I am around, because he knows our friendship is unconditional. I have seen him at his worse, and he has seen me at my worst, so we have no illusions about each other. It was an old school Hell Week; Tommy almost died. He had to be rushed to the hospital with dehydration and exhaustion," Dave told Sherry.

"What did his parents and the school do?" Sherry was horrified.

"Not much. Tommy was a legacy, so his dad went through the same thing. The school told the fraternity it had to change Hell Week, that's all," Dave answered.

Henry returned with a bottle of Cabernet and a baguette. "Dave told me a little about Hell Week. I am so glad he is here, and you guys can help each other through this next year." Sherry was getting a little buzzed on the wine.

A love story and social commentary

They ate dinner in a warm, friendly atmosphere complimented by an excellent Cabernet. When they finished eating, Henry took control.

"Sherry, I wanted Dave to come over so you could get to know him. I had hoped that would happen at the party, but it didn't. I knew my friend was vulnerable to the wiles of a beautiful woman, and I thought Sharon would like Dave too, but I had no idea they would reach critical mass and combust spontaneously." Henry smiled at Dave.

"I was surprised too. I was around Sharon when she was dating Bar. I thought she was an ice princess—beautiful, cold, and aloof. The way she was dressed, all the PDA, followed by the exit was surprising. She was always so reserved before," Sherry added.

"Also, I had lunch with Dave today, and he convinced me I should take you up on your offer and move in with you," Henry continued.

Sherry looked at Henry, then looked at Dave. "What?!"

"I am moving out of the Park house and moving in with you. Dave and I had a discussion today that sealed the deal for me," Henry told her.

Sherry got up, went around to Henry, hugged and kissed him. "That makes this a perfect evening." Then she searched Dave's face and looked into his eyes. Henry told her Dave saw himself as a sort of shaman, out to make everything better. She thought to herself, could it be true? Sharon almost fucked him in a room full of people, then he gets Henry to do something she had been trying to get him to do for months over lunch, and he changes her mind about him over dinner.

Henry looked around to make sure no one else could hear him. "Lastly, like I said, we want to do something this weekend. My cousin Jane sent me some LSD from San Francisco. Dave has taken mescaline before, so I asked him if he would take it with me since he has some experience with hallucinogens. Sharon wants to take it, and I want you to take it with us." Henry looked at Sherry.

"What?!" She looked at Dave.

"This did not come from Dave; it came from Cousin Jane. She wrote that I needed to expand my mind. She has taken the same thing we are going to take, and she convinced me to do it, not Dave. I want you with me on my first trip. If I am going to live with you, I want to do everything with you." Henry leveraged Sherry.

"Henry, are you sure it's safe? Are you sure you want to do this? It scares the hell out of me. I was so happy. Now I am terrified." Sherry looked stricken.

"Don't do it if you don't want to. I think you will have an amazing experience. There is that word again, but it has to be your decision and you have to do it because you want to, not to please Henry. I will look for a concert for us to go to. It enhances everything, and I do mean everything. You will have the most wonderful night together you have ever had. That is why Henry wants you to take it with him, so you don't miss that part," Dave reassured Sherry.

"I need to think about it. Let me sleep on it and decide tomorrow." Sherry relaxed a little and smiled again.

"I think you two have something to celebrate tonight, so I am going to take off. Here, put a little wu in the wu chang lang tonight, Henry." Dave got up and handed Henry the baggy with the half joint in it.

"What is wu chang lang?" Sherry asked.

"I will show you later, dear. Bye, guy." Henry and Sherry got up to say goodbye.

"I think I understand Sharon now and why you are Henry's best friend." Sherry gave Dave a little hug.

Dave thanked them both for dinner and drove back to his apartment to wait for Sharon to call. The phone rang around nine.

"Hi, Dave," Sharon said in a husky low voice that made him ache for her.

"Hi. How was your trip?" All she had to do was say hi, and he was lost.

"It sucked. The first leg to LA was fine. Then LAX was so crowded, we were held for over an hour. LAX's backup caused the whole West Coast to hold flights, disrupting connections. I just walked in, and I am dead tired," Sharon answered.

"Can I come over and tuck you in?" Dave hoped.

"I don't think you want to come over to tuck me in. I think you want to come over and fuck me in. You are welcome to come over and sleep here, but that's all. I am too tired for anything else. I like sleeping with you, and I especially like waking up with you." Sharon's voice was low and husky again.

"You're right. If I will come over, it won't be to sleep. Are you off the whole weekend?" Dave asked.

"I am off Saturday and Sunday, then I have a long trip with a layover on Monday and Tuesday followed by a turnaround on Wednesday. I need to get you a copy of my schedule," Sharon answered.

"So, can we spend the whole weekend together?" There was a touch of pleading in Dave's voice.

"Do you think you have to ask me like you are asking for a date?" Sharon answered.

"We just met, and I didn't know." She was unnerving him.

"Does it feel like we just met or that we don't know each about as intimately as two people can know each other?" Sharon voice was driving him up the wall.

"I know how I feel about you. I wasn't sure how you felt about me." Dave got it out without stumbling over his words.

"If you don't know how I feel about you, you are not as smart as I thought you were. What does a girl have to do?" Sharon said softly.

"You can open the doors of perception with me this weekend if you want." Dave relaxed. She had said it; she felt the same way about him as he felt about her. He was ecstatic.

"What?" Sharon voice was normal, and the sexy huskiness had disappeared.

"Just what I said. I have the keys to the doors of perception, and we are going to unlock them together tomorrow night." Dave was confident now.

"Are you saying what I think you are saying?" Sharon was excited.

"Yes." Dave was cautious because they were on the phone.

"You have to tell me more."

"I will tell you in the morning. I want you tan, rested, and ready, so take a hot bath and go to bed. Call me when you wake up. I will come over and bring your album back." Dave was as happy as a teenage boy with his first girlfriend.

"You have seen my skin; in fact, you have seen all my skin. Did you see any tan lines? I don't tan. My name is Sharon Kelly. I am Irish. I am very white, and the sun turns me bright red. I want you to keep the album at your place." Sharon sounded tired but happy.

"I have seen your skin; it's beautiful and flawless. But I also know something else that turns it bright red, and I intend to make you glow like a traffic light tomorrow night. Take that to your dreams," Dave said, turning the tables on her.

"You are a bad man, a very bad man, and I don't know why I like you. I will see you tomorrow." Sharon almost said more but stopped herself.

"It is because I am a bad man that you like me, and I intend to be a very bad man this weekend. Bye, I will see you tomorrow." Dave wanted to say more too but like Sharon, he didn't.

He walked down to the laundry room, got a paper from the newspaper rack there, and checked the entertainment section. There was a spread on a concert in the park on the 4th with the city symphony playing before and during a fireworks display. He kept looking. Santana was playing at the Civic Center Auditorium and tickets were still available at the box office after nine in the morning for as long as they lasted. Dave decided to call Henry in the morning to see if he could drive into the city to get the tickets since Sherry's place was closer. Dave went back to his apartment, turned on the TV, and watched *Twelve O'clock High*, an old movie about the B17 raids over Germany during the war. The movie disturbed him. It demonstrated that no matter how strong someone was, they could be broken by stress and responsibility. That made him think about what happened to his dad during the war, and thinking about his dad made him think about his sister.

He seldom thought about her. It was too painful. He kept her memory locked away deep inside him, but he thought about her and how the whole thing had affected his mother and father. His sister's death shattered his dad, and his mother was never the same after what she went through. It had altered his life too and was one of the reasons he became a doctor. What his family experienced with his sister motivated him to try to relieve suffering in others. He could not face those memories long. He shifted his thoughts back to his ability to get through the next year. Would he be able to handle the stress and responsibility, or would he be broken like Gregory Peck in the movie? He did not sleep well that night and woke up early.

He called Henry as soon as he woke up. Sherry answered.

"Sherry, this is Dave. Is Henry up? Can I talk to him?" Dave asked.

"Dave, you knowingly encouraged Henry to drug me and take advantage of me last night. It depends on what you mean by up. He was up earlier, but not anymore." She giggled. "He is still in bed. I am getting ready for work. Oh, by the way, I slept on it, and I am in." She giggled again.

Henry overheard Sherry and said, "I need to talk to Dave. I am sure it is about what we are going to do tonight." Henry took the phone.

"There's a Santana concert tonight. We can still get tickets, but you need to get to the Civic Center Auditorium box office ASAP. Can you make it, or should I go?" Dave told Henry.

"I got it. I am closer, and I can be there sooner," Henry replied.

"Let's meet in the zoom room at five thirty. The concert starts at eight, and all the tickets are general admission, so we need to be there early enough to get decent seats. Eat something before we get together," Dave continued.

"Five thirty in the zoom room. See you then," Henry confirmed.

"I will be at Sharon's if there are any problems." Dave hung up, ate a bowl of cereal, and drank some orange juice then waited for Sharon to call. When she hadn't called by nine, he showered, and got dressed.

He put on a pale blue work shirt with a three-mast, square-rigged sailing ship embroidered on the back. He had bought it from a vendor at a crafts fair on the beach the summer between college and medical school. He wore his jeans from Europe. They were straight-legged and had an American flag sewn on the back pocket. Dave doused himself in incense oils, put on his beads, tied his hair back in a pony tail with a bead on a leather thong, and slipped on his penny loafers; he had his concert uniform on, ready to rock and roll.

Sharon called.

"Hi, did you dream about traffic lights?" Dave asked.

"I just woke up, and I didn't dream about anything. I was dead tired. Can you tell me more about this weekend now?" Sharon asked.

"We are going to a Santana concert. I saw him at Woodstock, and he was great. I will tell you the rest when I see you," Dave answered.

"I have to have a new outfit! Bob and Phil's is having a 4th of July sale and they give me an extra discount. You can help me pick it out. I haven't been to a concert in forever. I feel like I am back in college." Sharon was wide awake now. "Give me about an hour to get ready."

"See you in an hour." Dave hung up.

3
The Concert

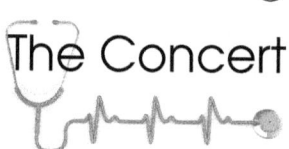

Dave put his shaving kit and a T-shirt in his on-call bag, drove to the bank and used the ATM to get cash, stopped for gas, and went to the market for a bottle of wine and a six-pack of beer. By the time he had done everything and driven to Sharon's house, an hour had passed. He went to Sharon's door and rang the bell. A pretty woman in a baby doll and fluffy slippers opened the door. "I am Dave Cameron. I am here for Sharon."

"I know who you are. I am Helen, one of Sharon's roommates. This is not a sorority house. It's the home of four grown women. Come in. I think you know where Sharon's room is," she said with a mischievous smile.

He had not met anyone at the party except Bob and Phil, yet everyone seemed to know him. "Are you all here today or are some of you flying?"

"We are all here, we were all at the party, and we are all a little curious about you. The others are having breakfast in the kitchen, and I know they would like to meet you." Helen studied him closely.

"Sure. I think I am a little early." Dave knew what was coming next; he was going to be scrutinized by the roommates.

Helen led Dave to the kitchen. "Here he is, girls. Dave, this is Audrey and Caroline." She indicated two attractive women sitting at the table. "We are friends, we went through training together, we live together, we bid our trips together, and we look out for each other."

"And some of us are half-naked in our lingerie with no robes. You could have warned me, Helen." Audrey frowned at Helen.

"I didn't think you would want to miss meeting him," Helen replied.

"It's OK. Don't worry, ladies, I am a doctor and a professional. I am used to it. Nice to meet you both." Dave extended his hand smiling.

"Oh, what the hell." Audrey took his hand.

"We know what kind of a doctor you are. We saw you operate at the party, and we know what you prescribed for Sharon," Caroline said dryly as she took his hand.

"Enough, girls. I know he is cute, but he is here for Sharon, and I have a feeling he is enjoying the view a little too much. None of us have much on. Oh, but I forgot he is a doctor, a professional, and he's used to it," Helen said sarcastically.

"A professional BSer," Audrey added.

"We are going to finish breakfast now, and Sharon is probably ready. Take one last look and say goodbye, Dave." Helen sat down with the other two at the table.

"Goodbye, ladies. It was great seeing you, and I look forward to seeing more of you in the future. I'm sorry, I couldn't resist." Dave continued to grin.

"You are right, Audrey, he is a BSer." Caroline picked up a blueberry and threw it at him.

As Dave walked down the hall and up the stairs, he heard them say, "He is so different from Bar." "I know, with that hair, those beads, and the embroidered shirt." "And a personality that is different from what I expected." "I like the way he looks. He is not some skinny nerd." "I just hope he is not another jerk. He seems really nice, and he is charming, but he may be a player." "She deserves a good guy for once, not a toxic jerk like Bar or another player just looking to score her."

Sharon opened the door in a bright yellow sundress. "I haven't been to a rock concert for so long I don't know what to wear."

"As soon as the band hits the stage, everyone's feet will hit the floor. Santana was great at Woodstock; he got half a million people up dancing." Dave put his hands on her waist. "We are going to take acid for the concert. That's what I was talking about on the phone—the doors of perception. Real, honest to God, lysergic acid diethylamide from San Francisco. Henry got it from his cousin Jane. We are going to have a cosmic night."

"I knew that was what you meant. I have to shop for a new outfit. I want it to be girly and flirty so I can spin." She did a little hop away from him and spun in place. The sun dress lifted out from her waist like a spinning pinwheel. *My god, she really is exquisite,* Dave thought as he grabbed her, and they fell on the bed together laughing. He pinned her arms. "I met your roommates downstairs, and I think they approve of me."

"That's why you are all revved up—you saw my roomies in their nighties. Well, you can put those thoughts out of your head. We are going shopping. Stop imagining doing all four of us together. I know how your devious little mind works." Sharon wiggled to try to get away from him.

"I was just imagining the three of them." Dave tried to hold her.

Sharon wiggled free. "Your play time is over. You can't expect me to be nice to you after a comment like that. All three, indeed—as if you could handle all three of them at once. You have an exaggerated opinion of yourself." She smiled. "So, my roommates turned you on, and you can't do anything about it. Serves you right." She stood up. "You can look, but you can't touch."

Dave sat on the bed and reached for her. "I said no touching until you redeem yourself by taking me shopping." She danced away. "Caroline and Audrey have boyfriends, and Helen has a different date every night. You are out of luck with them. I am your only hope of satisfying your lust, and I am not having it. I need a new outfit for tonight, so get up and let's go. We have the whole weekend together so let's make the most of it. You have orientation next week, and I have a two-day trip with a layover. Then I have a turn-around and you start your internship. We may not see each other for a while."

Dave frowned. She walked back and stood in front of him. "It will be fine. I have a copy of my schedule, and once you get your call schedule, we will work it out. I have a job, and you will be an intern, so it won't be perfect, but that's reality. We are in a kind of fantasy bubble right now, so let's go make the most of it."

"It's not that. It's the layover thing. Look at you. I'll bet you get hit on by every pilot, copilot, and first officer you fly with, not to mention the passengers. It's someone laying over you on the layover that's bothering me." Dave continued to frown.

"Are you jealous?" Sharon looked down at him.

"No, I am not jealous. If I were jealous, that would make me an insecure, pathetic loser. No one wants to be with an insecure, pathetic loser. I'm not jealous; I'm just concerned." Dave looked up at her.

"You are jealous." She pulled him up.

"OK, I am jealous, and I hate myself. Does that make you happy? See what you have done to me—you have turned me into a green monster. The thought of you sleeping with some pilot, first office, or passenger on a layover is killing me. I won't be able to sleep with you on a layover. I will be up all night worried about who is laying over you." He couldn't help the way he felt about her.

Sharon looked into his eyes. "Dave, listen to me—I guess I have to hit you over the head with it. I am not going to sleep with anyone else. I have never been happier than I am with you, and I don't want to fuck anyone else. If that changes, I will tell you. What do I have to do or say to prove the way I feel about you? All I want is the same commitment from you. I expect you to respect me enough to tell me if you are fucking someone else. That's all I need from you. Is that clear?"

Dave lay back on the bed and pulled her on top of him. "What guy in his right mind would want anyone else if he had you?" He kissed her. "Does this mean we are going steady? Do you want my class ring to wear around your neck on a gold chain?" Dave pulled off his medical school ring and held it out to her.

She sat up straddling him. "I don't know why I like you; I pour my heart out to you, and you make a joke about it. I should take it and wear it. I want to shop, but if you want to fuck, let's fuck. I am yours any time you want me." She said the last thing in the low husky voice she had used on the phone with him.

Sharon had left the door open, the other women had finished breakfast, and were on their way back to their rooms. As Helen walked by the door, she saw Sharon sitting on Dave, and heard. ".... let's fuck. I am yours any time you want me."

"If you are going to fuck, shouldn't you close the door?" Helen asked as she peered into the room.

"No, don't close the door. I want to watch," Audrey quipped as she joined Helen.

"Will she let us watch this time?" Caroline added walking up to the other two.

"Maybe, she has him pinned on the bed," Helen told the other two.

Sharon jumped up and went to the door. "You three are mean."

"Does that mean we can't watch?" Audrey said as they all three broke out laughing.

Sharon closed the door blushing. "After tonight, we stay at your place."

Dave got up and put his arms around her. "You are beautiful when you blush."

"Stop it. We are going shopping, and I mean now. If we don't leave right now, I will never live this down." She opened the door. "Let's go."

She bounded down the stairs and out the front door. Dave had to hustle to catch up to her. She was laughing when he got to her. "You are such a bad influence on me. They will never let this go."

"How is this my fault? You left the door open, sat on me, and talked dirty to me." Dave laughed.

"I intended to leave right away, but you became a pathetic, insecure loser. Your words, not mine, and I had to stop you from whining. I wanted to go shopping, and I still want to go shopping. If your head is finally on straight, can we go shopping? I can't believe we are actually going to take acid tonight. A new outfit, a concert, dancing, and I'm pretty sure I know how the night will end." She skipped to the car laughing.

They drove to the expressway and took it into the center of the city. Bob and Phil's Clothing for Discerning Men and Women was in the best part of the city surrounded by the most exclusive stores, shops, and eateries. Dave found a place to park, and Sharon led him to the store.

They went to the women's department, and she took her time looking at dresses, skirts, and tops. Dave followed her around commenting on the things she showed him. She picked a couple of dresses she liked, and the sales clerk took Sharon to one of the dressing rooms on the women's side and told her to push the button on the wall if she needed help. Dave waited for the clerk to leave, then went to Sharon's dressing room. She was pulling the sundress over her head when he entered.

"You're not supposed to be in here." He reached for her, but she shied away. "Don't even think about it. I see the look in your eyes. Go back to the fitting room and wait. Jesus you are so difficult."

He trapped her against the wall, pinned her wrist above her head, and kissed her. "You said anytime."

"I said anytime, not anywhere. Behave and I will reward later. God, you are like a child that I have to bribe to behave." Sharon tried to wiggle free.

"I don't want to do it. I just want to molest you a little." He let her wrist go and moved his hands down to cup her breast.

They heard a woman's voice. "Is there a man in there?"

Sharon pushed him a way and put her finger to her lips.

"I am going to get a manager. There aren't supposed to be any men on this side." They heard her leave.

"Get out." Sharon pushed him out the door. Dave went to the fitting room, sat down in one of the chairs, Sharon slipped on one of the dresses, and walked out to stand on the dais.

They heard a familiar voice. "Why am I not surprised it's you two?" They looked at the fitting room door and saw Phil standing there with a woman. "Don't worry, Mrs. Roberts, I will take it from here." The woman left and Phil walked into the fitting room. "Were you really going to do it in one of my dressing rooms? Why do you keep trying to do it in public?"

"I don't know what you are talking about, Phil. I am modeling outfits for Dave. I want something new because we're going to the Santana concert tonight," Sharon said innocently.

"You are a terrible liar, Gorgeous. And you, Dave, I told you to cherish her, not to bang her in public." Phil shook his head. Dave and Sharon could not hold back any longer, and they broke out laughing. "It's noon. Find something you like then I will take you to lunch. I can't be mad at you. Have you been apart since the night of the party?"

"Sharon had to fly one day," Dave answered.

"Have you done anything other than have sex?" Phil persisted.

"We listened to some music." Sharon looked at Dave. "We weren't going to have sex in your dressing room. I promise. We were only playing. Do you like this dress? Do you like it, Dave?"

"I like it, but I want to see the others. Sit down and help, Phil." Dave patted the chair next to him.

"She makes everything she puts on look good. What the hell, I have nothing better to do, like run a store, so I might as well waste time with you two. Maybe I can keep you out of trouble." Phil shook his head again.

Sharon tried on the dresses then asked, "Which one."

Dave and Phil both said. "The first one."

"I like that one too. So where are going for lunch?"

Phil took the dress from her, and gave it to the sales clerk. "Take this dress, ring it up as a no-charge, and bring it back. Then call Andre's and get me a table for three in fifteen minutes."

"You can't do that, Phil. That is an expensive dress, and Andre's for lunch!" Sharon was overwhelmed but excited.

"It's my store, so I can do what I want, and that is where I want to go for lunch. Come on, let's go. We can walk."

"This is going to be the best day ever; a new dress, lunch at Andre's, Santana tonight, and I have a feeling the after-party will be over the top. Thank you, Phil. You are the best." Sharon smiled at Phil.

The sales clerk brought the package to Sharon as they were walking out. Phil held Dave's arm to let Sharon walk ahead. "What have you done to her? She is a totally different person."

"You mean she is happy?" Dave looked at Phil.

"She has a bounce in her step and a joy about her that wasn't there before." Phil's eyes met Dave's.

"Let's just say she knows how to go woo, woo, woo now." Dave smiled at Phil.

"I thought so." Phil laughed. "So, you did do something to her."

"Yes, but she did the same thing to me. I have more than a bounce in my step. My feet don't even touch the ground. Phil, she is like no one I have ever met. She is my dream woman; she is my fantasy come to life, and I'm truly trying to do what you told me to do: cherish her" Dave gushed.

Sharon came back to them. "Why are you guys lagging? What's going on here? You did this at the party, Phil. What did you tell him this time?"

"It's not what I told him; it is what he told me," Phil answered Sharon.

Sharon took Dave's arm as they walked on. "What did you tell him?"

"He told me he was cherishing you," Phil responded for Dave. "Now let's eat."

Phil opened the door to Andre's, but Sharon hesitated for a moment and looked intently at Dave. She squeezed his arm. Knowing she was cherished aroused exceedingly strong emotions deep in Sharon for some reason and surprised her with their intensity.

Phil ordered a bottle of wine. "You two be careful tonight. Dave, your hair and dress may draw some verbal abuse or, God forbid, even something physical from some of our city's fine citizens. I probably don't need to remind you that there is a lot of tension in the streets, and don't think the cops will protect you. They will beat the hell out of you, Dave, and they'll have a great time groping you, Sharon." Phil looked worried.

"Yes, Daddy. We won't drink any gin and we will be in by ten," Sharon joked.

"Well, being an openly gay man in this city makes me paranoid, but I am sure you will be fine." Phil said, trying to lighten up.

The food arrived. "Thanks for lunch, Phil." Dave raised his glass in a toast to Phil.

After they drank, Phil continued with his discourse on society. "People support the civil rights movement, but what about gay rights? What about the civil rights for women? What about Catholics, Jews, and all the religious minorities in this country? Gays are harassed, beaten, and vilified as evil. Women are raped, forced into prostitution, forced to have sex to gain advancement, harassed, abused, and beaten. Straight male WASPs, like you, are the only group that isn't targeted in this country." Phil ate a few bites then nodded again at Dave. "You are too naïve; you see the world the way it should be, not the way it is. Your clothes and hair aren't a statement. They make you a target, the same way Bob and I are targets for being openly gay."

Once they'd finished their meals, Phil changed the subject. "Sharon, how many days a month do you fly?"

"Usually about sixteen. Why?" Sharon answered.

"Have you ever done any modeling?" Phil asked her.

"Not real modeling. When I was in college, I did some charity events. Why?" Sharon responded somewhat puzzled.

"Would you do some modeling for us when you are not flying? We use models for trade shows, the Apparel Mart, and advertising. You made everything you put on today look good," Phil told her.

"You must be kidding. I am not a model," Sharon scoffed.

"You could be. I saw that today. Plus, we pay a hundred dollars an hour for commercial work and five hundred a day for trade shows and the Apparel Mart. I am just asking you to think about it," Phil pleaded.

"We can work out the details later if you decide you want to try it. Just think about it for now." Phil answered.

"I don't like you anymore, Phil. We are going to have enough trouble being together with my schedule and her flying. Now you want to take more of her time, not to mention exposing her to a bunch of guys looking to score models." Dave frowned.

"You have got to stop being jealous. I thought we went over all that this morning. You have to trust me," Sharon said reassuringly.

"I trust you. It's other men I don't trust." Dave was not happy about the modeling thing.

"When I am flying, I say, 'Coffee or tea but not me.' I will say, 'You can have the clothes, but not me in or out of them.'" She laughed at her own joke.

Sharon showered before getting dressed for the concert, and Dave joined her. He washed Sharon's hair and saw that her hair was not really auburn but lighter with golden highlights. It was long and luxurious. He had been so taken with her eyes, her face, and of course her body, he had missed how extraordinary her hair was. "Do you color your hair, or is this it's natural color? It's beautiful."

"Of course not. Everything about me is natural. I am one hundred percent pure me." She leaned against him.

They got out of the shower and Sharon looked down. "I am woman, I am powerful. You know I could lead you around by this, and you couldn't do anything about it. You would just have to follow me." She walked to the bedroom holding him and laughing.

"You need to let go of me." Dave did not laugh.

"Why, am I making it hard on a guy?" She cracked herself up.

He grabbed her and threw her down on the bed as she continued laughing. "Goddammit, Sharon, you are letting this power thing go to your head."

"No, it is going to your head. Just look at you. I'm sorry, but knowing I can do something like that is so cool. I can't help myself." She threw her head back. "I am woman, and I love being woman."

"And I love being man. But you have to let me settle down. You know what you do to me, so stop doing it so we can get ready." Dave pinned her down.

"Let me up. I proved my point. But some Viking you are. Where is all the ravage stuff?" Sharon teased him.

"I will show what kind of Viking I am later, but we have wet hair, no clothes on, and we are going to be late if you don't stop." He let her up.

He combed out and dried her hair, marveling at how full it was. He put lotion on her, and she put incense oil on him. That almost caused another problem.

"Do you think Phil is right, and there might be trouble tonight?" She said, sounding worried. "I know they are out there—the deplorable despicables who are angry and consumed with hate. Their lives are dysfunctional, and they want to blame their miserable existence on something, so they look for a target—blacks, Latinos, gays, hippies, Jews, Catholics, the government, you name it. They don't have enough education or insight to understand their own deranged perception is causing their problems and the darkness in their lives. It is a darkness that permeates society and perpetuates the dark side of human nature. I don't want to see the darkness, so I try to deny they are there, but I know they are, so I try to see only the light and never acknowledge the darkness."

"Don't worry, there won't be any trouble tonight. This is not Altamont, and there are no Hells Angels so everything will be fine." Dave got his clothes to dress.

Sharon took the new dress and went to the bathroom. "You stay here. I don't want you to see me until I am the finished product. Jesus, did I just objectify myself?"

Sharon came out of the bathroom and twirled. The skirt lifted up just enough for Dave to see a flash of black bikini panties. Dave thought of the line from the song, "Black panties and an angel's face."

He had already seen the dress; it was chic and expensive looking. It fit her perfectly, accentuating her body, her long legs, and in her high-heel ankle boots, she was eye to eye with him.

"You look magnificent." Her hair was shining, and she had created deep waves in it. Her makeup drew attention to her eyes with glitter in her eye shadow, and her lipstick was redder than usual.

Dave slid his arm around her waist and took her hand as she put her arm over his shoulder; they waltzed around the room cheek-to-cheek to no music. He stopped but continued to hold her. She pulled back from him. "Dave, I am a little frightened. I know I talked about wanting to try LSD, but now that it is about to happen, I'm not so sure. What if something happens? People have bad trips. We could run into trouble, like Phil said. I am not as brave now as I was when we were just talking about it."

"We will be fine. Bad drugs cause bad trips, and no one is going to bother us. But if you don't want to do it, don't. I told Sherry the same thing. You have to want to take this trip, you have to want to open the doors of perception and see what's on the other side, you have to want to explore yourself and expand your mind. If you don't want to, then let's not. It is up to you." Dave looked straight into her eyes.

"Will you be with me the whole time?" Sharon asked.

"I will be with you the whole time," Dave answered.

"I trust you, Dave Cameron. I don't know why, because you are a risk-taker and you scare me, but if you are with me, for some reason, I know I will be alright. Let's go." Sharon untangled herself from his arms, and they left for the house next door.

As they were walking to the other house, they saw Henry drive up and park. Sherry had on a short, tight, black dress with heels, and Henry had on slacks, an expensive dress shirt, and loafers. They walked into the house as Harven was coming out of the kitchen with a beer. "Wow, where are you ladies going? Jesus, you both look great!"

"We are going to a concert. Where is Connie?" Sherry looked around.

"She is working the three-to-eleven shift. I am going over to her place later for some midnight madness after she gets off. Who are you going to see?" Harven answered.

"Santana. Where is George?" Sharon asked.

"He is upstairs getting ready; he has a date with a grad student he met at the lab where he works." Harven continued.

"Dave, this is Harven Watson. We went to prep school together." Henry introduced Dave to Harven.

"I met Harven. Hi, Harven. Who is Connie?" Dave asked.

"She is an ICU nurse I am dating," Harven replied.

"You didn't tell me you were dating a nurse." Mike came out of the kitchen with a beer and walked up to the group.

Mike was standing close to Sharon looking at her in a way that was making her uncomfortable, so Dave moved up beside her and put his arm around her protectively.

"Mike, I don't think you had a chance to meet Sharon the other night. Sharon Kelly, this is Mike Detrick; he was my roommate for two years in medical school." Sharon had been looking down because Mike's stare made her uneasy. She looked up at him and put her hand out.

"My God, you're beautiful. You have the most amazing eyes I have ever seen." Mike took Sharon's hand.

"I think she may have heard that before." Dave hugged Sharon, and she looked down again to avoid Mike's eyes as he took her hand.

"I saw you when you were leaving the party, but I didn't get a chance to meet you because Dave was intent on keeping you all to himself. I'm Mike."

Sharon shifted her weight toward Dave leaning against him. "It's is nice to meet you. I guess you already know Sherry." Sharon tried to divert his focus.

"Hi, Sherry, nice to see you again." But Mike continued to stare at Sharon as he acknowledged Sherry.

Henry intervened. "We are going to have a little pre-party in the zoom room, if that's OK with you guys."

"Mi casa es su casa, because it is su casa. Don't worry, we won't bother you. Mike and I were going to have a beer and watch the ball game." They went to the front room.

"See you guys later." Henry started down the hall to the zoom room with everyone following him.

"That little man was so crude at the Bar party. Sharon, you should have heard what he said about you," Sherry exclaimed.

"I think he's creepy. He kept staring at me. Guys stare at me, but he made me feel uneasy." Sharon took Dave's arm.

"Enough about Mike. No bummers and no negative thoughts. Let us spend the evening with Mister Natural," Dave said, trying to redirect the two women.

"Henry, I know you have a flask, but drinking only makes you feel bad the next day when you trip. I have done mescaline, but this is LSD. We need to follow Cousin Jane's directions. She said to put the tab on your tongue and let it dissolve and rub your tongue on the roof of your mouth until it is all gone. If it is like mescaline, you get a strange metallic taste in your mouth when it starts coming on. I can't describe the taste, but you will know it when you taste it. We took capsules of mescaline, so it took about half an hour for it to come on. This may come on faster because it is absorbed in your mouth. It can be intense when it first starts coming on, so just hang on until it gets manageable." He gave each one of them a tab to put on their finger.

"This is the point of no return. Once you do this, you can't undo it. If you have any doubts, don't do it."

Dave turned to Sharon and she said, "I am ready."

"Kiss me then put your tab on my tongue, and I will put mine on yours. I want to start this trip with a kiss."

Sharon kissed him lightly and put her tab on his tongue, then put her tongue out. Sherry and Henry mimicked them.

"Well, the game is afoot. Do you guys want to listen to some music?" Dave asked.

"Let's go to the park. I can't sit on the floor in this dress," Sherry answered.

They walked to the park and found two benches with views of the gardens and lake.

"What a lovely day. I am glad we are all together to do this. For some reason, it feels right for the four of us to be together," Sherry said dreamily.

"Sherry, do you have any kind of taste in your mouth?" Dave looked at Sherry, and he could see it in her eyes.

"Why yes. My God, did you see that butterfly? Its wings were a foot across. Look at the flowers, they are so big and bright. What a wonderful day," Sherry continued.

"Sherry is off. Sharon do you have any kind of taste in your mouth?" She took Dave's hand but did not say anything. "Are you alright?"

"Wow, what a rush. Just hold onto me," Sharon replied.

Dave put his arm around her as he tasted it and started to feel it. It was much more intense than the mescaline, and it was taking him for a ride. He wondered how Sherry and Sharon were really doing since they were both lighter and drugs are weight-dose-related. They had to be soaring. "This stuff is righteous. Do you think you can drive, Henry?"

"Hell, I can teleport." Henry was fucked up too.

"Let's take a walk first. Look at the sky, the trees, the flowers, and the grass. I want to walk around and see everything." Sharon got up and turned in a circle with her arms out. Through the lens of the LSD, all the flowers were a bright day glow color, the sky was an intense blue that was hard to look at, and the grass was a sea of varying shades of green. "Come on, Dave." She held out her hand. The trees seemed to be giant beings standing guard over all the bounty of nature below them. They walked further into the park holding hands. Sherry and Henry followed them.

"It just keeps going. When does it top out?" Henry asked.

"I hope we peak at the concert," Dave answered.

A love story and social commentary

"I think I will be in outer space by then," Sherry added.

Dave saw a bush with long stalks growing from it. The stalks were tipped with large fluffy white balls. He took out his pocket knife and cut two at their base. "Here girls, nature's paint brush or a magic wand, whatever you want it to be."

There were roses planted along the path, so Sherry and Sharon touched them with the fluffy tips of the stalks singing, "We are painting the rose red." They waved their wands at everything, laughing and acting like little girls as they walked through the park.

Dave looked at his watch. "We need to go. Henry, are you sure you can drive."

"I got it. Let's go." They followed Henry to his car while the women continued to touch things with their wands and laugh.

They got in Henry's Mercedes coup and started for the city center. Dave and Sharon cuddled in the back seat with Sharon touching the window with her wand as they passed things. Sherry touched Henry on the top of his head with her wand from time to time, laughing at something only she knew.

"Fuck it. I can't drive anymore." Henry pulled over on the expressway. "Can you drive, Dave? I'm too fucked up. A pair of hands came over my shoulders, took the wheel, and started driving. I let go the wheel and let them drive until I realized I wasn't steering the car. I am through." Henry didn't realize that the hands driving the car were his hands, and he had hallucinated about them coming over his shoulders to take the wheel, but that didn't matter. Henry was right. He was definitely too fucked up to drive.

"I have driven high before but not on acid." The four of them traded places. Dave drove the rest of the way to the Civic Center, parked in the public parking garage, and they joined the diverse group of people walking along the path from the parking garage to the auditorium. It was a colorful procession strung out along the path in all types of attire, like a moving impressionistic multicolored ribbon. There were lines at the entrance to the building, so they picked the shortest line and waited. Some Latinos were calling out "Carlos" from time to time and chattering away in Spanish. They were surrounded by the smell of weed. A black guy in the line next to them said, "Somebody's smoking some good shit."

"People will head for the front when the doors open, but a lot of them will get shut out and start back to find seats. If we go for the middle, we will get good seats without a scramble. Everyone will be on their feet in front of the stage as soon as they start playing anyway," Dave told the others.

"Don't let me get lost in the crowd, Henry. Everyone, stay close. I don't want to get separated." Sherry was the smallest person in the line.

A guy in the line next to them said, "Don't worry, Little Mama. If you get lost, I will take care of you." His buddies laughed. Sherry moved against Henry, and he put his arm around her. As the excitement continued to build, more cries of "Carlos" rang out from the crowd.

Sharon was looking around at all the people. "How many people do you think are here? This auditorium is not very big."

"There are probably a few thousand. Not much of a crowd for a rock concert, right Dave? How many did Santana play for at Woodstock?" Henry answered.

"I think the peak was around five hundred thousand. Arlo Guthrie announced it was half a million on Friday night, and that was the figure they used to declare us a disaster area. There must have been about that many when Santana played Saturday afternoon," Dave answered.

A yell went up from the front of the line, and they began to move forward. Henry handed everyone a ticket. "Hold on to my belt from behind, Sherry. You do the same with Dave, Sharon. Here we go."

The line moved quickly as they walked single file through the doors and handed their tickets to the attendant. Henry led the way through the rush to four seats on the aisle about a third of the way back from the stage. The house lights were up, and through their acid-altered eyes, everything seemed to glow in their brilliant glare. A lot of the girls had flowers in their hair, and some in peasant dresses were spinning around making huge bubbles. Beach balls had appeared from nowhere and were being batted around over everyone's heads.

The smell of pot permeated the atmosphere, and a guy walked by with a pipe. "It's a happening, man. Can you dig it? It's rock and roll, man. It's far out. You want a toke?" He offered the pipe to Henry who declined saying he was far too fucked up for grass to have any effect on him. "Wow! Are you riding the rainbow, man? I can dig it. Better living through chemistry." He walked on.

It was a city venue so there was no alcohol being sold, but vendors were hawking sodas, waters, and snacks. Henry bought some waters for them. They sipped their waters and watched the show being performed by the crowd unfold around them. Several girls decked out in Gypsy costumes were dancing through the aisles banging on tambourines while others played wooden flutes. They could feel the tension building as the auditorium filled up and the audience started to anticipate the start of the concert.

It was well after eight o'clock when the house lights went down. In the total darkness that followed, a voice came over the PA system. "Ladies and gentleman, all the way from San Francisco, California, please welcome Santana!"

The stage lights went up, the band walked on stage, and Santana picked up his guitar. The crowd screamed and yelled as he hit a long cord that sliced through the auditorium, followed by a solid wall of sound as the rest of the band joined in. The people in front rushed the stage, pushing the chairs aside as they went.

"Let's go," Dave yelled at the others as he got up. Sherry hung back, freaked out by the crowd, so Henry picked her up and put her on his shoulders. Her tight dress rode up to her waist as her legs slid over Henry's shoulders, but she did not care, because now she could see, and she was above the mass of people. She began to bounce to the music and wave her arms in the air with a huge smile on her face.

Dave held Sharon's hand as they worked their way to a good spot. She was swaying with the music as Dave leaned over and yelled, "Can you dig it?"

The music took them away. It felt as if Santana had lifted the whole building off the earth, and they were flying through the time-space continuum, at one with the cosmos. The crowd was moving to the music, screaming and going wild as each song ended. Sharon swayed beside Dave for a while, and then she yelled in his ear "I need room to move."

They worked their way back through the crowd. Everyone was standing, either in the crowd at the front of the stage, or in the back of the room where other couples were dancing. Sharon put her hands above her head and begin to move. The music took control of her. She was unaware of anything else as the music moved her body as if it were being played like an instrument by Santana. Her body connected

Sex, Drugs, and Scrubs

directly to the music, and everything she had learned as a dancer was triggered by the music steaming through her. As the acid peaked, she became one with the music. It was sensual and beautiful.

They were dancing next to a black couple, and the black woman was an excellent dancer too. A circle began to form around them. No one in the circle stopped dancing, but they watched the two women as they danced.

Between songs, the black man leaned over to Dave. "Your woman can move."

"So can yours," Dave responded.

"Yeah." The black man laughed. "Can she do more than dance?"

"She can do more than dance."

The black man held out his hand grinning and they slapped skin up and down.

Santana played for over two hours, and then Carlos stepped to the front of the stage, and all the stage lights went off except for a single spot on him. The band stopped playing, the crowd went silent, and the dancers stopped dancing. There was total silence and total darkness except for the single spot on Santana. He played a guitar solo for about fifteen minutes as Sharon and Dave stood mesmerized with their arms around each other's waists. When he finished, the wall of sound slammed through the crowd again as all the lights came up. A bank of spotlights at the front of the stage played across the audience as the band tore into the song. Dave had chills as he put his head back and let the sound wash over him. Then the band did an encore. The whole auditorium shook with everyone dancing and shouting as the spotlights continued to play across the crowd.

When Santana finally left the stage, Sharon wrapped her arms around Dave's neck, hooked one leg behind his knees, pulled herself against him, and kissed him passionately. The black man put his arm around his partner as he looked at Dave and Sharon. "She's running hot. She's got the fever. You better take her home quick and treat it."

Sharon broke the kiss and leaned back looking into Dave's eyes. "I think he is right." Sharon had a mischievous smile on her face. Her hair was down around her face, and her skin was glowing and glistening with sweat from dancing. She leaned forward, bit Dave's ear, and whispered, "You know what dancing is, don't you? It's foreplay." Dave crushed her to him as she ground against him. He was so turned on and wanted her so badly, he fairly ached for her.

"Hey, like I said, you better get her home and treat that fever, but if you like to dance, there is a club not far from here called Mother's Blues. The house band is great, and a lot of white people go there. You'll be alright. Check it out." He pulled his partner closer. "But I think you better do something about that fever now. It looks like it is getting worse." The black woman nodded to Sharon. The black man held his hand down; he and Dave slapped up and down again, and they left.

Henry and Sherry showed up beside them with Sherry still on Henry's shoulders. "I want my wand. I am queen of the world, and I need my wand."

"You need to get down now. Atlas got tired of holding up the world, and I am tired of holding up its queen." Henry tried to take her down.

"I am never getting down. I like it up here. I am the queen of the world. I am taller than everybody, and I am above the masses where a queen should be." Henry took her by the waist and hauled her down.

"Man, when the spots hit us at the end, I completely lost it. What an experience, what a concert, wow! Are you guys ready?" Henry looked at Sharon and Dave. "What a stupid question. Of course you are ready. Do you think you can wait until we get home?"

"Do you think you can drive?" Dave and Sharon broke their embrace and held hands.

"Not only can I drive, but I can't wait to drive. I am on top of this shit now. I am in control. I am going to drive my car, and then I am going to drive you, my dear." Henry reached for Sherry.

"Don't be crass, Henry," Sherry said as he enfolded her in his arms.

As they walked along the path back to the parking garage holding hands, Sharon sang in a clear voice that rang out. "I could have danced all night, I could have danced all night, and still have begged for more. I could have spread my wings and done a thousand things."

Henry turned to her. "We just heard one of the best guitarists in the world playing some amazing shit, and you break into show tunes. You should be singing Black Magic Woman. Carlos!" Henry finished with a yell, then they all four yelled, "Carlos." There were multiple echoes of Carlos along the path back to the garage.

"I danced with a black magic woman tonight," Sharon responded.

"What are you talking about?" Sherry asked.

"Sharon and a black woman put on a dance clinic during the concert. We went further back so we could dance and ended up dancing next to a black couple. Sharon and the woman became a part of the show," Dave explained to Sherry.

"So that's what got you worked up. Dancing girls will do it every time," Henry interjected.

"I am not a dancing girl Henry, you chauvinist. I wasn't dancing for Dave; I was dancing with him. We are equal partners in this relationship." Sharon corrected Henry.

"You two are in a relationship? How long have you known each other?" Sherry asked Sharon.

Sharon hugged Dave's arm. "We have known each other all our lives."

"Honestly, I can see how that might be true. I am not a chauvinist, Sharon, but I can tell you that watching a beautiful woman dance turns a guy on, and there is no way to get around that with some feminist bull shit," Henry told Sharon as they walked along.

"Sharon is my white magic woman." Dave put his arm around her.

"You are in a relationship because Sharon is a white magic woman who dances for you and you have known each other all your lives? I am completely lost." Sherry looked confused.

They got to the car. "Buckle your seat belts, ladies and gentlemen. Henry is at the wheel." Henry drove back to the Park house as if he were driving the Grand Prix at Monaco as Sharon as Dave cuddled in the back seat, and Sherry used her wand to move cars out of Henry's way. Dave was too engrossed in Sharon's body to care how Henry drove. They flew through the cosmos back to the Park house at hyper speed in Henry's Mercedes.

They got out of the car and stood in wonder as they watched the full moon rise over the trees in the park. The acid had stared to mellow, so their consciousness was no longer being torn and ripped by the initial rush and peak of the drug. They were still tripping, but the mind-shearing, enhanced sensory overload was beginning to burn out. They were in control again. Before, the acid had control of them, but now they controlled the acid. Things were still enhanced on this part of the trip, but the mind, intellect, and emotions were stimulated as well as the senses.

"Come on, Sherry, I want to take a little stroll through the park." Henry took Sherry's hand. "See you guys tomorrow. What a great concert. Take off your shoes if you are worried about walking in those heels in the dark."

Sherry took off her shoes. They all four hugged and said good night, and then Henry and Sherry started into the park with Sherry complaining about the gravel hurting her feet and wanting Henry to carry her on his shoulders again. She still had her wand.

Sharon put her arms around Dave's neck and leaned her head back. "Best day ever! I have never had so much fun."

"That could have something to do with riding a few hundred micrograms of lysergic acid diethylamide." Dave hugged her.

"I know it's the acid, but it is more than that. It's you, the last few days, everything, but mainly it's because I seemed to have found some things that were missing in my life," Sharon said seriously.

"Like being able to go woo, woo, woo?" Dave teased her.

"Yes." She laughed. "But other things too. Things like joy. I feel like I am finally free to be who I really am. It's hard to explain. We can talk about it in the morning. Right now, I want you to take me in and make me go, woo, woo, woo." She jumped up and wrapped her legs around his waist, kissed him, and nibbled on his ear, as he carried her to the house.

At the door, Dave put Sharon down. "I wish you could make love to me in the soft grass under the full moon."

It was not lost on Dave that she said make love, not have sex or fuck, but she said make love.

When they were inside the door, Dave unzipped her dress and took it off. Sharon stood in front of him in the black panties and ankle boots as Dave kicked off his shoes, took off his shirt, stripped off his jeans, and threw his clothes in a pile on the floor with the dress. He pulled her up into his arms with her arms around his neck and her legs around his waist again and carried her upstairs to her room.

There is no way to describe sex on LSD. Sex is the most intense, pleasurable sensation a human can experience; LSD enhances and magnifies that sensation massively. It creates a euphoria while eliminating inhibitions and restraints as the neurotransmitters in the brain are released at peak levels. Dave and Sharon experienced sex on LSD to its fullest. Dave pushed Sharon's moments of ecstasy past being bearable until she reached a mindless state unaware of anything other than the pleasure pulsing through her body. Dave had exquisitely intensified periods, each one greater in magnitude than the one before.

Sharon's room was not big enough to hold them; she got a blanket, and they moved outside to the lawn between the two houses under the full moon. Dave felt as if he was watching as well as participating in his own pornographic movie. When they were finally completely satiated, they bathed in the light of the moon and talked.

Sharon told him how her eyes, he thought were so beautiful, had caused her to be bullied as a child. "My eyes caused me a lot of pain when I was young. My mother and father both have emerald green eyes, the color of the rings around the outside of my irises. The doctors said I had a mutation that caused the cells in my irises to fail to produce pigment. That's why they are so light. There is green pigment around the edges but not much in the body of the iris itself. My skin is very light too, so people thought I was an albino. Children can be so cruel. They made fun of me, called me names, and wouldn't play with me. But the adults were worse; they thought there was something really wrong with me. The Evangelical Christians told their children I was evil, and my eyes were the mark of the devil. Others said I was a witch, and they wouldn't let their kids near me. I am sure I would have been burned at the stake in an earlier century. When I matured, the same boys who tormented me when I was young couldn't stay away from me; the athletes and the most popular boys in school wanted to go out with me. I was everything in high school: home coming queen, prom queen, most beautiful, and top of my class. Those boys acted as if I would just shine on what they did to me when we were young. Well, I didn't. I gravitated to the nerds. They had been bullied too, so they knew how it felt, and I felt safe with them. All of that has carried over and influenced my later relationships with men."

Dave cradled her in his arms. "I worship your eyes."

Dave felt he needed to tell her about his sister. She had the courage to tell him about the bullying, so he needed to man up and tell her about his sister. "I have a brother who is in college. I had a sister who was born between us. She was born with severe deformities that were not compatible with life, but she lived for over two years. I went to her room and visited her every day during those years." He had to stop to compose himself because talking about it brought back the pain.

"I felt so sorry for her because I know she suffered a lot. She had a pretty face, but the rest of her was hard to look at. I was just a child when she was born, and I couldn't understand why God would do something like that to a baby. She was just an innocent little baby. Why did she have to suffer; why couldn't she be normal?" He almost broke down. "My sister's death broke my dad's spirit, and my mother was never the same again. I don't know how my mother had the courage to have another child. But my parents wanted the American dream. They wanted the house in suburbia with a two-car garage and the standard two children, a boy and a girl. My mother really wanted a girl with her last pregnancy, but she got my brother instead."

Dave went on to the worst part. "My sister's death hit me hard. After the funeral, I still went to her room every day, but she wasn't there. That was very difficult for me. Where was she? What was death? I was a kid, and I didn't understand, so her death was very hard on me. She is one of the reasons I became a doctor. I want to prevent that kind of pain and suffering in others, but most of all, I want to prevent death."

Sharon had no idea he hid so much emotion and was so vulnerable. She realized he had a deep tormented soul, and he had to help others in order to ease his own pain. He was called upon by his own experience with suffering to administer to others who were suffering. He was compelled to be a doctor; there was no choice for him.

They understood each other now. They held each other on the blanket in the moonlight, knowing that they were not alone any more. Sharon did not tell Dave about Bar or her father. She knew she would tell him eventually, but not now; nor did she tell him how she felt about marriage and children. There was no need for that yet. Dave did not tell Sharon about his insecurities regarding his upcoming internship or his concern about his ability to meet its challenges. He thought that was something he had to deal with on his own.

Sharon's and Dave's young lives were the products of their experiences. Sharon's dealings with men were guided by her childhood traumas, and her feelings about marriage and children were based on her parents' troubled marriage. Her relationship with Bar had left an indelible imprint on her psyche. Dave's career choice had been shaped by his sister's birth and death. His need to resolve conflicts physically harkened back to his participation in contact sports where he could get instant results. The solution was simple: hit the other guy first, before he could hit you, and hit him harder.

They viewed everything through the lens of their past. Their exposure to the significant events of their lives formed a paradigm through which they evaluated, judged, and analyzed everything. Their brains had been programmed to respond in certain ways to the situations that confronted them. The acid trip reflected all of that back to them in a manner that let them gain insight into themselves they could never have gained without the drug. Their defense mechanisms and personality traits would have prevented them from seeing themselves clearly, but the drug broke all of that down and forced open the doors of perception. They both suffered childhood traumas and experiences that had shaped their personalities, but the acid allowed them to reevaluate and share them in a way that led to a better understanding of themselves and of each other.

Coming down allowed them to see how bittersweet life was. They saw the pathos of the human condition in its stark, unvarnished reality, stripped of any and all illusions. Life, death, the cycle of everything, including the universe that will also eventually end, its vastness, the impossibility of understanding its complexity—all of it came flooding in like a torrent. But they were buoyed up and carried along on the tide of increased perception by their connection to each other.

Dave and Sharon felt more at peace with themselves and more comfortable with who they were than they ever had. They also formed a unique bond during the acid trip that was sealed by the mental, emotional, and physical connection that had developed between them. They went to Sharon's room and fell asleep.

4
Falling in Love

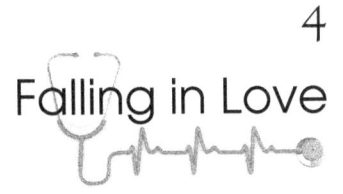

They slept late and lounged in bed after they woke up. "Wow, did we do everything I think we did last night?"

"Yes, and we definitely overdid one thing and did it almost all night long," Sharon answered and laughed.

"What a night, and I don't mean only that part of it, but the whole night, the concert, Santana, your dancing, lying in the moonlight, everything. Sleeping beside you and feeling you close to me, then waking up and seeing you. I don't want you to fly away, and I don't want to start at the hospital." Dave pulled her closer.

Sharon faced him. "Maybe we won't go to a party, smoke Jamaican weed, make fantastic love, eat Chinese, listen to music, smoke more Jamaican weed, make fantastic love again, go shopping, get caught in the women's dressing room, take LSD, go to a concert, dance, make cosmic love all night long, moon bathe, share our innermost thoughts, and be with each other almost constantly, but we will go on. Even with me flying and you at the hospital, we will go on. David Cameron, you are one intense young man. Do you always go at life full-tilt boogey with the pedal to the metal? Are you always the last man standing, taking it to the limit one more time?"

"Let's take a bath and get something to eat." Dave hugged her.

They bathed together in very hot water, sitting in the tub for some time. They dressed and went down to eat. It was almost noon when they walked into the park, found a nice quiet secluded bench, and sat down to talk.

"I had lunch with Henry while you were gone, and we talked about the stress and responsibility we will have to deal with at the hospital. There is something else along with the fatigue, long hours, and lack of sleep; it's the damage of what we are exposed to—what it does to us and how it changes us. I think it is like what happened to my dad in Europe during the war. He saw things he couldn't unsee, he was exposed to things no one should be exposed to, he was involved in things that left him with psychological scars." Dave shifted his position on the bench to face her.

"Let me give you an example. If we are going to be together, you need to know a little about what it's like." He took her hand. "I did an elective in neurosurgery last year. I will tell you about one case, not just the medical part, but the whole story we pieced together from the EMTs, the cops, and her girlfriends, then we are never going to talk about what I do or the hospital again, understand?" Sharon nodded. "Good. She was eighteen years old, just old enough to work in a club, with a drug-dealing older boyfriend who hooked her on heroin. She worked every night in the club, gave him all her money, and he kept her strung-out on heroin. If she didn't work or didn't give him everything she made, he wouldn't give her any heroin. He wanted more money out of her, so he tried to turn her out to do tricks, and when she refused to prostitute herself, he cut her off. Her friends said she suffered terrible withdrawal symptoms with severe stomach pains, and when she couldn't take it any longer, she got a gun, went out in the alley behind the club, and shot herself." Sharon looked horrified. "She put the gun to her temple and pulled the trigger, but it was aimed too low and too far forward, so it just blew out her eyes."

Sharon gasped.

"This is too much for you." But Sharon looked determined and demanded he finish. "We operated on her, debrided the wounds, and patched the meninges, the coverings of the brain and neuro tissue, but spinal fluid continued to leak from the area. She had to have a spinal tap every day to remove all her spinal fluid to relieve the pressure on the meninges so they would heal. That's where I came in. I was the only stud on the neurosurgery service, so I had to do a spinal tap on her every day."

Sharon asked why he was called a stud.

"A medical student is a STUD, short for student. Not only did I have to tap her every day, but I also had to change the dressings and look into those two cavities in her face where her eyes used to be. She wanted to die. She screamed, pulled out her IVs, tore at her bandages, and fought, so she had to be put in four-point restraints. She thrashed around and fought the restraints. We tried to keep her sedated to prevent withdrawal, to treat the pain, and to calm her down, but she would come out of it and start screaming and fighting. I can still hear those screams and the awful sounds she made. The nurses had to hold her in position for the spinal taps, and even though she was sedated, she was still awake. I was a student, so it would take me a couple of attempts to get in, while she was fighting, screaming, and making those sounds the whole time. By the time I finished, I would be shaking and covered with sweat. She hated the taps and she hated me. She started screaming every morning when I got there. The nurses tried to stay on top of it and sedate her, but she fought the sedation. The EMTs said they found blood trails and patches of blood in the alley where she crawled around trying to find the gun so she could finish the job. The other women she worked with said she was very pretty and popular with the customers at the club. Well, she wasn't pretty anymore, and one of the things that got me was the way everyone talked about her. She was a just a junkie whore to them. They made fun of her, said she was a one-bagger and laughed. She was someone's baby girl. My mother would have given anything to have had a daughter. I couldn't do anything to help her; in fact, I was adding to her suffering by tapping her every day. The shrink told me she would kill herself the first chance she got. I could have given her fifty milligrams of IV potassium, but even having a thought like that scared the hell out of me. What do you do with a thought like that? What do you do about something that makes you have a thought like that? They tell you to compartmentalize it, to put in a box, and to store the box. I actually thought about taking her life. How do you put something like that in a box? It damages you. I can still see her, see the room, hear her screams, and smell the old dressings.

"That was only one case from my clinical years of med school. How many cases like that does it take until you wall off your humanity, losing yourself and the reason you became a physician in the first place? I don't want to end up like my father, spending all my mental energy keeping the things I have experienced suppressed. I don't want to lose who I am, to become what I want to be. But you have to be trained and properly trained, you have to be the doctor in charge, you need to be in a city/county hospital where you see everything and in a good program where you are taught how to deal with what you see."

Sharon put her arms around him. "Didn't you have anyone you could talk to? Don't they provide some type of therapy to help you cope with experiences like that? No one should be expected to deal with that kind of horror without some sort of support."

"Not where I went to med school. It was guts, balls, trial by fire, and survival of the fittest. You are right though—sometimes I wanted to do a Joseph Conrad and scream, 'The horror, the horror.' I deal with it by distracting myself, and that's why I need to be doing something all the time," Dave answered.

"I understand now, so let's go do something fun to distract you." Sharon kissed him.

"We can go to my place, spend the rest of the day at the pool, listen to some music, and get into some serious distracting later tonight. Don't worry about your skin or getting burned; I will slather you in layers of sunblock. I think smearing that lovely body of yours with sunscreen will be a lot of fun and very distracting." Dave stood up, pulled her up, and took her in his arms. "You can bring your case and uniform with you and spend the night at my place. You will be gone on a layover tomorrow night, and like you said, I will be working by the time you get back, so this could be the last night we have together for a while."

"OK, but no distracting in the morning. I have two long hard days ahead of me, and I have to be at the airport early. I can't be late, because you can get fired for being late or missing a trip. I want to spend the night with you, but we have to get our distracting done tonight." She kissed him, and they walked back to the house.

When they got back to Sharon's room, she packed her flight bag, put her uniform in a hanging bag, and changed. "I only have one bathing suit, and it is a little risqué. I got it at a resort in Cancun on a layover." She put on a white string bikini top that did not come close to covering her breasts, a white string bikini bottom with a Brazilian back, and a white mesh cover-up. She looked so hot, they almost didn't make it out of her room.

They drove in separate cars to Dave's apartment. He changed into a bathing suit, got two towels, a bottle of sunblock, and put two beers with two waters in a small cooler. The pool was crowded; after all, it was a single's apartment in a large city on a sunny Southern summer Sunday. Sharon needed shade, so Dave pulled two lounge chairs close to a table with an umbrella. He was busy getting everything ready and didn't notice that every man at the pool, whether they were with someone or not, was looking at Sharon. When he finished, Dave sat down on one of the lounge chairs and watched Sharon take off her cover-up. It was only then that he realized he was not the only one watching her. *God*, he thought, *she must stop traffic when she walks down the street.* He smiled. *She certainly stops my traffic.*

Sharon lay back on the lounge chair. "Time for sunblock. I can already feel the burn." She seemed oblivious to the stares and Dave thought, *she is so used to it, she ignores it.*

Dave stood up with the sunblock. "As a doctor, I know the proper way to apply lotion to the human body."

Sharon looked at him warily. "You don't need to prove anything to other men out here."

"Yes, I do. Look around you. There are guys out here who will be on you like a duck on a June bug, even though you are sitting with me. I am going to take immense pleasure in rubbing every inch of your body with lotion, and letting them know you are taken; otherwise, I guarantee you, one of them will make a move on you right in front of me."

Dave applied the sunscreen, let the lotion dry for a while, then repeated the whole process two more times. When he was finished, Sharon lay back with her eyes closed. "I will call you from New York City tomorrow night when our crew gets to the hotel so you don't worry about someone laying over me, but you have to stop being jealous."

Dave sat up. "Let's go for a swim."

Sharon stood up, left Dave sitting there, walked confidently to the diving board with her head up and a smile on her face, stepped on to the diving board, looked back at Dave, tossed her hair back still smiling, walked forward, hit the diving board like a professional diver, and made a perfect dive into the water with hardly any ripple. When she came up treading water, Dave made a running dive from the side of the pool and came up in front of her. "I thought you weren't a water person."

Sharon put her arms around his neck and her legs around his waist making him tread water for both of them. "There are clubs that have pools, golf courses, tennis courts, and places to eat that some families belong to. Some have indoor pools where you can swim all year round."

Dave let them sink so she had to swim for herself, and they swam to the shallow end of the pool where they could stand up. She wrapped her arms and legs around him again. He said, "So, you are a country club brat."

She looked a little sad for a moment then laughed. "Only until I went to college, and look who's talking, frat rat."

"Spoiled country club brats who are stuck-up sorority girls don't get to call fraternity men frat rats unless they can breathe under water." Dave went under with her wrapped around him.

She came up for air. "If you drown me, I won't be able to distract you later." They continued to play in the pool until Dave swam to the ladder, climbed out, and waited for Sharon. As she climbed out, she held on to the ladder and put her head back in the water to let her hair stream down her back, then she stood on the ladder, brought her hair around over her shoulder, twisted it to get the water out, and let it fall over her breast.

In Dave's mind she appeared to be the goddess Venus rising form the ocean foam. As she stood on the ladder, she was more beautiful than any rendition of Venus Rising he had ever seen. It began the minute he saw her; it grew as they talked and got to know each other, accelerated with the sex, and expanded exponentially with the acid trip; now it exploded in him with an overwhelming force. He didn't recognize it at first because he had never felt it before. Then he realized what it was.

Jesus Christ, I'm in love with her. I am in love with a woman who is more goddess than woman. I love her for her perfect body, her beautiful face, those marvelous eyes, her intelligence, her wit, her kindness, her gentleness, her purity, but most of all, I love her for that intangible quality she has that makes her different from anyone I have ever known.

He had been infatuated many times before, but he had never been in love. He would never forget this moment, and he would be able to picture her standing on the pool ladder looking like Venus rising from the ocean foam for the rest of his life. *I hope she loves me too, God please let her love me.*

Sharon looked at him as she stood on the ladder. "What?" When he did not answer, she looked down at her swimsuit. "What, am I coming out of my bathing suit?" She climbed out of the pool, adjusted her top, and walked up to him. He picked up a towel and wrapped it around her like the cherubs wrapped the cloth around Venus in Botticelli's painting. "What? Did all that sunblock slathering and pool frolicking get you all worked up? I have on three layers of sunblock with no burn, and I am having fun, so you will just have to cool your engine for a while."

Dave hugged her after wrapping her in the towel. "That's not it. Well, it is in a way. It's that I love you. I know we have known each other less than a week, but I love Sharon."

Sharon pulled back and looked into his eyes. "I love you too, Dave. What do you think I have been saying? I am yours; you can have me anytime. I don't want anyone but you. Like I said, what does a girl have to do? What do you think we have been doing if it wasn't falling in love? I don't care how long we have known each other; I love you. I have never been in love before, but I know this is love. Phil was right, you can be so dumb sometimes." Dave crushed her to him. "Like drowning me, if you crush the life out of me, I won't be able to show you that I love you later." Sharon freed herself and handed Dave the other towel. "I think we are causing a scene." Almost everyone at the pool was looking at them.

They went back to their lounge chairs, lay down, and Sharon took Dave's hand. "When we go in, I need to tell you something about myself."

Dave squeezed her hand. "You can tell me anything you want; it won't change how I feel about you. I love you."

They spent the rest of the afternoon in and out of the pool, reveling in the joy of their newly expressed love.

"I need to wash my hair; besides, I don't want to burn. I have to remember to bring a hat and sunglasses next time. This has been so much fun, and I want to do it again, so let's not spoil it with too much sun."

They gathered up everything and went back to the apartment. When they were inside, Dave grabbed her and fell into one of the beanbags with her. "Does this mean you need distracting now?" Sharon maneuvered so they were face to face, smiled, and touched his lips with her fingertip. "First, I need to tell you something important."

Dave kissed her finger. "Nothing you tell me will change how I feel about you, but if it is important to you, then it is important to me, so go ahead."

Sharon repositioned herself in the beanbag. "Dave, you need to know something about me. I am never going to marry or have children.

I will stay with you and remain committed to you, but I will not marry you or have a child with you. I want you to know that before we go any further with this relationship."

Dave looked into her eyes. "I don't care if we are married, as long as we are together, and I have never even thought about children."

Sharon searched his face. "You may say that now, but what about when you have a practice and people know you are living with someone you are not married to, or you want a son to carry on your name? You need to think long and hard about this."

Dave sat up. "I don't have to think about it at all. I want to be with you. I love you. I don't care about marriage or children. I love you, and you love me. That's all that matters. We belong together."

Sharon sat up beside him and put her arms around him. "I guess we both have a little baggage to bring into this relationship. I am fine with yours, and it seems you are fine with mine, so I guess we are going steady. Can I have your class ring now?" She laughed then became serious. "You deserve to know why. My dad is a lawyer, my mom is a stay-at-home mom who never worked, and I am an only child. My dad is very good looking—I mean movie-star good looking. My mom is pretty, but my looks come from my dad. He makes a lot money, and we had it all: the country club, nice cars, nice house, and I had anything I wanted. You are right, I was a little spoiled until high school. It started when I was about sixteen. He cheated on my mom. She caught him time after time, but he kept seeing other women. They pursued him because he was handsome and had plenty of money to spend on them. It went on until I started college, and then they got a divorce my freshman year. They had been married for twenty years, and my mom had no way to support herself, but my dad did not want to give her any money. They fought in court for another year. Being a lawyer, he knew all the tricks. When I was eighteen, he said he was no longer responsible for me, so he stopped paying child support, and managed to decrease what he was paying my mom to the bare minimum. My mom paid for my college, the sorority, and saw that I had what I needed on the amount of support he paid her and the settlement. I worked in the summers and tutored during the school year to help out, but I know she went without sometimes. I have seen firsthand what can happen with marriage. I am never giving up my name or my freedom by signing a contract to tie myself to someone who can leave me and take everything. I don't want to bring a child into this world to suffer the way I have."

"I am not your father, but no matter, no contracts, no marriage, keep your name and your freedom. I get it about children because of my sister, so we are on the same page there. It is obvious your father, not just the bullying, had a lot to do with your feelings about men. Regardless, I am fine with it. If you are not going to be my wife, what do you want to be—my mistress, my concubine, my significant other, my old lady? It's up to you." Dave pulled her down with him.

Sharon snuggled against him. "I think I want to be your mistress. It sounds sexy. Everyone will know we are together, that it's a permanent situation, and that we are in love." She looked at him and smiled mischievously. "And they will know we are fucking. Is that why you love me, Dr. Cameron, because I am a good fuck?"

Dave went after the strings of her bikini. "Maybe, I don't know. Let's test you and see how good you really are. Dirty talk is cheap; I judge performance."

They made love in the beanbag. At one-point, Dave paused, and she opened her eyes to look at him. "I want to stay inside you with you wrapped around me like this all the time." Sharon pulled his head down and kissed him.

Later, they were lying on the floor side by side. "I know you have been with a lot of other girls, but I don't want to think about that. I don't want to think about you doing what we do with anyone else. I want to think I am the first and only girl you have ever been with. But you didn't learn how to do what you do, the way you do it, on your own, and I don't think it was divine inspiration. The other women you have been with taught you. And although I hate them, and I never want to think about them or talk about them, in a way, I am grateful to them. I love you for a lot of reasons, Dave Cameron, not the least of which is the way you make love to me."

Dave turned on his side, rested on his elbow looking at her, and lightly ran his hand over her body. "You are right, there were some very hedonistic pleasure-seeking women focused on sex and their own gratification who taught me a lot. Plus, I am a doctor, so I know about the lady parts and what to do with them; we actually had a class on human sexuality in med school. But I learned that sex simply for pleasure is just a form of pornography; sex with someone you connect with is much better, and now I know making love to someone you are in love with is the most wonderful thing in the world. I have to admit I had a great time learning, but this is where it all comes together, no pun intended, in making love to you."

Sharon rolled toward him and pushed his hand away. "You can be such an asshole. Don't touch me anymore. I told you thinking about your other women upsets me. Then you give me a blow-by-blow account. You are cut off until further notice. I have to get the picture of you enjoying your lessons with your teachers out of my head before I let you touch me again."

Dave reached out, pulled her to him, and tried to hug her, but she wiggled free. "No, you are on the naughty bench for a time-out until you learn how to behave and not be hurtful."

Dave lay back with his hands behind his head. "OK, but while I am on the naughty bench, you can tell me about Bar. I told you about the women I have been with, so you can tell me about Bar. I don't understand why you stayed with someone who treated you that way."

Sharon sat up. "No, I don't want to."

Dave persisted. "That tells me I need to know about him. Come on, Sharon, I don't have any secrets from you, and I will never lie to you. I love you too much to jeopardize your trust. Tell me about Bar."

Sharon locked her arms around her knees and hugged them to her as she sat beside him. "Fine, but you have to promise me that no matter what I say, you will let it go and never do anything about it."

Dave sat up beside her. "I promise."

Sharon put her head down on her knees. "He hit me."

Dave put his arms around her. "That mother fucker. I will pound his ass to a bloody pulp."

Sharon pulled back and looked directly into Dave's eyes. She had tears in her eyes that were starting to run down her cheek. "No, you will not. You promised. I knew you would react this way. That's why I didn't want to tell you. You have to keep your promise."

Dave held her by her shoulders and looked directly into her eyes. "Why would you want to protect someone who hit you and abused you? You have to understand if anyone ever hurts you, I will go after them, and God help them when I get my hands on them." The storm she saw in Dave's eyes frightened her, and she knew that if that storm ever broke on someone, they would need God's help. The look on his face told her that all her concerns about that side of his nature were true. Sharon shrugged off his hands and put her arms around his neck. "I am not protecting him. I am protecting you. You have a violent side despite all your tenderness and sensitivity. I have known that since the first moment I saw you, and I am afraid of what you would do to him, not for his sake, but for yours. You could end up in jail with your career ruined. His family is very powerful. They would never allow someone to hurt their golden child. They would retaliate. If anything happened to you because of me, it would break my heart, and if our future were ruined because of me, I wouldn't be able to live with myself. Please let it go, he is not worth it. Keep your promise for your sake, for my sake, for our sake, not his."

Dave was silent; he was so angry, he couldn't talk. Regardless of what he promised Sharon or what she said about Bar's family, he knew he would not be able to control his anger if he ever encountered him. He would unleash it on him with a vengeance and Sharon was right, he would hurt him; he would hurt him bad. As Sharon held him waiting for him to cool off, she could feel the tension in his body. Dave was buff, not pumped-up like a body builder, but cut and muscular. Holding him, Sharon could feel the power in his body, and she was sure she was right; he could do serious damage to someone like Bar.

"Let me tell you about it, and then we can put it behind us and never speak of it again. I will block out your women, and you can block out what happened with Bar. Both things are in our past. It is what is in our future that is important."

She sat back with her arms around her knees again. "I need to start from the beginning for you to understand. I didn't lose my virginity until I was a senior in college. I had been dating this guy for a while, and I thought it was time, so I let him do it. After that first time, I didn't have sex again until I met Bar. You are right, I get hit on all the time, especially on the plane, not just by crew members, but by passengers too, mainly in first class. We are not supposed to date passengers, but everybody does. The men I dated wanted to fuck me, but I didn't fuck them because I knew that's all they wanted, just to fuck me. I had sex with Bar occasionally during the six months I dated him, but you have been with a lot of women and had sex with them I don't know how many times. I don't want to think about how many women you have been with or how many times you fucked them, because it upsets me, but I am supposed to be OK with it because you are a man. If a man fucks a lot of women, he is a stud, but if a woman fucks a lot of guys, she is a slut. That stupid double standard is why I was so worried you would think I was a slut after our first time."

"I am sorry, but thinking about you with someone else drives me crazy," Dave interjected. He was insanely jealous of no one in particular and everyone in general.

"Ditto, Dave, and it is much worse for me. So, I dated a lot of guys but said good night at the door. I was having a great time, and I never had to worry about buying food because some guy took me out to dinner every night. Then when med school started last September, the guys moved in next door and came over right away to introduce themselves. Bar pursued me relentlessly until I finally went out with him."

Sharon touched his lips with her fingertip. "Listen, don't say anything, and when I am finished, it is over, never to be spoken of again and you will do nothing about it. Dave, I need that commitment from you."

Dave nodded yes, but he knew if he ever met Bar, he would beat the hell out of him, no matter what he promised. It was bad enough for any man to hit any woman, but for some Ichabod Crane jerk to hit Sharon was far beyond anything Dave could ignore.

"Everything was great at first, and I thought I had found my perfect man. He is the smartest person I have ever met; he is charming, witty, and well-mannered. His family is very prominent, and his father was the governor at one time. He took me around, showing me off to all the people in his family's circle, so I was flattered and got caught up in the glamour of it all. I started on the pill, but Bar and I hardly ever had sex, and when we did, it was like he was preforming a duty. Before I met you, I thought sex was just for the guy, and the woman was only there for him to bounce up and down on until he got off and that was it. I thought there was nothing in it for the woman; she was there just to gratify the guy." Dave started to say something, but Sharon put her fingertip to his lips.

"Then he started putting me down and humiliating me in front of our friends, never in front of his parents, their friends, or anyone he knew through his parents, but in front of his buddies or people I knew. I got tired of it and told him I was through with him. He told me I couldn't reject him; I was his, and he hit me. He hit me hard in the face with his fist, and it hurt like hell. He is a wimp, but it still left a red mark then a bruise. I called the police, but when they found out who he was, they wouldn't charge him. He kept calling me and coming over, but I dropped him flat, hung up on him when he called, and refused to see him when he came over. He told people he was moving to Boston and wasn't going to take me with him, so he broke up with me. I told people he was an asshole and a jerk, so I dropped him. His friends believed him, and mine believed me. So now you know." Sharon looked directly into his eyes. "Does it matter anyway? No, so that is the end of it."

Dave cuddled her in his arms. "No one will ever hit you again."

She snuggled against him. "I had such a poor track record with men. That's why I was excited and maybe a little desperate to meet someone decent. Based on what Henry told me about you, I think I started to fall in love with you before I met you."

Dave held her. "I will tell you something if you don't laugh at me. When I was in the shower getting ready for the party, I sang 'Tonight' from *West Side Story*. I think we fell in love for a lot of reasons, but one was because we were both ready."

Sharon hugged him. "You were just like Henry described you, but at first I was a little frightened of you, then you almost blew it with your macho Hemingway shit. You know that, don't you?"

They cuddled on the floor a while, and then Dave got up and put Fleetwood Mac on the turntable. "We can listen to some music, and then clean up. I will wash and blow out your hair, lotion you, powder you, and put you to bed. We can order a pizza for dinner."

Sharon laughed, got up, walked up to him, and put her arms around his neck. "Does that mean we aren't finished?"

"I don't know. Come sit with me, and we will see." Dave sat in one of the beanbags. Sharon joined him, and they smoked a joint. After Fleetwood Mac, Dave played Steely Dan and the Eagles. Those three groups and their songs became Dave and Sharon's music. They would do their dance of love to that music on many more nights.

Sharon was in the beanbag with Dave. "You do have a bed, you know. We could try using it instead of the floor or this beanbag."

"This from the girl who fucked me in the yard beside her house and almost fucked me in a room full of people," Dave said and laughed at her.

"That was when we were fucking. Now we are making love, and I want to enjoy it in a bed. You said it yourself—it is a whole new kind of wonderful. The lust and passion are still there, and if you want to be spontaneous, I won't stop you, but when we are in a loving mood, I would prefer the comfort of a bed." Sharon put her arms around his neck and kissed him.

The day they declared their love for each other became a pattern for the next two months. On the weekends Sharon wasn't flying and Dave wasn't on call, they would spend the afternoon at the pool, smoke some weed, spend the evening making love to their music, shower, get something to eat, listen to more music, go to bed, make love again, and go to sleep. They spent the nights Dave was not at the hospital at Dave's, and Sharon spent the nights he was on call at her house.

5
Dr. Sheffield

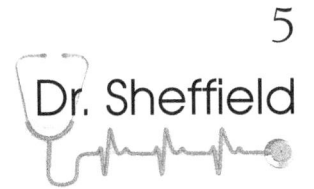

Orientation is critical to a teaching hospital staffed by physicians in training. The process is a well-orchestrated seamless transition. It is a choreographed realignment that occurs every June in every teaching hospital in the country. The incoming interns and residents take over the functions of the hospital from the old house staff and step into their new roles on day one. Every summer, there is a migration of physicians in the United States, as graduate medical students move to the location of their internships, interns move to the location of their residencies, residents move to take fellowships, and trained physicians move to where they are going to practice.

Dave found the main conference room on the first floor of the hospital and sat down with Mike and Henry. Henry looked serious.

"I have been thinking about what I want to do after my residency. I realized I don't want to do patient care. I am going to apply for a fellowship in infectious disease at Hopkins, then do research at the CDC. I don't want to teach either; I just want to do straight research. The more I think about it, the more I am sure that is what I want to do."

Dave smiled. "Something has changed for me too. Sharon and I are in love."

"In love? You have only known her for a week! She is just using that body of hers to catch a doctor, and you fell for it." Mike's jealousy was showing.

Henry congratulated Dave. "Sharon has her mighty strong man, and you have the best collection of estrogen-induced secondary sex characteristics I have ever seen."

The hospital administrator took the podium, and their first day as interns began. He welcomed them, gave a brief history of the hospital and medical school, praised the attending staff and mentioned their two Nobel Laureates. He introduced the department heads for Medicine, Surgery, Obstetrics and Gynecology, and Pediatrics. The director of nursing, the head of the nursing school, the head dietician, and the manager of the laundry joined him on the podium.

The director of nursing talked about the quality of nursing at the hospital and the need to interact with the nursing staff in a professional manner. The head of the nursing school gave a brief history of the nursing school followed by the guidelines for working with student nurses.

The hospital administrator added, "We understand boys will be boys and girls will be girls, but not on the hospital campus. First rule, no unwanted advances. No means no. Second rule, we understand you are consenting adults, but while you are on this campus, you will conduct yourselves in a professional manner at all times. Third rule, the only people allowed on this campus are staff, patients, and patient visitors—no wives, girlfriends, boyfriends, or dates. If something comes up and they need to see you for a legitimate reason, they need to go to the office and get a visitor's pass. Random people are not allowed in the hospital for any reason. Last rule, this should not have to be said, but we know from past experience we have to go over it: these same rules also apply to the interaction between physicians. No mixed couples in call rooms at night."

The dietician was next on the agenda. "Everything that has been said about the code of conduct between the sexes applies to dieticians and our students as well. Your meals are free as long as you are in the hospital. Everyone gets breakfast and lunch. You get dinner if you are on call or working late. Show up with your ID, and we will feed you. We discourage coming to the hospital for meals if you are not working, but if you are hungry, show up and we will feed you." Then she talked about the role of dieticians on the wards and finished with general information about meals and meal planning.

The last speaker was the head of the laundry. He told them their lab coats and OR shoes were in the laundry in packages labeled with their name. "Scrubs don't leave the hospital. If you take scrubs out of the hospital, you will be charged for them, and it will come out of your salary. When your lab coat is dirty, turn it in to the laundry. Scrubs can be worn with your OR shoes and lab coat in the ED, Surgery, L and D, the Nursery, and if you are on call. On the wards and in the clinics, you are required to wear a dress shirt, tie, dress pants, and dress shoes with your lab coat. Women doctors need to dress accordingly. Since it is required that you wear a shirt, tie, and pants, you can turn them in to the laundry under your name for service also. The same goes for women and their dresses."

The administrator ended with, "Please pass your paperwork forward before you leave, and if your contact information has changed, stop by the office and update it. Now, go to the conference room of your service. Rotators, go to the room of your first rotation. Thank you, welcome to University Hospital, and good luck."

Everyone filed out of the conference room. Mike and Henry were straight Medicine interns and Dave was starting his rotations on the Medicine wards, so they walked to the Medicine conference room together.

Henry turned to Mike. "I almost forgot. Harven wanted me to tell you Connie checked with her nursing friends about a date for you. One nurse knows a physical therapist who just moved here from somewhere in the Midwest. Connie can set you up with her if you are interested."

"Does Connie know anything about her, or would this be a double-blind date?" Mike caught up to Henry.

"I think it is a double-blind date, but Connie wouldn't offer unless her friend said good things about the therapist." They found the Medicine conference room.

The room looked like a high school classroom with student desks and a black board at the front of the room. Dr. Sheffield was a tall, nice-looking man in a lab coat, dark slacks, a dress shirt, and a blue tie. He was standing at the front of the room with a younger man dressed the same way.

"Come in and find a seat near the front. I want to welcome you. I am Dr. Sheffield, and this is Dr. Jeffery the chief resident for this year. I know all of you, but you do not know each other, so starting here, please introduce yourself to your fellow interns." One by one they all said their name. "I know you will not remember everyone's name, but soon you will get to know each other. Dr. Jeffery will pass out a packet with some very important information in it, not the least of which is the call schedule for the wards for the next three months and your team assignments. He will go over all that information with you, and then I want to talk to you. Afterwards, Dr. Jeffery will take you on a tour of the hospital. When the tour is finished, you are free to go, but report back to your ward or the ED by ten in the morning to start taking over from the outgoing teams. Dr. Jeffery they are all yours." Dr. Sheffield was an icon of medical education. He had produced several Nobel

Laureates and convinced two of them to stay on to lecture and do research in his department. He was known at the NIH, CDC, and all the top Medicine Departments in the country for turning out excellent physicians for private practice, teaching, and research.

"Doctors, check your team assignments. There are three teams on the wards and four in the ED. Ward teams consist of two interns, a junior resident, and a senior resident, and when the studs get here in September, four studs will be assigned to each team. There are four ED teams with two interns and a junior resident on each team with one senior resident assigned to the ED each day. Again, when the studs get here, four studs will be assigned to each team. Call is every third night on the wards, rotating from Team 1 to Team 3, so Team 1 is on call first. In the ED, teams one and two rotate with teams three and four every other day, with the teams alternating between Major Medicine and Minor Medicine. Major Medicine goes from seven AM to seven AM. Minor Medicine goes from seven AM until seven PM with everyone out of Minor Medicine by nine PM. Anyone left after nine PM will be transferred to Major Medicine. The senior resident of the ED will help clear any back log. Now check your schedules. Teams in the ED are not expected to attend any conferences or to meet with staff; they are expected to be available in the ED at all times. On the wards, the studs start at six AM doing scut work, rounds start at seven AM, and you meet with your attending at ten AM. Rounds with the chief are at eleven AM, and the team on call the day before will have their charts ready. Lunch is at twelve with clinic starting at one PM and ending at four PM. Follow-up rounds are at four PM. You should be out of the hospital by six or seven at the latest."

The chief resident looked around for questions; there were none. "There are seven holidays. Only the team on call or working the ED that day has to come in. The team on call will round for the other teams, and there will be no meetings or conferences. If the holiday is on a Saturday, the team on Sunday will round for everyone so they are the only ones who have to come in the day after the holiday. Grand rounds are on Saturday at eleven AM; attendance is not mandatory but encouraged. Rounds on Saturday and Sunday are at nine AM, and there are no meetings or conferences on Sunday. You get one week of vacation, from Monday to Monday, and we encourage you to take it on an easy rotation since your fellow interns will have to cover for you.

Well, I think that covers about everything. Are there any questions?"

Again, there were no questions.

"You do not sign out an unstable patient. You stay with your patient until that patient is stable. You do not call in sick. You come in, and we will decide if you are fit to work or not. You will average about a hundred hours a week in the hospital, so get ready to put your social life on hold. Dr. Sheffield."

"Doctors, that's what you are now. You have been granted that title along with the great privilege of spending your life as a physician. You earned the title with four years of college, four years of medical school, countless hours of study, and a lot of hard work. Now you are one of us; you are a doctor, and you will spend the rest of your life in one of the most rewarding, fulfilling, and satisfying callings one can have. Make no mistake about it—it is a calling. If you were not called to be a physician, you do not belong here, and you should get up and leave right now. If you are here because you want a good income, because your father or mother is a doctor, because your parents or grandparents want you to be a doctor, because you want the profession to benefit you in some way, or because it seemed like a good idea, you should get up and leave right now, because you do not belong here. But if you have been called to serve humanity, and if you are driven and compelled to relieve suffering, prevent disability, and prolong life in your fellow man, then welcome to University Hospital and the Department of Medicine.

"I want you to describe yourself in one sentence. Who are you, what is your philosophy of life—everything about you in one sentence. Go ahead, I will give you a little time." Sheffield paused. "OK, go over the sentence in your mind. If you did not begin the sentence with, 'I am a physician,' you need to re-evaluate who you are, because being a physician needs to define you. What does being a physician mean? It means your primary goal in life is to relieve suffering, prevent disability, and prolong life. Think about that. Your life will be dedicated to relieving suffering, preventing disability, and prolonging life in your patients, or for all mankind if you do research or teach. What higher calling can there be? This next year will prepare you to do just that, but make no mistake about it—it will be tough. It will challenge you to your very core. You will suffer from lack of sleep. The stress will be overwhelming, and the demands will be beyond what you think you can endure, but when you finish your internship here, you will be well trained and ready to be a physician. Thank you for your time. Now Dr. Jeffery will take over again."

Jeffery held up two notebooks. "These are your Bibles. One is your guidebook, and the other is the notebook you will fill in with pearls of information. Write everything down at first; later, you will learn what you need to write down and what you don't. You don't have to write down a lot of stuff anymore, because we have created this guidebook with all the numbers, facts, conversions, and formulas you need in it. It was compiled from the notebooks of a lot of past interns by a past chief resident. Now, follow me and we will tour the hospital, including the call rooms, the doctors' lounges, locker rooms and showers for the wards and ED."

As they walked out of the conference room, Mike scoffed. "That was a little over the top."

Henry stopped and looked at him. "I agree with and believe every word Sheffield said." Henry could do or be anything he wanted, and he had chosen to be a physician.

"So do I," Dave added. They walked away from Mike and followed Jeffery more closely. Dr. Sheffield had touched, motivated, and inspired them, and now they were ready for what they had to face, including never failing to live up to his expectations.

Jeffery led them through the hospital. He introduced them to their counterparts on the current teams and to the nursing staff, who were mainly young, dedicated, hardworking women. They finished in the early afternoon, and Jeffery dismissed them with the admonishment to be back by ten AM to work with their counterpart to assure a smooth transition. They all noticed how thin, pale, and stressed the current interns looked. That would be them in a year.

"How about a beer?" Mike wanted back in the fold.

"Sure, let's go to The Pub and get some Guinness drafts. Dave, you know where it is. Mike, I will give you directions." Henry gave Mike directions, they left the hospital, and met at The Pub.

They found a table and ordered three drafts. When the beers came, Henry raised his glass. "Well here's to surviving, because that's about all we can hope for."

"We are off on the 4th, so tell Connie to set me up with the double-blind date, and let's have a party." Mike wanted to be a part of the group again.

"I'll talk to Sherry, and she will organize a picnic for the concert and fireworks. Sharon can talk to the girls she lives with. I will contact Bob and Phil, and you talk to George and Harven. We'll have an old-fashioned picnic, listen to the concert, watch the fireworks, and have a party afterwards." Henry always took charge of things.

They finished their beers and Dave got up to leave. "Sharon is going to call me when she gets to New York City, and I don't want to miss her call, so I will see you guys tomorrow." He left some money for the beer. Henry and Mike ordered another round and talked a while longer. Henry told Mike about the acid trip and the concert. When Mike left, he didn't leave any money for the beers.

Dave got to his apartment, put Marshall Tucker on the stereo, smoked a joint, and waited for Sharon to call. The phone rang in the early evening; he answered and heard her low husky voice. "How was the first day of orientation?"

The sound of her voice made him yearn for her. "I miss you. I hate layovers, I hate whoever invented layovers, and I hate the airline for having layovers. It was fine. The good news is Henry and I are on the same team; the bad news is I will be at the hospital every day and spending every third night there for two months. With your schedule and mine, I think we will be lucky to be able to be together about half the time. I want to be with you every night. I want to be with you right now. I don't want you on a layover; I want to be laying over you."

Sharon dropped her voice another octave and made it huskier. "Do you want me to tell you what we would do if I were there with you right now?"

"Jesus, no, that would only make it worse. That's just cruel," Dave responded.

"You know, I like the power I have over you. I can control a certain part of your body and the majority of your mind with it," Sharon purred.

"Now you are just being mean." Dave tried to laughed.

But Sharon was not through. Her voice turned to honey. "If I were there right now, I would love you all over."

Dave warned her. "Goddammit, Sharon, if you don't stop, I will show you who has the power, and I won't have any mercy on you."

But Sharon ignored his admonishments. She had the upper hand, she knew it, and she was enjoying playing it for all it was worth. "Oh, please don't, unless of course you absolutely have to. If you absolutely have to and you aren't going to show me any mercy, I guess I will just have to take it."

"If you keep this up, I won't be able to sleep tonight. It is hard enough to sleep without you as it is," Dave pleaded.

The low, husky voice came back. "That is just what I want. I want it hard on you. I want you so turned on, you tear my clothes off and fuck me to the wall the minute you see me."

"Don't worry, you'll get what you want." Dave decided he would do just that.

Sharon spoke in her normal voice. "Dave, this is going to be a tough year, but we will make it work. We will make every moment we are together special, and even when we are apart, I am with you and you are with me; we will always be together."

They were silent for a while, holding each other in their hearts. Sharon spoke first. "When are you on call, and when can I see you? I don't want all that verbal foreplay wasted."

"I am on the third of July and every third night after that for two months. I have the weekend of the 4th off, so if you are not flying, we can have the whole weekend together," Dave told her.

"I am off. I always try to avoid flying on a holiday weekend. Are you not going to have any mercy on me for two whole days?" Sharon's voice was husky and low again.

"Everyone is going to a picnic in the park for the concert and fireworks on the 4th. The girls you live with and their dates are invited too. Don't worry, we will have plenty of time for you to pay for all this teasing. Can we spend the night at my apartment when you get back tomorrow?" Dave asked.

"What time do you want me to come over? I get back at five," Sharon answered.

"As soon as you can get here." They talked for a while longer then said good night.

Dave made himself a ham sandwich with a glass of milk for dinner. He ate, put some more music on, and tried to settle down, but his yearning for Sharon was more than just physical; she was right, she had a powerful hold over him mentally as well as emotionally. He finally fell asleep that night with images of her in his head.

A love story and social commentary

He woke up the next morning, ate a bowl of cereal, showered, dressed, and drove to the hospital. Dave and Henry met the two outgoing team-three interns on the wards. Both interns had ten patients on their services before any discharges, but they would admit another six to eight before their shift was over. The outgoing interns introduced Dave and Henry to their current patients then the four of them went to breakfast. Henry and Dave planned to go back after breakfast, review their patients' charts, then make rounds on all their current patients. Tomorrow, they would come in early to pick up any patients admitted overnight, round on the remaining patients and meet with their attending at ten.

At breakfast, they learned their attending would be Dr. Finkelstein, an endocrinologist and head of the Department of Endocrinology. He hated interns, especially rotating interns. He felt the internship year should be eliminated and residency should start right after graduation from medical school. He was tough and not altogether fair. Henry knew him by reputation only. They were told it was hard to get a decent recommendation from him, but it was Sheffield who tracked the performance and wrote the recommendations for the Medicine service for rotators.

Dave worked hard and completed his day by five. He drove to his apartment, showered, doused his body with incense oil, and dressed. He lit all the candles and incense sticks, put Steely Dan on the turntable, rolled a joint from the Jamaican weed, and waited for Sharon to arrive.

He heard her at the door before the doorbell rang. He got up, tripped the turntable, and opened the door. She was standing at the door holding her travel case and her hanging bag. He had been picturing her in his mind for two days, but her reality far exceeded his memory of her. Her long hair was down around her face and over her shoulders. She had on a light green top with darker green shorts and sandals with wedge heels.

"I have to stop coming over when the guys that live here are getting home from work. More followed me today." Dave looked down the stairs to see a couple of guys looking up. Without saying a word, he pulled her in, shut the door behind her, and kissed her passionately. She dropped her travel case and hanging bag. He broke the kiss, pulled her top over her head and off, throwing it aside. "Dave!" He found the zipper for her shorts, unzipped them and pulled them down to her ankles but not off. "Dave!" While he was bent over, he put his arms behind her knees and his shoulder into her midriff hoisting her onto his shoulder in a fireman's care. "Dave, what are you doing!" He carried her into the bedroom and flipped her down on the bed. "Dave!" He pulled her shorts and thong off, stripped off his T-shirt and dropped his jeans.

He pinned her down, kissing her mouth, ears, neck, breast, midriff, and on down as she moaned "Dave." It wasn't long before she wasn't moaning "Dave" any longer but crying out and convulsing violently. As she lay trembling all over, he moved his hands to her rear, lifting her as he stood up. He needed no encouragement sliding easily into her as she gave a sharp intake of breath and wrapped her legs around him.

He turned around and walked to the wall beside the bed with her attached to him. He pushed her against the wall, took her arms from around his neck, and pinned them against the wall above her head. He pushed into her as deep as he could. She dropped her feet to the floor, but remained basically impaled and suspended on him. He continued to push deeper into to her, lifting her as he forced her harder against the wall. She began to shake uncontrollably as she called out for God and used a few profane words in connection with Dave's name. Dave wanted to go on to show her he was the one in control, but he couldn't.

They were still joined as he carried her back to the bed, laid her down, and looked straight into her beautiful eyes. "Is that what you had in mind?"

"Pretty much."

"Did it meet your expectations?"

"Pretty much."

"Did you accomplish what you set out to do on the phone last night?"

"Pretty much."

"Do you still think you are the one with the power?"

"Pretty much."

Dave raised up on his hands in a push-up position over her. "What?"

"Do I really have to explain to you that I orchestrated what just happened? I got just what I wanted—oh excuse me, what I deserved." She smiled hugely and kissed him long and passionately. "Oh Dave,

A love story and social commentary

I missed you and it was only two days, and I missed making love to you. I couldn't wait to be back in your arms again, and when I was, it was better than I hoped it would be. That was incredibly intense. What we have is almost too much. I love you, and I love the way you make love to me. The 'fuck me to the wall' was a metaphor. I never expected you to take me literally and actually fuck me to the wall. I am just glad I didn't say fuck my brains out." She laughed. "Obviously, I have never experienced being fucked to the wall before. I liked it. Being suspended on you put a lot of pressure on my trigger. I don't think I could take it all the time because it is too intense, but occasionally, I want you to fuck me to the wall." She laughed and rolled on top of him, straddling him, and kissed him.

Dave rolled her back. "You do realize I made you call on the Lord."

Sharon smiled. "I was calling on the Lord to help you." She wiggled free and got on his back wrapping her legs and arms around him from behind. They rolled around in the bed struggling with each other until the bed was a complete wreck. They ended up cuddled together in the pile of bedding. "Are we going to eat something tonight?" Sharon sat up.

Dave sat up beside her. "There is a family-run Mexican place only a few blocks away. It's a quiet neighborhood spot."

When Sharon was dressed, all Dave could do was stare at her with his mouth open. Sharon sensed his thought and shook her head. "Don't objectify me. I objectify myself enough. I know how I look, and I admit I use my looks. I used them and I continue to use them on you. But I put too much of my self-worth in my looks, and that worries me. Objectifying myself worries me. I know this sounds counterintuitive, but the way I look gets in my way. Men don't take me seriously and only want to fuck me. Women hate me and are jealous."

Dave came up behind her and kissed her neck. "I get it. But please don't stop objectifying yourself. I love your beauty. But you are much more than that, and you should not put all your self-worth in your looks. You are intelligent and educated, sophisticated and well read, accomplished and stylish; you have character and integrity. Your inner beauty far exceeds your outer beauty."

—∞—

Dave could hardly keep his hand off Sharon's thigh long enough to shift gears in the four-speed 240Z as he drove. Every man in the restaurant looked at Sharon as she walked to the table.

The smiling little man pulled her chair out for her and leaned over her shoulder as he gave her the menu and put her napkin in her lap. Sharon asked Dave, "Are they still looking?"

"Four boys are turned around in their chairs, and I am sure you will occupy their dreams tonight. The mothers are looking at the fathers, and the fathers are trying not to look at you while their wives are looking at them. All and all, you caused quite a stir." Dave smiled at her and took her hands across the table and kissed them one at a time.

After dinner, they drove back to Dave's apartment and smoked a Jamaican bud. "Stay here, I will be right back." Sharon took her travel case and went to the bedroom as Dave lay back in the beanbag very stoned and drifting on the weed.

Sharon entered the front room, walked in front of Dave, and stopped. She had brushed her hair, touched up her makeup, and put on a black filmy negligee. It was so light, it billowed away from her as she walked.

Dave was high, so he thought he had fallen asleep and was dreaming. "Oh my God." Sharon turned and the negligee flowed around her body. "From Saks 5th Avenue in New York. Now who is calling on the Lord?" Dave stood up to face her. They were both very high.

Sharon put her arms around his neck. "I am wrapped up in a package just for you."

"Phil is right, you could be a model. You look like you walked right off the pages of *Cosmo*." Dave put his hands on her waist and looked into her eyes.

"Do you want me to walk around in a negligee in front of other men?" Sharon asked.

"No, of course not. But you can model for Bob and Phil," Dave responded as he held her.

They cuddled in one of the beanbags listening to Buffalo Springfield with Dave fondling her as they lay in each other's arms feeling the music.

Sharon thought about the coming year. She knew she was stronger than Dave. Dave was a gentle, vulnerable soul. She knew his shoulders, arms, and the violent side of his nature came from playing football, but that wasn't who he was. He was too idealistic for the harsh realities he would have to face in the coming year. She would need to be there for him to lean on, and she would have to use her strength to bolster him. She smiled as Dave stroked her body through the negligee. She was idealistic too, maybe even more than Dave. Like Dave, she had been searching for a great love, but the love she found was nothing like her fantasy. She pictured her true love as a white knight and thought he would be a Shelly or a Keats—reserved, intelligent, educated, sensitive, cultured, and completely consumed by his love for her. Dave was not what she had pictured. He was a Shelly or a Keats—gentle, intelligent, educated, sensitive, cultured, and completely consumed by his love for her, but he was a man who lived by a code she did not completely understand, and he was different from her fantasy in so many ways. She never dreamed that she needed a love that consumed her with passion and made her cry out in carnal pleasure, rather than a pure knightly love.

They listened to a few more songs and then went to bed. Sharon took off the negligee, and they made love one more time, but it was sweet, caring, and giving. Their passion had been spent earlier, and they just wanted to express their love for each other. Sharon fell asleep in his arms almost immediately after their lovemaking, but Dave lay awake for a while thinking.

He had only known her for a week, yet he couldn't imagine life without her. He could feel her warm body and hear her soft quiet breathing as she slept next to him. His idea of a great love had been based on all the books he had read, and the woman he had pictured was a combination of expectations derived from fiction. Sharon was so much more than that. Her reality far exceeded his fantasy, and his love for her far exceeded his dream of a great love. He fell asleep and slept soundly because he knew he was as ready as he was ever going to be for the coming year.

Part 2: Internal Medicine

6
The Wards

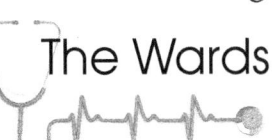

Dave woke up and slipped out of bed, making sure not to wake Sharon. She was flying a turnaround with a later departure time. After he was dressed, he went back to the bedroom to look at Sharon sleeping peacefully. He crept to her side and kissed her lightly on the cheek, then thought to himself as he looked down on her shadowy beauty in the dark, *Here I go, Baby. Wish me luck in your dreams.*

Dave left the apartment and walked to his car knowing he would always remember his first day as a doctor. All the previous days of his life were in preparation for this day. Most of his life had pointed to this moment, and he had spent a great deal of his youth working to reach it. Now, it was finally here, and he felt the thrill of accomplishment coupled with a huge sense of pride and satisfaction. He had achieved his goals; he was a physician, he had the love of a beautiful woman, and their future was spread out before him like a wide, majestic, open landscape devoid of any boundaries.

He joined the early morning commute traffic on the expressway going into the city. It was dark, and Dave could see the other driver's faces in the glow of their dashboard lights as he passed them, and he thought, *Am I one of them? I am going to work, like they are, only this is the first day of my life as a doctor, and I left a beautiful woman sleeping in my bed, so does that make me different? I want to be different; I want my life to be different, I want to live an exceptional, well-lived, full life.* The thoughts rushed through his mind like the cars rushing along the expressway.

Dave hated getting up early, but he liked driving in the early morning hours just before dawn. He had done it for two years during the clinical years of med school, and he had gotten used to the fresh clean feeling of the beginning of a new day. He saw the predawn as a heralding of a new beginning—a new beginning in which anything was possible.

Dave listened to the FM radio station as he drove, and he recalled the station where he went to school; it played recordings of Dr. King's sermons and speeches on Sunday mornings. In his post Woodstock consciousness, those sermons and speeches rang like a bell in his mind, making him aware of the civil rights movement, racism, bigotry, and intolerance. Those Sunday mornings had shaped his understanding of the need for changes in society. Listening to Dr. King had given him a social conscience. He smiled to himself as he thought how different his views had been before Woodstock and Dr. King's teachings.

His last thoughts before he reached the hospital were of Sharon. He pictured her lying on the bed in the black negligee and heard her voice telling him to trust and believe in himself. Dave spoke out loud as he left the car and walked toward the hospital, "OK, Baby, here I go. "

The campus of University Hospital was all lit up and brimming with activity in the early morning darkness. When the automatic doors of the ED opened, he was hit with the sounds of a busy ED in a busy city/county hospital. He felt an adrenaline rush as he walked past the triage desk, nodded at the triage nurse, showed her his ID, and started down the hall for the elevators. He was back in it, and the intensity felt good to him. He took the elevator up to the Medicine wards with his heart beating a little faster and feeling the flush he used to feel before an athletic event. He smiled. *It's game time, and I am in the starting lineup.* He stepped off the elevator and walked to the nursing station ready for his first day as a doctor.

Dave was the first one of his team to check in at the nurse's station on Medicine 3, but it wasn't long before Henry joined him.

"Hey, Poncho!"

"Hey, Cisco!" Dave responded.

"We be in it now! The first day we be the real doctors, RDs! Can you dig it!" Henry had a huge grin on his face. "How is Sharon? Does she know about the 4th? I am surprised you could tear yourself away from her exceptional assets long enough to join us here today."

"She is great, sleeping soundly in my bed while I am here stomping out disease and saving lives. She knows about the picnic and will tell her roommates. I tore myself away from my warm bed because it's game time, and we got to get it done." Dave could tell Henry was approaching his first day as a doctor the same way he was, like it was an athletic event, and he was just as keyed up with the adrenaline flowing.

They had picked up their lab coats yesterday. They put their stethoscopes, notebooks, reflex hammers, dividers, and tuning forks in the pockets of one, and left it hanging in the doctor's station on Medicine 3. Now, they put on their coats for the first time. They were more than a little cocky as they donned the mantel of their profession to begin their career as doctors.

"Well, Poncho and Cisco, are you ready to stomp out disease and save lives now, or do I need to wait a little longer until you two finish working out your social calendar and high-fiving one another because you be in it and you be the real doctors now? It is good to know your names are Poncho and Cisco. I thought you were Dr. Tarkington and Dr. Cameron." The nurses in the nurse's station giggled, but the charge nurse who was standing in the door of the doctor's station looked at them without the slightest hint of a smile. She was young, neat, prim and proper with her whole being screaming tough, competent, and no nonsense.

Dave and Henry looked at each other, and something told them ex-military, probably Vietnam, which meant she was an excellent nurse who knew what she was doing. They both answered together, "Yes, ma'am, we're ready."

The faintest hint of a smile appeared at the corners of her mouth, because she knew they were nice, polite, and well-mannered, not a couple of rowdies like she had first thought. "I am one of four charge nurses on Medicine 3. You met one of my counterparts yesterday, and you will meet the other two as you rotate through your call schedules and they rotate through their shifts. The interns' desks are the ones next to the chart rack. Poncho, you are on the right; Cisco, you are on the left."

She established control and dominance by using their nicknames. They were Poncho and Cisco from now on. "I expect you to address all the nurses with respect, like Mrs. Jane Pauley, who pulled all your charts and filed your labs and reports for you today. In the future, your labs and reports will be in the baskets on your desk, and you will have to pull your own charts and file your own labs and reports. Dr. Tarkington went to school here, so he can help you get to know the routine, Dr. Cameron. We are changing shifts, and we need to give report, so Mrs. Pauley will answer any other questions you have."

Nurse Jane Pauley was standing behind the charge nurse. She was older, slightly overweight, friendly, and the interns' ally. "You can call me Jane; I like that better than Mrs. Pauley, which makes me sound like an old lady. I act as the liaison between the house staff and the nurses, so if you have any problems or questions, come to me first."

Dave and Henry dubbed her Nurse Jane Fuzzy Wuzzy. They soon grew to like, respect, and depend on her.

"Poncho, you picked up two admissions overnight, and you picked up three, Cisco, so with the discharges from yesterday, you each have twelve patients on your services. Poncho, since Cisco got the last admission, you will be up for the first admission when you are on call on the third. Cisco, I remember you as a student, and I am happy to see you again. Unless you have any questions, I suggest you both get to work."

"Thanks, Jane. I remember you too, and I am glad you are here to help us, because I know we are going to need all help we can get."

Henry and Dave sat down at their desks and began their first day.

Jane came back with two cups of coffee and a handful of condiments. "Don't expect this again either. Like having your charts pulled, your labs and reports filed, this is a one-time thing. I know you need coffee and don't have time to go to the break room, so I got you some. That's my last contribution to your first day." She smiled.

Dave and Henry found their new admissions on top of their pile of charts with their new admits' old charts next to the pile. They reviewed the new patients' charts first then made rounds on those patients. They finished rounding and charting on the new patients by seven, so they were caught up and ready to round on the other patients when the junior resident walked into the station.

He was thin, pale, shy and socially awkward, with intelligent eyes behind rimless glasses, and a shock of unkempt brown hair. Dave and Henry looked at each other and almost burst out laughing because he was the worst dresser they had ever seen. He had on a crumpled tattersall shirt with a knit tie, wrinkled khaki pants, and scuffed brown loafers.

"I am James McDonald, but everyone calls me Jay. I am the junior resident, and you are..."

"Poncho and Cisco," a loud female voice came from the nursing station. The nurses' station and the doctors' station had a large opening between them where the rotating chart rack and order boxes sat on a wide shelf.

"What? I thought your first names were Henry and David." Jay looked confused and off balance.

Henry stood up and put out his hand. "I am Henry, and that hippie over there is Dave. We are old friends and call each other Cisco and Poncho like in the TV show, *The Cisco Kid*. The nurses picked up on it." Henry took Jay's hand and shook it.

Dave stood up and took Jay's hand from Henry. "I'm Dave or Poncho; he really is the Cisco Kid. We were college roommates, fraternity brothers, and are best friends, so we tend to be pretty loose with each other, but we can act like professionals if it is absolutely necessary." Dave smiled at Jay as he shook his hand.

Jay was saved from further confusion by the charge nurse. "Dr. McDonald, I was glad to hear you were going to be our resident. It is good to see you again. I hope you are doing well." The charge nurse was in the door again.

Jay became more awkward. "It is good to be back, and it is nice to see you again, Carol."

The charge nurse's face had softened, and she was smiling at Jay in a way that revealed she was more attractive and younger than Dave thought. She was in her mid-twenties and for all her toughness, she was demonstrating she had a softer side too. "Well, I need to get home and get some sleep. I just wanted to say hello and welcome you before I left." She walked away briskly.

As soon as she left, the senior resident took her place in the door. "Hi Jay, I know who Henry is, so you must be David. I am Ed Walker, the senior resident." He shook their hands in turn, giving Jay the opportunity to regain his composure and put the Poncho and Cisco confusion behind him. Ed was a nice-looking, well-dressed young man of average height and build, with a smooth, confident manner that made people like him instantly. "It is after seven, so I suggest you get started. Henry and Dave, when you are finished with your charts and the nurses have taken off your orders, Jay and I will write our notes. The nurses know to give us the charts after they are finished, so as my grandpappy used to say, daylight is a-burning."

Dave rounded on his other patients, wrote notes and orders, and formulated a treatment plan for each of them. Dave's service was typical for a university hospital. His had patients with congestive heart failure, chronic obstructive pulmonary disease, a diabetic with keto-acidosis, one with DTs, a drug over dose, pancreatitis, pneumonia with sepsis, end-stage cancer with organ failure, failure to thrive, stasis dermatitis with cellulitis, liver failure, and asthma. All twelve were admitted because they would not have survived without hospitalization. Dave felt he could get the OD, asthma patient, DKA, elderly patient, the one with DTs, and the COPD patient out in three days, so he would start call with six. Not bad, but five would be better, but that depended on the patient with pancreatitis. The CHF patient had myocardiopathy, the liver failure patient had ascites, the cancer patient was terminal, and the cellulitis patient was chronic, so they were in for the long haul and would be with him for a while.

    Dave and Henry went down for some breakfast before meeting with their attending. "Man, my service is a train wreck with five or six patients I am going to have for a while. How about you?" Henry was still keyed up.

    The adrenaline and excitement had faded for Dave, and he was settling in to the reality of the situation. "I think I can get it down to five or six before call. I don't think you have a train wreck; I think this is the way it is going to be. We are going to get six to eight admits per call and have six to eight left, so I think we are going to carry twelve to sixteen patients all the time." Henry began to settle down and come to grips with what Dave said. "Jesus, I am going to need roller skates to get through rounds by ten o'clock with that many patients."

    "Yeah, and we have to wait until seven to start because of the nurse's shift change. You can't get anything done between six and seven with the shift change and report going on. We are going to have to be here and be ready to get on our horse at seven to be finished by ten. That's only ten to fifteen minutes per patient, so I think the thing to do is to get a lot done the night before, so everything is set up for morning rounds. That will mean staying late and eating dinner here. I am going to try to go from seven to seven on the days we are not on call, so with weekends, that's about a hundred hours a week, like Jeffery said. I don't think there is any way to do everything in less time than that, and if we have an unstable patient or a lot of patients on the weekend, it will be more than a hundred hours a week. I can get up at six and be here before seven, so with six hours of sleep, that leaves five hours a night to be with Sharon when I am not on call and she is not flying. " Dave had worked it all out.

Henry looked at Dave with a slight smile. "Don't you have your priorities backwards? You are scheduling your Medicine rotation around Sharon. Shouldn't you be scheduling your time with Sharon around your Medicine rotation?"

"I am balancing Sharon with my Medicine rotation." Dave had come up with the best solution he could under the circumstances.

They got eggs, bacon, toast, juice and coffee for breakfast, showed their IDs at the register, and found a table alone. "Henry, I have never known you to be dishonest. Why are you keeping the room at the Park house and not telling Sherry?"

"I know. I feel bad about it, but it's complicated. I have made up my mind about an infectious disease fellowship and doing research at the CDC as a career. Sherry has visions of a prestigious private practice with her as my wife. I am not going to marry her or go into private practice, so we are not on the same page. I think when she finds that out, she will break up with me, so I am keeping the room at the Park house for when she kicks me out. The bottom line is, I like having a woman, and I don't have the time to find a new one. I am not being dishonest; I am just keeping my plans to myself." Henry didn't meet Dave's eyes as he spoke.

"So, you are using her until you can find someone else." Dave kept eating as he talked.

"Look who is talking. How many women have you used? From what I have heard, you had a harem at one time in med school." Henry was more annoyed with himself than he was with Dave.

"Hey, I am not criticizing. As your friend, I am only pointing it out to you. How many times have you done that for me? You are right, I used a lot of women, and I ended up feeling pretty bad about it. I don't want you to compromise your integrity and then hate yourself for it," Dave added.

"I know." Henry and Dave finished eating as the two residents arrived. Dave was amazed at the contrast they presented as they walked to the table.

"We finished our rounds, notes, and chart review. I liked what I saw, and I think we have a good team. Now all we have to do is convince Finkelstein of that," Ed told them and laughed. "Jay and I are going to grab a bite to eat, so we will see you back up there."

When they got back to the station, Dave called his number hoping Sharon was still at his apartment, would know it was him, and would pick up.

"Dave?" Her voice on the phone always drove him to distraction. "Hi, Baby, I can't talk. I wanted to let you know I will be home around seven and that I am going to eat at the hospital."

"I am just leaving for the airport. And hey, since when am I your baby?" Her voice was so enticing.

"You've been my baby since the minute I met you." Dave forgot the nurses were listening. "I have to go. I will see you tonight."

"When you get home, what do you want—coffee, tea, or just me?" Sharon laughed.

"Just you, Baby. I have to go now, bye."

"Poncho, what you going to do to your baby when you get home tonight?" It was another female voice, but it was plain their nicknames were being passed around among the nurses.

Dave thought, *My dick is getting in the way, and I can't let that happen. Henry is right; I need to get my priorities straight.* He refused to look at Henry.

The residents got back to the station, but Dr. Finkelstein did not arrive until after ten thirty. As they waited, Ed and Jay reinforced what Dave and Henry knew about their attending—he was an arrogant opinionated ass.

Dr. Finkelstein filled the room with his personality when he arrived. "Doctors, I am Dr. Finkelstein. I know who you are so we can dispense with introductions. I am a full professor of medicine and head of the Endocrinology Department." His arrogance was palpable. He continued, "First, I would like to use this time to get acquainted. Let's start with you, Ed. What are you going to do when you finish your residency?"

Ed was looking into private practice opportunities in the city. "I like it here, and my wife has already started her career here, so we want to stay, raise a family, and become a part of the community. I also would like to volunteer to supervise residents in the Medicine clinic here."

It was a good answer and Finkelstein liked it, especially the part about volunteering to work in the clinic to supervise the house staff. Dave wondered if Ed threw that in because he knew it would go over well.

"Jay, what about you? What are you going to do when you finish?"

"Academic medicine. I will look for an entry-level teaching position at a medical school where there is room for advancement." Jay liked academics because it was the one place he felt comfortable.

"Henry, what about you?"

"I am going to apply for a fellowship in Infectious Disease with the goal of doing pure research at the CDC." Another good by Finkelstein's standards.

He finally turned to Dave. "And you, David? Why did you apply for a rotating internship, and what do you plan to do with it?"

"Actually, there are two reasons I applied for a rotating internship. First, I like Medicine, but I also like Surgery. I thought doing a rotating internship would give me a chance to further evaluate both. Second, to get a straight internship at a top institution, I had to be in the top ten percent of my class and the top ten percent on the National Boards. I was in the top fifty percent of my class and the top twenty percent on the National Boards. By doing a rotating internship, I could get a position at a top institution, and work my way into a better residency."

Finkelstein looked intrigued. Dave had given him a good reason for doing a rotating internship.

"Two questions, David. The discrepancy between your position in your class and your National Board scores tells me something. What does it tell me? What are you going to do after you finish this better residency?" Finkelstein leaned forward toward Dave.

"I was immature. I needed to grow up and focus on my career instead of enjoying myself. The National Boards were a better measure. I want to practice in a small town in an area with clean air, clean water, and where I can be close to nature. I want to serve and be a part of a small community where everyone knows everyone and is interdependent on one another." Dave was honest about his plans.

"Good, now you all know what you want to do, so you can direct your efforts toward gaining the skills you will need in your future endeavors. A doctor in an urban, university-connected private practice will need different skills from one who practices in an isolated, rural area. An academic and a researcher will need different skills from someone in patient care. This service currently has twenty-four patients, and those twenty-four patients are your priority, but your approach to that priority can vary as long as those patients remain your priority. Is that clear? Tomorrow, we will start discussing your care of those patients. I will meet with you at ten to go over all the patients on the service. I expect your performance to be excellent, and I will accept nothing less than excellence." He left without saying another word.

No one said anything as they filed out to go to rounds with the chief. Their attending had lived up to his reputation. Dave and Henry lagged behind the two residents.

Henry turned to Dave. "That was sobering. For a minute, I thought you were going to say you underperformed because of sex, drugs, and rock and roll." They both laughed. "I think you gave a good answer on the rotating internship question. He was prepared to climb all over you, but how could he argue with what you said? I don't think he had ever considered that doing a rotating internship could improve the quality of your residency. He wanted to attack you, but you shut him down with that answer, so I think you are OK for now, but he is going to pick on you again."

"Let's face it, he is going to pick on all of us, because it is in his nature to fuck with people under him. It is going to be a miserable two months with him breathing down our necks."

They got to the Medicine conference room and took their places in the front row with the charts of their new admits stacked on their school desks. The rest of the interns and residents on the wards filed in and took their seats quietly. Sheffield stood at the front of the room, rocking back and forth on his feet in a stylish gray suit with a white shirt and gray tie.

"Are we all here? Good, let's start. I want to discuss a case from last spring, because it illustrates something I think is very important and a lesson I want you to learn on your first day. This is the case of a forty-year-old Hispanic woman admitted in extremis with symptoms involving multiple organ systems. She was admitted by a good intern, two excellent residents, and one of our best attendings. By the time of this conference, the working diagnosis was Addison's disease, hypothyroidism, and diabetes. Now, I have only one question and since you two are up," he looked at Dave and Henry, "what organ is involved in all functions of the endocrine system?"

Dave and Henry both answered, "The pituitary."

"Correct, she had panhypopituitarism. She had a million-dollar work up with four doctors involved, but the only one who made the correct diagnosis was the student. How did he make the diagnosis? He made it by taking a detailed history. All the doctors took a history, but they failed to ask one question. Why did the student ask the question? Because he was doing a thorough job. All the doctors asked about her pregnancies; she had five pregnancies and five children. The question the student asked, that the others failed to ask, was did she have any problems with any of her pregnancies? The answer was yes; she bled heavily with the last delivery, the bleeding couldn't be stopped, and she had to be transfused. So, what happened, Team 3?"

Dave and Henry shared the answer.

"The blood supply to her pituitary was compromised."

"It was knocked out by the ischemia."

"Correct. The lesson to be learned here is that ninety percent of your diagnoses can be made by history. Talk to your patients, be thorough, and they will tell you what is wrong with them. You don't need labs, imaging studies, and technology if you talk to your patients and use your clinical skills. A thorough history by the intern on this case could have saved thousands of dollars and prevented delay in the patient's treatment. Remember, your main purpose is to relieve suffering, to prevent disability, and to prolong life. Don't treat the chart; treat the patient. Don't rely solely on technology; evaluate the patient's clinical picture. Base your treatment on the patient, and don't change the treatment if the patient is improving. Don't change the antibiotic because of the culture and sensitivity if the patient is responding to the current antibiotic. Many patients improve in spite of our intervention, not because of it. Less is more a lot of the time, especially in elderly patients. Talk to and relate to your patients. Yes, you are dealing with a complex biological organism, but you are also dealing with a human being. Never leave the human factor out of the equation. The doctor-patient relationship is part of the process. Patients who trust and rely on their doctors have better outcomes. Don't be the eager beaver and jump on every new technology or treatment that comes along before it is thoroughly tested and proven. On the other hand, don't lag behind new advancements that can enhance the quality of your care. Never be the first and never be the last, and your patient will never suffer because of you. But again, the lesson of this case is, talk to your patients, get to know them, and treat them as human beings, not just as cases or diagnoses. Healing is an art as well as a science. Your interaction with your patients is a part of your treatment and integral part of that art of healing. Depend on your clinical skills and your humanity, as much as you depend on technology in your approach to patient care. Thank you for your time. Tomorrow, we will begin in earnest."

Tom and Jay were waiting for Dave and Henry at the door. "Do you guys want to catch some lunch before clinic? We have plenty of time."

Dave declined. "I'm going back to the station to go over all my patients and their charts again. I'm going to set things up for morning rounds before I leave tonight. I have no illusions; our convivial attending intends to be up my ass with track shoes tomorrow morning. In his eyes, I am far from excellent; I have long hair, I am a rotator, I have low ambitions, and I am not a ten percenter. He doesn't think I belong here, and he is going to make my life a living hell. I am going to have to keep my head down, try to stay below his radar, and make sure he doesn't come down on me any harder than he already is."

"Don't overreact. You can handle yourself, and his bark is worse than his bite. Do a good job for Sheffield, and don't worry about him. I am going to get lunch. I will bring you a sandwich and a Coke you can wolf it down in clinic." But Henry knew Dave was right; they were all in for it from Finkelstein, but Dave would catch the worst of it.

Dave went back to the doctor's station and ground his way through his patient's treatment plans again, making notes of the things he needed to do on afternoon rounds. He rushed to clinic, gobbled the ham sandwich and chugged the Coke Henry brought him. Most of the patients he saw in clinic were hospital follow-ups or long-term patients with chronic diseases. He saw fifteen patients and still managed to get back to the floor by four thirty. He completed all the tasks in his notes by six thirty, signed out to his counterpart on Team 1, grabbed some dinner, and was home by seven thirty. He was physically exhausted and emotionally drained when he walked into his apartment.

Sharon was standing inside the door waiting for him. She had on a cropped white T-shirt that just covered her breasts, tight faded jeans, and she was barefoot. "Wow, Dave, I have never seen you dressed up. You are a very nice-looking man. No wonder you had all those little Florence Nightingales fluttering around you when you were a student."

Dave was dressed in tan designer slacks, a white Gant button-down shirt, a solid brown silk tie knotted perfectly, brown Florsheim cap-toed shoes and matching belt. His hair was pulled back in a ponytail, so from the front, it looked like he had short hair.

"You look totally different and so professional. I like it." She jumped up and locked her legs around his waist, put her arms around his neck, and kissed him.

She looked like a barefoot beauty, and when he felt her body pressed against him, smelled her perfume and tasted her kiss, all the fatigue, stress, and mental duress of the day melted away. It no longer mattered that his service was too big. It wasn't important that he had four or five patients who would probably never leave the hospital in his lifetime. So what if his attending was one of the biggest assholes he had ever met. Who cares if University Hospital was a huge pressure-cooker that drained him dry—he could come home to her. Dave crushed her to him and buried his face in her neck and shoulder.

"Dave, I do have to breathe. Was it that bad?" Sharon could feel the tenseness in his body as he held her.

"Worse." Dave leaned back from her.

"Tell me about it." Sharon looked into his eyes.

"Never."

"Dave, you need to talk about the things that trouble you. You can't bottle them up inside. I am here for you." Sharon dropped down and stood in front of him.

"Not with you. I have Henry. I want to leave that toxicity at the door and never bring it into our world. I want our world to remain clean and pure. If you want to be there for me, help me make a place where I can forget the hospital. I want a fantasy world to come home to, and I want to enjoy that world with you." Dave kissed her lightly. "Now, I need a shower because I am very grungy and a beer—no, I need about forty-seven beers."

"I don't see forty-seven beers in the fridge, so one will have to do. Is there anything else I can do for you to help create our fantasy world?" Sharon laughed from the kitchen as she got two beers.

"You bet. I will show you later." Dave took one of the beers and headed for the shower.

Sharon went to the turntable and put the Four Tops on. As Dave was undressing, he heard, "You know that I love you, Baby. I love you and nobody else." *It is going to be alright,* he thought, *because no matter how bad it is at the hospital, I have this to counter it, and it doesn't get any better than this.*

Dave finished his beer, showered, and cleaned up as quickly as he could. Sharon was in one of the beanbags when he got back. She had all the candles and incense sticks going. He sat in the other beanbag and rolled a small joint. After they smoked the number, Dave got up and changed the record, and more soft R and B sounds filled the room. He joined Sharon in her beanbag; they cuddled and nuzzled in the comfort of each other's arms as the music played. Dave was finally relaxed on weed, beer, and Sharon's warm body. He was in the cocoon of his apartment protected from the harshness of the outside world and in the arms of the woman he loved. They were insulated from the rest of the universe, immersed in their love and focused on each other.

Dave woke with the alarm at six. He turned the light on since Sharon was flying early and had to get up too. She stayed in bed, propped up on her elbow, and watched him dress. "Phil was right, you do have a cute tush."

"So do you." Dave looked at her wondering how anyone could have such a perfect body.

"Dave, you look so different when your hair is pulled back. I think people would respond differently to you if your hair were short and you dressed like that more often. You really are quite a handsome man." Sharon sat up in bed exposing her breasts.

"I was voted most handsome in high school." Dave gazed longingly at her.

"I was most beautiful, Homecoming Queen, and Prom Queen." Sharon smiled because she knew he was looking at her breasts.

"I was a National Merit Scholar, All-District in football and All-Regional in track. You are so competitive." Dave knew she knew he was looking at her breasts.

A love story and social commentary

"I have to be competitive; I am a woman," Sharon got out of bed and stood in front of him nude with her hands on her hips. "I was a National Merit Scholar too, and as for all those all-this and all-that, I am all you can handle."

Dave walked over and pulled her to him. "You can't do this to me. I have to get to the hospital."

"I know. When will you be back?" She put her arms around him.

Every fiber of his being wanted to throw her down on the bed. "I will call you when I am ready to leave the hospital. I will try for seven, but I have no control over when it will be."

Dave kissed her goodbye and willed himself to go. *Don't let your dick get in the way*, he kept telling himself over and over as he walked to his car. He was happy as he got in his car and drove to the hospital.

When Dave got to Medicine 3, Jay was talking to the young charge nurse from the eleven-to-seven shift, and Henry was pulling charts to get ready for rounds.

"Did you get delayed by Baby this morning?" Henry smiled.

"Just a little, but I got a lot done last night with no one around, so I have things under control. But it took all the discipline and self-control I have to walk out of my apartment this morning. God, Henry, she is so beautiful, so sweet and loving. I want to be with her all the time. It is torture for me to leave her." Dave started pulling his charts from the list he had in his notebook.

"I hear you; she is something." Henry had a faraway look in his eyes for a moment. "Jay told me the senior resident is here for oversight only. He is available if we need him; he sees the patients, reviews all the charts, and writes notes daily, but he comes and goes as he pleases. The service is Jay, you, and me. And here is the good news: the attending shows up for a while to make sure we can handle things then stops meeting with us until the students start. He reviews the charts and checks with the senior resident, that's all. So, the quicker we get on top of things, the quicker we get rid of Finkelstein."

"Well let's get 'er done, Cisco." Dave started going through his labs and reports. Jay came back in the station. "Hey, Jay what's up with you and that charge nurse? What's her story?"

Jay blushed a bit. "She was asking if you were giving me a hard time like some of the guys did when I was an intern. I told her you guys were treating me fine."

Dave and Henry looked at each other. "Do you think maybe she likes you? Are you single? Is she single?" Dave looked at Henry as he spoke, not at Jay, but Henry frowned.

Jay looked down at the floor. "She is way out of my league. She is pretty, smart, and a real hero. Besides, she is engaged. She is just being nice. She is nice to everyone "

Dave continued. "A hero? What do you mean?"

Jay looked up. "Jane told me about her. Jane got the story from the director of nursing. Jane said Carol never talks about it and acts embarrassed if anyone brings it up, but she has some kind of citation for bravery, some kind of star. She joined the military right out of nursing school and did two tours of duty in Vietnam as a Trauma nurse. What Jane told me is that during TET, her facility was under fire, being shelled or attacked with rockets, mortars, or something, I am not sure. But she risked her life to save the lives of the patients. They gave her a citation for bravery."

Dave and Henry were looking at each other, and Henry wasn't frowning anymore. "Wow," they both said.

Dave concentrated on the four patients clogging up his service. The patient with CHF had a myocardiopathy and was waiting for cardiology to decide what to do with him. He would eventually get on their list for a transplant or be moved to a skilled nursing facility for long-term care. In the meantime, there was nothing Dave could do about him. The patient with liver failure and ascites was terminal. Dave would have to approach the family about his care. That left the patient with cellulitis and the patient with terminal cancer.

Because of his moribund obesity, the cellulitis patient required total care as well as treatment for his stasis dermatitis and the cellulitis. Since the amount of care he required was all that was keeping him in the hospital, Dave approached Home Health Service to see if they could deliver the care with frequent home visits. He was not a candidate for a skilled nursing facility because of the amount of acute care he needed. After an evaluation from the Home Health team, they concluded they could offer him morning, afternoon, and evening visits. So, Dave discharged him to Home Health and arranged for an ambulance. If the amylase came down on the patient with pancreatitis, he could be down to four patients before he started getting new patients on Friday.

A love story and social commentary

The cancer patient was a young single mother on welfare with metastatic cancer of the ovary. She had two children in middle school, and her husband left her with the children when he found out she had cancer. She was terminal but refused any morphine to ease the pain because she thought it might kill her in her weakened condition and she still needed to figure out who could take care of her children. Her parents were dead, and her sister was taking care of her children. The sister and her husband had three children of their own, and they didn't have the resources to take care of her children permanently, so when she died, they would go into foster care unless the husband could be found. She was willing herself to stay alive until the husband was found. She was in foster care as a child and had been abused, so she was fighting to stay alive to protect her children from what she had experienced. Dave was so amazed by her courage and will power, he was determined to help her. There was nothing he could do for her medically, but he could help find the husband so she could die peacefully without pain.

Dave met with Social Services to see what he could do to help. They had exhausted all their approaches, given up on finding the husband, and were setting the children up for foster care. The patient told Dave her husband was an oilfield worker, so was his father, and they often worked jobs together. Dave directed Social Services to look for the husband's father instead of the husband. They found the father's wife living near the city. She told them her husband was in West Texas working on a drilling rig. Social Services called the number the wife gave them and got the husband's father. The father told them his son was in California working on a pipe line and gave them his number. It took all day, but by early evening, the husband was on his way back from California to take care of his children.

The woman broke down in tears when she heard, then she agreed to take morphine to ease the pain if she could see her children first. The sister brought the children in. She spent time with them, talked about their future living with their father, and told them goodbye. She died shortly after the first dose of IV morphine. Dave pronounced her with mixed emotions. He had helped her keep her children out of foster care, relieved her pain, and helped her die peacefully, but he knew giving her morphine was what had killed her. He knew he would write many more orders for morphine in the years to come, and by doing so, he would be partly responsible for many more deaths.

When he finished the day, Dave sat in his car trying to control his emotions. It didn't matter that he had taken a grilling from Finkelstein. It didn't matter that he had solved the problem of the cellulitis patient. It did not matter that he had sent other patients home with their illness resolved or controlled. For the first time, he had written an order that took a human life. Granted, it was not meant to kill her but only to relieve her pain. Granted, she was terminal, and she probably gave up and died when she knew her children were safe. But it was still his hand that had written the order. There was another reason he was upset. It was because things like this kept happening, and there was nothing he could do about it. Not for the first time and certainly not for the last time, Dave questioned how a caring God could let things like this happen. Dave pulled himself together and drove home with a heavy heart. He had set out in his career to save lives, and now he had lost his first patient, and it was by his own hand. He not only lost a patient; he lost a part of himself as well. He would help other patients die peacefully and painlessly in the future without any emotion because of this case. The experience changed him in a fundamental way and made it possible for him to write orders for morphine on terminal patients without it touching him because that part of him was gone. Dave grieved for his patient, but he also grieved for the loss of a part of himself. He would never be the same, and he knew there would be many more cases that would affect him the same way. Once again, he asked himself if he wanted to make that kind of sacrifice to be a doctor.

The question brought him back to the struggle of good versus evil and the reality that good was often consumed in the process. Did he have the courage to be consumed in process of accomplishing good? What bothered him most, was wondering if it even made a difference in the overall scheme of things. Would his sacrifice be in vain? Could he make a difference against such an overwhelming mass of pathos, or would he just be collateral damage?

Dave called Sharon when he was ready to leave the hospital, but he sat in his car for a while before driving home, so he knew Sharon would be waiting for him. When he opened the door, she was there in

A love story and social commentary

her faded jeans and T-shirt, with classical music playing and all the candles and incenses burning. Dave felt like he had a heavy overcoat on that contained everything he had dealt with that day in its pockets. He shrugged the coat off and left it on the ground as he crossed the threshold into his apartment. But unlike yesterday, he was different, and he could not shrug that difference off. He carried it with him into the apartment, and when he saw her standing in front of him, that realization overcame him. He pulled her to him and buried his face in her neck and shoulder, smelling her perfume and holding her body against his.

Sharon hugged him back, not saying anything, letting him hold her until he kissed her. Dave stepped back and slid his hands under her cropped T-shirt and cupped her breast. "How are the girls? I thought about them all day and hoped they would be free when I got home." As he caressed her breast, he kissed her again. "Beer, shower, and you, in that order."

Sharon noticed a sadness in him. "Is the music OK or is it too sad? I thought you might need something soothing. Should I change it?"

"No. The music is perfect, and you are perfect." Dave needed a lot to counter what he had dealt with today. He got himself a beer and poured Sharon a glass of wine.

Sharon came to him in the kitchen. "Dave, I know what you said about not talking about the hospital and your work, but you can't lock me out. I don't need or want details, but I want to be included in the things that affect you the way something is affecting you tonight. Talk to me. Don't shut me out. I love you, and I want to help."

"It is nothing new. It is the same thing that has been nagging me. I don't know if I can do this, and what is more, I don't know if I want to do it. That's a hell of a realization after what I have been through to get here. I thought I could use our world to balance the stuff at the hospital, but those things make changes in you that become a part of you. Because they are a part of me, I can't leave them at the door." For some reason, Dave felt better after he talked to her about his dilemma.

Sharon was prepared to help him. She took the beer and wine from him and sat them on the counter. "I am here for you. Whatever you decide to do, I will support your decision. I want you to be happy. I want us to be happy. You have to decide what to do about your career, and you need to think long and hard before you give up on your dream.

You have just started. Give it some time before you make a decision, and make sure it is not an emotional decision but an objective one you have thought through carefully and completely."

Dave hugged her. He felt the weight that was weighing on his heart lift a little and some joy seep back into his life. Sharon smiled as he held her and put her arms around him gently. "Go shower. I can see you need distracting in a big way tonight, so don't dawdle."

When Dave came out of the bathroom, it was dark, the curtains were closed, and the only light in the apartment was the light from the candles. Otis Redding was playing softly, and he smelled her perfume before he saw her standing silhouetted in the bedroom door with nothing on. He dropped his towel, picked her up, and carried her to the bed. Dave lost himself in their lovemaking, slipping away from reality in the intensity and ecstasy they experienced every time they made love.

They lay in each other's arms for a while until Dave fell asleep. Sharon looked at him sleeping as she lay next to him. The fact he had fallen asleep so quickly and was sleeping so soundly told her she had been successful. Sharon smiled as she watched him sleep. *Well*, she thought, *if that is all it takes every night to keep him on track, it is all right with me*. In fact, she couldn't think of anything she would rather do every night. Sharon fell asleep content in the knowledge that Dave would be alright with her help.

The alarm went off at six, and they followed the same routine as the day before, only Sharon stayed in bed watching Dave get dressed until he was ready to go rather than getting out of bed to tease him. She marveled at the transition he went through. Dressed for the hospital with his hair pulled back, he looked like a well-dressed professional.

Dave came to the edge of the bed, got down on one knee, and took her hand. "I am going to miss you tonight, but I will see you tomorrow. I don't know how to say this, so I am just going to say it. I don't only love you; I need you. I didn't know that until last night. I have never needed anyone in my life, but I need you." He stood up, bent down, and kissed her. She threw her arms around his neck, pulled herself up and kissed him passionately. It would be alright; her love would see him though.

Dave's adrenaline was up as he drove to the hospital, but it was not the excitement of a few days ago; it was a more mature, controlled elevation. It was his first day on call, and he had work to do before he got his first admission. He knew from past experience as a student you had to get amped up for being on call. Being on call was like being in the batter's box; you had to hit every pitch that was thrown at you. The stress and pressure of call at a big city/county teaching hospital was huge and required a maximum effort. Dave was pumped up for that effort as he walked to the doctor's station.

Henry and Jay were already in the station when Dave arrived.

Jay said, "Here are your beepers. The number you call will appear on top. It will be one of the Medicine floors or the ED. If it is the ED, it is an admission. As the call team, we are also the code team. Since this is our first call, I will be the code leader, but in the future, we will rotate. But no matter who is code leader, we all respond along with anesthesia, the EKG tech, the respiratory therapy tech, and the charge nurse with the crash cart. We do not respond to codes in the ED, OR, or Land D, and we do not respond to Pedi codes; they handle their own codes. We respond to all floor codes and all codes in the common areas of the hospital. And by respond, I mean you run to the code site. You will hear Code Blue and the location overhead and the announcement will repeat until all members of the code team respond.

"It is going to be a long tough day, so I suggest you get to work and don't waste time. One last thing: rest and sleep any chance you get. If you need me or need help, beep me. I am here to help you, answer your questions, and help you solve any problems." It was obvious Jay was hyped up too. "It is almost seven, and we are in the box at seven. If there are any hold-overs, we could get an admission immediately. Good luck."

The night charge nurse stuck her head in the door. "Good luck, I will see you tonight." She was followed by the day charge nurse and Jane. "Remember, we are a team, and the nursing staff is here to help you. Don't hesitate to call on us. Let us do our jobs, and it will make your jobs easier. If things get crazy, and they do sometimes, we may get behind, but don't worry. We will catch up."

Jane smiled at them. "Remember come to me first if you -have a problem."

"Jesus, everyone acts like we are going into combat or something." Henry laughed nervously.

"We are, only the battle is out there, and we are in here taking care of the causalities." Jay sat down at his desk.

Dave and Henry began the routine of their morning rounds. The amylase was down on Dave's pancreatitis patient, so he wrote discharge orders on him and dictated his discharge summary. Things had improved for Henry as well, and he was down to five patients after morning rounds. Jay checked the ED, and it was clean with no hold-overs. There were no rounds with their attending when they were on call, so they didn't have to deal with Finkelstein, and by the time they went to rounds with the chief, Dave had everything under control. The patient with sepsis and pneumonia had a normal temp, so if it stayed down for twenty-four hours, he could go home tomorrow on oral antibiotics. The patient with liver failure was stable and could go to a nursing home in a few days. Cardiology told him they were almost through with their evaluation of the patient with myocardiopathy, and they would make a decision soon about his candidacy for a transplant.

Walking to lunch with Henry and Jay, Dave realized he had put everything that happened yesterday behind him; he felt good and was ready for today. They loaded their trays and found a table. Jay was a good guy and a good doctor, and he didn't deserve to be treated badly. Dave thought about what Sharon said to him about the way he dressed, and its effect on others. If Jay dressed well and took care of his appearance, it might make a difference for him.

"Jay, I am curious, why don't you follow the dress code?"

"What dress code?" Jay looked anxiously at Dave.

"You don't know about the dress code? We can wear scrubs when we are on call. I am going to change after lunch. Do you ever wear scrubs when you are on call?" It looked as if Jay had slept in the clothes he had on.

"I don't like scrubs; they make me look skinny." Jay looked troubled. He didn't know where this conversation was going.

"Do you know what we are supposed to wear when we are not on call?" *He is totally clueless,* Dave thought.

"A tie." Now Jay was definitely worried.

"We are supposed to wear a dress shirt and tie with dress pants and shoes." Dave took a deep breath and continued. "I think you would get less flak from people if you followed the dress code. "Henry is going to give you a note to take to Bob and Phil's Clothing downtown. They will help you buy the right clothes to wear on the wards."

"I am?" Henry looked up from his lunch.

"I don't buy clothes." Jay looked more than worried; he looked frightened.

"Take my advice and do this. Plus, get a good haircut, start combing your hair, and use some decent products," Dave added.

"I cut my own hair." Jay looked from one of them to the other. He was totally off balance now.

"Why am I not surprised? I think if you follow my advice, it will make a difference in the way people treat you," Dave finished.

Henry pulled out his notebook, tore out a page, scribbled on it, and gave it to Jay. "There is a good barber just down the street from the clothing store. Give this to one of the store owners, not a clerk or manager, but one of the owners. He will take care of you. I have to agree with Dave. Buy some clothes and get a haircut. I am going to go change and lay down until I get an admission."

"Me too." They left Jay sitting at the table with the piece of paper in his hand and an unsure look on his face.

Dave got his first admission around two o'clock that afternoon. It was an easy one, a rule-out Ml. The man was playing golf and had chest pains with shortness of breath while walking the course. His EKG in the ED was normal, as were his first set of cardiac enzymes, and his pain resolved with rest, oxygen, and nitroglycerin. He was admitted for daily EKGs and enzymes to rule out a subendocardial myocardial infraction. If he ruled in, he would get a cardiology consult and be transferred to their service for a cardiac cath, if he ruled out, he would get a treadmill and go home if it was negative. If it was positive, the same process would be followed as if he had ruled in. Dave got six more admissions and finished his last work-up a little after three in the morning. He slept for a few hours then got up to round on the other team's patients and his own service. There were no rounds with the chief, so after he finished, he ate lunch, signed out, and drove home exhausted. He was hoping for four more hours of sleep.

Two things happened on his first call; he participated in a code and the night charge nurse spent some time talking with him. He had finished the work-up on his last patient and was about to go to the call room when she came to the doctor's station.

"Are you finished with your admission?" She was standing in the door again, as if she were not allowed in the doctors' station for some reason.

"I'm finished and was on my way to get some sleep." Dave looked up at her.

"Oh well, good night then." She looked down and started to leave.

"You didn't come over here to check on whether I had finished my last admission and tell me good night. Come in and sit down. What's on your mind?" Dave motioned her to Henry's chair at the other desk.

"No, you need to get some rest." But she did not leave.

Dave pulled the chair out and held his hand down toward it. "Sit down, I am so far gone that a few more minutes won't make any difference. Do you want some coffee, or can I get you something else, like orange juice?"

"I think I just need to talk to someone." She sat down and looked directly at him. "You remind me of my fiancé, and I thought it might help if I talked to you since I can't talk to him." She looked down again.

"Is he still over in Vietnam? Are you worried about him?" Dave rolled his chair next to her.

"God yes. I miss him so much and I am so scared." Dave saw a tear roll down one cheek as she looked up. "He is a surgeon I worked with on my last tour. It started because we worked so well together, then we started doing everything together. The next thing I knew, we were in love. He is from here and is coming back when he is finished with the military. I am so worried about him, and it is hard to be without him. It is like a part of me is missing. I am sorry, but you remind me of him in some ways, and I thought talking to you might help."

She started to stand up, but Dave put his hand out to stop her. "I am in love too. I can't stand to be away from her for long, and it would drive me crazy if she were in any danger."

The way he looked at her told her he understood. "Until TET, I thought medical personnel were safe. I was in a tertiary care hospital in the middle of a major compound in Saigon. The rounds started landing in our wing of the hospital without warning. Patients and staff were wounded and killed. He is still there, and it could happen again." She broke down and Dave held her while she cried it out.

"I am so sorry. You have enough on your plate. You certainly don't need me unloading on you. I didn't intend to; I just wanted to talk. I thought it would help. I didn't mean to cry all over you. You need to go get some rest now. Thanks for listening."

Dave held her to keep her from getting up. "Jay told us a little about you, and I asked Jane about you. You are a very brave woman, so please don't apologize for being human and worrying about someone you love. I wish I could say something to make it better, but I respect you too much to patronize you. All I can do is be here for you anytime you need to talk or if you feel lonely. Please, don't hesitate, because talking to someone helps. I learned that last night. I can't be him or take his place, but I can support you as best I can when you need someone."

She stood up. "Thank you. Talking and getting it out did help, but I am not brave. I did what anyone would have done in the same circumstances, and you have no idea how scared I was or how scared I am for him now. I just want him home and out of harm's way."

As Dave watched her leave, it struck him again how young she was. Jane told him what her citation said. She got patients out of the wing that was under fire, moving them to gurneys and wheeling them to safety, returning time after time until they were all out of danger. She used her body to shield them from flying glass, falling masonry, and shrapnel by lying over them on the gurney when the rounds hit. She was wounded several times in the back but continued despite her wounds until all the patients were safe. She received a Silver Star and a Purple Heart. It didn't matter what you called it—bravery, character, integrity, a sense of duty, a sense of responsibility, or just concern for others. She had made a difference in the lives of others. She was a significant person. That is what Dave wanted to be—a significant person who made a difference in people's lives.

All three of them were in the doctor's station when the code was called. They heard, "Code Blue, Medicine 1." Jay was the first out the door with Dave and Henry right behind him. The Medicine 1 charge nurse was waiting for them with the crash cart when they got to the room.

Jay ran the code, Henry put a CVP line in, and Dave tubed the patient. The patient was in ventricular fibrillation, so Jay shocked him right away. He went back into sinus rhythm after being shocked, and his vital signs were stable by the time everyone on the code team got there. The patient had coded with the nurse's aide in the room and was only down for a few minutes. The anesthesiologist took over the tube along with a respiratory therapist. The nurses managed the lines and meds, so there was nothing more for Dave and Henry to do. They went back to Medicine 3, the patient was transferred to the CCU, and Jay stayed to write the transfer orders and the note since he had run the code.

"How did you learn to intubate like that? I turned my head to get the CVP line and when I looked back you already had him tubed." Henry was impressed.

"I learned one night in the Medicine ER when I was a stud. Mike and I were on together. A troll came in under CPR. Mike and I tried to tube the guy but failed, and the resident called the code, not because we couldn't tube the patient, but because he was fixed and dilated. He was found on the street and no one knew how long he had been down, but since the EMTs had started CPR, the resident was obligated to go through the motions. After he pronounced the patient, the resident told us we needed to learn how to intubate. He had us take the guy to the last bed in the back of the ER and tube him over and over until he was satisfied we were proficient at intubation. This guy was a full-on troll who had been living under an overpass somewhere drinking wine, pissing and shitting himself for God knows how long. I had never smelled anything so bad in my life. I think Mike threw up, and I know I threw up in my mouth a few times. His teeth were rotten, so we broke and dislodged a bunch of them, then at one point, I think we dislocated his jaw. We must have tubed him a hundred times. The resident came back to check our technique from time to time but made us keep at it all night. Mike was mad about the whole thing, but I realized the resident and intern were doing extra work so we could become proficient at intubation. That morning the resident told me his resident had done the same thing to him when he was a student, and he thanked him mentally every time he had to tube a patient. The whole experience taught me something besides how to intubate. It is not the old 'see one, do one, teach one' thing. It's about repetition and doing or seeing something over and over; like practicing a sport or a musical instrument. You have to do it or see it over and over, practicing until you get good. That's why we have to see so many patients. It's not about how much time we spend learning our craft; it's about the number of patients we see, practicing what we do over and over until we have perfected our abilities. It is not a time game; it's a numbers game." Dave smiled. "I just wish there was an easier way to go about it."

"Man, do I hear that. Dave, you have changed in the last few days. You're more mature and serious. Are you finally growing up and joining the rest of us here in the real world?" Henry's protective nature came out as he looked at his best friend, thinking, *Don't change or grow up too much, Dave; the world needs dreamers too.*

"I came to grips with the things bothering me. You have to give up putting yourself first to make a difference in this fucked-up world. That's my dream: to make a difference. Sharon made me realize I would regret it if I gave up on that dream. A case broke me of putting myself first. To make a difference as a physician, you have to put the needs of your patients first. The night charge nurse showed me you have to be willing to sacrifice yourself to make a difference in the lives of others. I understand now, and I am ready to do what it takes. I was afraid to give up who I was, to become who I want to be, but I am ready now," Dave said, opening up to Henry.

"Like I said, you have grown up and joined us in the real world, but don't let becoming what you want to be change you too much. The world needs people like you too, Dave," Henry said.

Dave called Sharon as soon as he got to his apartment. "Hi, Baby. I am home, and I am going to sleep for a few hours. I will see you at four, and we can go to the picnic." Dave said goodbye, went to bed, and set the alarm for three.

He struggled to wake up. The only thing that kept him from turning off the alarm and going back to sleep was knowing Sharon was waiting for him. He dragged himself out of bed, got ready, then drove to Sharon's house.

Sharon answered the door. She was dressed for the Fourth of July in white shorts, a red silk blouse, a long blue silk scarf tied at the side her neck, and strappy wedge sandals.

"Can we skip the picnic?" Dave put his arms around her.

She twisted away. "No, I spent a lot of time getting ready, and I am not going to let you get me unready. We are going to the picnic, the concert, the fireworks, and the party, then we can do that all night if you want."

"You bet. I'm for that all-night thing, I'm just not sure I can wait with the way you look." Dave tried to hold her, but she pushed him away. "And I intend to continue to look this way. Now, let's go. Everyone is already next-door. It's the Fourth of July, and I have a lot to celebrate besides the founding of the country. I intend enjoy myself with food, music, fireworks, dancing, and a cute guy if he plays his cards right." She brushed past him.

Dave followed her as she started for the house next door. "I be playing them cards right, you bet. I am all over them cards, you just wait and see. I be the cute guy wants to be doing that all-night thing." Dave caught up to her, took her hand, and they walked to the house next door.

The door was open, and they could hear people talking and laughing as they walked in.

Sharon said to Dave, "I was lonely last night without you. I have gotten used to sleeping with you, and the bed felt empty without you. I know you were busy, but I wish you had called me. When you are on call, can you try to call me, if only to say good night?"

"You bet," Dave said as they walked in the door.

Phil and Bob were standing in the entryway talking to two women. Phil saw them and exclaimed, "Gorgeous, you look absolutely radiant; you are positively glowing. Hi, Dave. From the way she looks, I would assume the good doctor's treatment is agreeing with my beautiful friend. These are our friends Rachael and Samantha. Rachael and Sam, this is Sharon and Dave." Phil and Bob hugged Sharon. "Rachael and Sam are our friends who like Bob and I, are in a long-term relationship, and like Bob and I, they should be married, but as we all know, that is against the law in our fair state. So, we have to say they are partners, like they are in business together. But look at you two: the perfect couple. Gorgeous, looking at you makes me wish I were straight, and then I look at Dave and I am glad I am not." Phil laughed at his own joke.

"Don't start with your stand-up gay comedy routine. Is everyone here? Are we the last ones?" Sharon smiled at Phil.

Phil looked around briefly. "Everyone but Sherry and Henry."

"Henry and I were on call last night. I finished my last patient around three, and I know he got one after me." Dave had barely finished talking when Sherry and Henry walked in.

A love story and social commentary

"Hi, everyone, let's get this party started." Every man there was dressed like Dave in shorts and a T-shirt, polo shirt, or casual shirt with athletic shoes. All the women had followed the same motif as Sharon: shorts, a top, and sandals in a red, white, and blue color scheme. Not Henry; he had on khaki pants, a white dress shirt, and loafers. That was as casual as Henry ever got for anything. Sherry was dressed in slacks, a blouse, and sandals.

"Hey, Cisco, are you alright? I know you got less sleep than I did," Dave said to Henry.

"I am running on empty, but I am running, and I have enough gas for the rest of the day." Henry showed Dave his flask. "Most of us know each other, but since some of us don't, let's go around and everyone can introduce themselves. I am Henry, and this is my paramour, Sherry."

Sherry pushed Henry and laughed. There were twenty of them, and they would become known as the gang: Bob and Phil, Rachael and Samantha, Henry and Sherry, Dave and Sharon, Mike and Janice the physical therapist, Harven and Connie, George and the grad student from the lab where he worked, Audrey and Jake the pilot, Caroline and Ron the financial advisor, and Helen with her current date. Dave looked and listened as the self-introductions went around the room. He introduced Sharon as his mistress. The physical therapist with Mike was cute, but she was short and built like an adolescent boy. The woman with George was like George—average in every way. The pilot looked like a pilot; he was handsome, rugged, and manly. The financial advisor looked slick, and there was an older guy with Helen who looked like money. They were the gang.

As they were leaving, Mike and his date walked up. "This is Janice, a physical therapist who moved here from Missouri recently. She just started work at the hospital."

Sharon, who was always nice to everyone, greeted Janice warmly. "I suppose Mike told you he and Dave roomed together in medical school."

"Yeah, until Dave traded me in for Sharon, and I think you can see why. He definitely traded up." Mike's gaze was fixed on the swell of Sharon's breasts exposed in the opening of her top.

Janice was bubbly and perky. "He told me about Dave but not you. Are you a model? You are so tall." Sharon's wedge sandals had three-inch heels, and Dave's Nikes raised him about an inch, so they were both a little over six feet tall. Barefooted, Sharon was a little over five nine and Dave was a little under six feet.

"I'm sorry to disappoint you, but I'm a flight attendant." Sharon wondered if Mike's date noticed where he was looking.

"Well, I was on call last night and I am desperate for a beer. Mike, weren't you on in the ED? Did you get any sleep? Aren't you thirsty?" Dave put his arm around Sharon's waist. "My mistress and I are going to find some beer."

Sharon leaned into Dave. "Your mistress is far too classy for beer, but some good white wine would be nice."

"I didn't get any sleep last night, but I slept from eight this morning until three this afternoon, so I am fine, but I could use a beer." Mike, ever the mimic, put his arm around Janice's waist, and they walked to the park together.

Sherry had taken care of everything with help from Connie, Harven, and George. They had staked out three tables on the edge of the open area in front of the stage with lawn chairs and blankets in front of the tables. The tables had paper tablecloths clipped to them, with plastic plates, wine glasses, knives, and forks on them. At the end of each table were platters covered with foil that contained beans, coleslaw, potato salad, ribs, barbecued chicken, brisket, and cornbread. A small cake was on each table with an American flag in the icing along with containers of chips and dip. Beer, white wine, and bottled water were in a wash tub with ice and there were a couple of bottles of red wine on the tables.

Sherry considered this her party, and if it was her party, it was going to be done right. She went around and collected twenty-five dollars from each couple. Mike told her he did not have any cash with him and would pay her later. Sherry looked at Mike and moved on to the next couple. Sherry only collected for the food, beer, and wine. She had paid for everything else. Now, she had also paid for Mike and his date. It wasn't that Sherry couldn't afford it; she could have paid for everything easily. It was the idea that he thought she should pay for him. *Oh well*, she thought, *I'm certainly not going let him spoil my day or my party.* Sherry gave Henry the money to put in his pocket and took charge of her party.

A love story and social commentary

"Harven and George brought a couple of Frisbees and a football over for you boys to play with. There is beer for the boys, white wine for the ladies, and water if you need it. The concert starts at seven thirty and the fireworks at nine, so we will eat around six. That leaves a couple of hours for the boys to play and drink, and for the ladies to just drink." She laughed and went on. "After the fireworks, we will throw everything in the trash bags and carry them, the wash tub, and any left-over food back to the house. Harven has set up some speakers in the front room, and we moved the furniture to the walls so we can dance. We will put the wash tub and any left-over food in the dining room, and then dance in the front room." Sherry was very proud of herself.

Sharon was the first to compliment her. "What a perfect party on a perfect day. I can't wait to dance." She twirled in place beside Dave and leaned into his arms laughing.

Phil was standing next to them. He bumped Sharon's arm. "And I have some killer Jamaican herb." He showed her some joints he had in his shirt pocket. She could smell how strong they were. "We be having a little smoke before de concert starts, man, and then we go to de zoom room for another little smoke before for de dancing be starting. Arrry man, one hit and de world turns round."

"You have the worse Jamaican accent I have ever heard. Put those away, I can smell them from here and they are not even lit. People will smell it if we smoke out here. Do you want to get us busted? You know there are cops here for crowd and traffic control. I can see the headlines: *Doctors and young professionals busted for smoking pot while partying with a bunch of stewardesses at 4th of July concert*. We would probably even make the tabloids." Sharon put her hands on her hips and looked hard at Phil.

"We can go off in the trees. It doesn't matter if people smell it; they won't know where it is coming from. It's you who should worry since you take your clothes off and try to fornicate in public when you smoke this shit. You are the ones most likely to get arrested and make the tabloids. *Young doctor and hot stewardess arrested for getting busy at fourth of July concert in front of a thousand people*. There would probably even be some pictures with blurred-out body parts." Phil starting laughing.

Dave watched the whole exchange with amusement. "We will fornicate tonight but not in public. I am having a lot of impure thoughts about her in that outfit but what we do, I want to do in private."

"I don't like either of you. I am going to get some wine and find someone with pure thoughts to talk to." Sharon walked away.

"Good luck in this crowd," Phil called after her. She turned and stuck her tongue out at him.

Dave got a beer, and Phil poured himself some white wine. Dave was about to take a sip of beer when a football flew at him. He caught it with his left hand and looked up to see who had thrown it.

"Your mistress told me you played a little ball." The pilot was standing with Sharon and Audrey smiling at him. "I was looking for someone to play catch with."

"As long as it doesn't interfere with my beer drinking." He threw the ball back, took a sip of beer, and moved away from Phil as the pilot motioned the girls back a little. He picked up his beer, took a sip, then fired the ball back at Dave, but Dave had his right hand free now and caught it easily. The pilot had a good arm, so they moved further apart and continued to throw the ball back and forth. The pilot began to bare down and really cut loose with some fastballs, but Dave simply reached out and snagged them, took a sip of beer, and tossed the ball back.

"He has really soft hands," the pilot said to no one in particular.

"How soft are his hands, Sharon?" Audrey teased.

"Is there anyone at this party who doesn't have impure thoughts? There has to be someone here who has a clean mind." Sharon laughed.

"Not a chance. If that's what you are looking far, you need to find a different group people." Audrey clinked Sharon's wine glass with her own. Helen joined them, and they took a sip together. "Don't leave me out." Caroline ran over and the four friends repeated their toast. Then they all hugged in a circle laughing.

Dave and the pilot stopped playing catch, and Dave walked over to the pilot. "Why do women always do that when they are excited? When they are young, they jump up and down, and squeal. At least when they get older, they stop squealing."

"Why do men throw a funny-shaped pointy ball around to show how hard they can throw it or how easily they can catch it."

A love story and social commentary

Sharon walked over to Dave and whispered in his ear. "I want you to show me just how soft those hands are later." She bit his ear, then skipped back to her girlfriends. The girls looked at the pilot and Dave, and laughed at some private joke they didn't have to say out loud to share.

"That's some gun you have; you are obviously a quarterback. Did you pitch too? My brother is a pitcher, and he has a gun like that." Dave handed the pilot the ball.

"I played quarterback in high school and college. You have great hands." They walked back to get another beer.

They were standing beside the beer tub when they heard Henry yell, "The macho men are back. Are you guys up for a real man's game, or are you afraid of a little Frisbee—a game of finesse and skill where your brute strength will do you no good?"

Henry and Harven were tossing a Frisbee back and forth in the open field. The pilot and Dave looked at each other then ran into the field. Dave was in a dead run when he jumped up and intercepted the Frisbee, turned in midair, and threw it to the pilot who set his feet and launched it over Harven's head. George suddenly appeared running behind Harven and caught the Frisbees and threw it back to Henry. What ensued drew everyone's attention. The five women attached to the five men playing with the Frisbee sat down in the lawn chairs to watch a demonstration of skill by young men who had spent many wasted hours and days at the beach throwing and catching a Frisbee.

Dave was fast and could jump. After all, he had been a sprinter and a long jumper. Jake was a college quarterback with a great arm. Harven was an excellent tennis player. George had played everything in high school, and of course, Henry had been a world-class swimmer. They were all good athletes who loved to play no matter what the game was, and they were all good at throwing and catching a Frisbee.

They were totally unaware anyone was watching them, even when the things they did led to comments from the women. They were just boys focused on playing and thoroughly enjoying themselves, but it all ended when a flash of brown fur caught the Frisbee in midflight and without hesitation ran into the wooded part of the park. "Hey, dog, bring my Frisbee back!" Harven yelled as he ran after the dog to no avail. "That flipping dog stole my Frisbee." Harven walked back out of breath and put his hands on his knees.

They came together in front of the girls, laughing and wise-cracking, teasing Harven about being slower than a dog. "That dog probably saved us all from a lot of sore muscles tomorrow." Henry had his hands on his hips. "I need a beer. Where is my concubine? Ah, there you are. Woman, fetch me a beer and come sooth my aching body after my manly exercise."

Sherry stood up. "I am no one's concubine, nor do I fetch. If you want a beer, get it yourself, and if you keep showing off for your friends, that's not all you will be doing for yourself." Sherry turned to the other women. "He goes off, does some male-bonding ritual, and thinks that makes him special because he is a man and does manly things." She turned to Henry. " You were playing Frisbee for God's sake. That doesn't qualify as a manly activity."

Henry looked at the other guys. "We should never have liberated them. Look what it has led to."

Sherry held up her fist and yelled, "Lysistrata! No sex for men who go off to play Frisbee then act like assholes."

Henry grabbed her, picked her up and sat down in the chair with her on his lap. She put her arms around his neck. "You can be such an asshole."

"No Lysistrata," Henry said to the other guys.

Harven got the other Frisbee from the table. "Look, we are destroying our Frisbee. We will never play Frisbee again. Frisbee is evil and keeps us from our women." He dropped the Frisbee on the ground and stomped on it. Everyone laughed.

Dave pulled Sharon up from her chair and hugged her. "I don't want any Lysistrata. Remember, I did not say a word. I be playing my cards right for that all-night thing later."

Sharon kissed him. "Don't worry. I want to see how soft your hands are."

"You two didn't even make dark this time." Harven had been in the zoom room the night of the party.

Connie slapped Harven on the back of the head. "Behave yourself." Connie had been in the zoom room too.

A love story and social commentary

They all sat around drinking and talking before dinner. Dave got to know Jake, the pilot dating Audrey. He was in ROTC at college and went straight into the Air Force when he graduated. He became a fighter pilot, did one tour in Vietnam, and served out the rest of his time in the Air Force getting multiengine time. When he got out, he applied to the airlines. No one asked about his time in Vietnam or about the war. His only comment about it was that he flew an F-4. He was in his late twenties and a little older than most of them, except for Rachael and Sam, who were in their mid-thirties, like Bob who was ten years younger than Phil, the oldest at forty-five.

When he had a chance, Jake leaned over to Audrey and said quietly, "I really like your friends. I like the guys lot. They remind of my friends from school. Why haven't we hung out with them more often?"

Audrey looked at him. "You always want to stay at your place and do things with people you know from work. I would love to spend more time with my friends."

"Ouch, do I detect a little Lysistrata?"

Audrey shook her head. "Of course not, I am glad you want to be more a part of my world." Jake had already decided he was going to ask her to marry him.

They ate with eight at one table because the four flight attendants refused to be separated, and two tables of six each. Henry and Sherry, Bob and Phil, Rachael and Sam sat at one table. Harven and Connie, Mike and Janice, George and his date sat at the other table.

Connie was a smart, pretty, breezy, happy blonde who was very well endowed. Today, her endowments were encased in a red tube top that augmented them significantly, much to Harven's delight. He seemed to constantly find ways to become involved with them, which caused Connie to have to take measures to ward him off. Connie was between Mike and Harven at the picnic table. She had seen the way Mike was looking at Sharon in the house, and now he could hardly take his eyes off her chest long enough to take a bite of food. Connie decided to have a little fun with him; if he wanted to look, she would give him a good look. She purposely leaned over to get something in front of Mike, putting the contents of the red tube top only inches from Mike's nose.

Harven said, "Stop that. I know what you're doing."

Mike asked what they were talking about. Connie looked at Mike. "Oh, we were talking about Georgia peaches, how big, sweet, and juicy they are." Connie was from Georgia. Connie and Harven started laughing.

"I don't get it." Janice didn't get a lot of things.

George, who had been watching quietly, as he always did, made a comment, which he almost never did. "Harven is partial to Georgia peaches." Connie and Harven laughed harder.

"Where is the cafeteria monitor? That table over there is out of control, the table with the young ones. They are disturbing our dinner. Something needs to be done about those children; they are having too much fun." Henry threw a piece of corn bread at Connie and Harven.

"Act your age, Henry. You are not in the fraternity house, and you are not going to start a food fight at my party;" Sherry smacked the hand that had thrown the cornbread. Henry threw another piece of cornbread at Harven and Connie. "You are disturbing your elders. Stop having fun."

Mike knew he was the object of the laughter. Connie had teased him with her breasts then they had all made fun of him. It never occurred to him it had started with him leering at Sharon, but Sharon was so beautiful, and her body was so perfect, he couldn't help looking at her. Looking at her always gave him an ache inside, especially when he thought about what she did with Dave.

They finished eating, cleared everything away, filled the garbage bags, and moved the chairs to face the stage. There had been a lot of people in the park when they arrived, but there were a lot more now, with more filing in all the time.

Half the gang walked back to the house with the garbage bags and food. The other half stayed behind to made sure the growing crowd didn't infringe on their space. Mike had a feeling he was being left out and wanted to go with them, but Janice was chattering away to anyone who would listen to her.

When they all got to the house, they dumped the garbage bags out back and set the food up in the dining room. Phil started a joint, and passed it. "I will light a second one. Take a hit if you want or pass it. Bob and I never take more than a couple of hits of this stuff. One hit will get you high, two will fuck you up, and three will put you out."

A love story and social commentary

"Don't I know it. One hit and the world turns round. Two hits and you forget where you are in the world." Sharon was very high on the weed combined with the wine she had been drinking. Everyone laughed. Almost everyone took one more hit.

They were loose and loaded when they sat down to hear the concert. "I won't ask what took you so long because I can smell what took you so long. Jesus, Sharon, I am getting high just sitting next to you." Helen looked at Sharon and laughed.

The open area in front of the stage was full of people on blankets and in lawn chairs, all the tables were full, and the city symphony was set up on the stage.

The university ROTC color guard stood on the front of the stage, and the symphony played the national anthem. Everyone in the park stood with their hands over their hearts and sang along to the end, then cheered and shouted. Dave noticed that Jake and Sam saluted rather than putting their hands over their hearts, so Sam was ex-military too. The war had gone on for so long and so many had served; there were members of the military at any gathering.

The concert consisted of rousing patriotic songs and folk favorites, like "America the Beautiful" and "This Land Is Your Land." They were songs everyone knew, so they sang along, cheering and shouting when each song finished. It was a joyful concert that lifted the crowd's spirits and filled everyone with good cheer. The music ended as the sun was starting to set. People began to reposition their chairs and blankets for the fireworks, which were going to be set off at the other end of the park over the lake.

The three couples talked as they lay waiting for the fireworks. The guys got to know each other better, and everyone got to know the financial advisor. Ron was from back East. He was polite, well mannered, conservative, and reserved. He was a really nice guy who was completely devoted to Caroline, who was outgoing, fun loving, and friendly; she was his complete opposite in many ways. He was Ivy League, with a degree in finance and an MBA. He worked at the local branch of a large financial institution.

After the fireworks they went back to the house and Harven started the party tape he had made.

Like every occasion or holiday, there were multiple parties in the houses that lined the Park Area. The young, hip crowd who lived there went from house to house staying for a while, or permanently if they liked the vibe. College students, grad students, and young professionals began to wander in and out of the house as the party tape played on. At times, there were up to fifty people crowded into the two front rooms.

Dave and Sharon were dancing next to Connie and Harven as the Rolling Stones sang, "She can make a dead man cum." Harven nodded at Connie and Sharon, who dancing side by side, leaned over to Dave, and yelled, "Man, ain't it the truth!" Dave and Harven bumped hips laughing.

"Oh, if you want to dance with Dave, I will dance with Sharon." Connie turned to Sharon and they danced together.

Dave and Harven watched them, until Harven put his head back, looked up, and said, "God, it's good to be alive." They moved between the girls and resumed dancing.

It was close to twelve when the party tape ended with two slow songs: Otis Redding's, "Try a little Tenderness" and Boz Scagg's "Slow Dancer."

Everyone danced, swaying and moving their feet to the music, but there was more hugging, kissing, groping, and handsy activity than real dancing. They sang along with "Hold her, squeeze her, don't ever leave her, you gotta, you gotta, try a little tenderness." But with "Slow Dancer," there was complete silence, and they simply swayed tenderly to the music in each other's arms.

Sharon whispered in Dave's ear as they held each other, "Have you had enough foreplay? Are you ready for that all-night thing?" It was the perfect way to end the day and the party.

Dave and Sharon saw flashing red lights outside as they were leaving, and a policeman appeared at the door. It was midnight and the police were going around the Park, shutting down the house parties.

Sherry was very tipsy, but she managed to totter over to the door. "Is it night-night time?"

"Yes, and I hope everyone at this party lives near here, because if we see anyone from this party get in a car, they are going straight to jail." The policeman was serious.

Sherry turned to the group. "The nice policeman said it is night-night time and no driving, so go find a place to sleep..." Sherry giggled, "...or whatever." The cops left and everyone who was not staying in the house began to file out.

A love story and social commentary

Sharon and Dave waited on the front porch for Audrey, Caroline, Jake, and Ron so they could all walk back to the other house together. Sharon said, "Best day ever," and it was echoed by, "Best 4th ever," from the other two girls.

When they enter the house, they saw Helen's date sprawled on the couch in the front room snoring loudly. They said good night to each other and went to their separate rooms.

The next two months played out for them pretty much as they had planned. Sharon scheduled her trips to coincide with Dave's call schedule in order to give them as much time together as possible. When Dave was on call, Sharon bid layovers, and she tried to bid turnarounds for the nights they spent at Dave's apartment. On the weekends Dave was not on call, they went out with their friends on Saturday night and spent the afternoons at the pool. Sharon informed Dave early on she did not cook for herself and would not be cooking for them. "I never learned to cook, and I never intend to learn to cook. It is smelly, nasty, and dirty. I can make bacon and eggs for breakfast, and that's it."

On the nights they were together, they listened to music, smoked weed, and never went to sleep without making love. When Dave spent the night in the hospital and Sharon was not on a layover, he always called to tell her good night, and they would spend a few minutes talking. The nurses listened, and began to ask from the nurse's station, "How is Baby tonight, Poncho?" They liked Dave and were touched by the snippets they heard from Dave's side of those conversations.

The other thing that happened on his call night was his conversations with Carol continued. In essence, they acted as therapists for each other. Dave discussed his most emotionally challenging patients with her, and she told him about her fears for her fiancé and her loneliness. They listened to each other with respect and care, always bringing things back to a positive place before they said good night. The other nurses heard that as well, and it made them like Dave even more. He began to find coffee waiting for him on his desk, along with his charts with the labs and reports filed in them every morning. Henry asked Jane about it and she told him they all had developed a soft spot for Poncho and Baby, so for him not to take it personally. Henry told Jane he had a soft spot for Dave and Sharon too, so he understood.

Finkelstein tormented Dave and Henry for a few weeks after the 4th, then stopped coming, leaving the three of them to run the service with oversight from Ed. Rounds with Sheffield however became more and more intense each time they were on call. He would use his favorite admonishments, "You can't not know that!" "You can't make that kind of a mistake!" "When you make a mistake, it affects your patient, not you!" "You are here for your patient, to relieve pain and suffering, to prevent disability and death, nothing else. Never forget that!" God help the intern who let the potassium fall or overshot the blood sugar while treating a DKA. Oxygen saturations that were not maintained treating pulmonary patients led to tirades in French or Russian. Rounds with the chief were brutal but fair, and Sheffield handed out praise as well as criticism, always focused on teaching, motivating, and inspiring.

Dave admitted one hundred and fifty patients in the two months he was on the Medicine wards covering the gambit of infirmities adults suffer that require hospitalization, and he became proficient at treating those common ailments. He managed a litany of chronic and acute illnesses with the six hundred clinic visits he did. His confidence and ability, along with his clinical skills, grew day by day as he ground out the work. He may not have reached Finkelstein's demand for excellence, but he became good at what he did, and he was proud of the quality of care he provided.

There were cases that affected him deeply, and each one left its mark on him, but they also prepared him to deal with such cases better the next time he encountered one. The patients he had the most difficulty with were young individuals with cancer admitted for terminal care. There were no words to describe the anguish these cases produced in Dave; his heart ached for them, but there was nothing he could do. Over and over, Dave questioned why such pain and suffering happened. What possible purpose could it serve? Where was a benevolent caring God in all this?

By the end of two months on the Medicine wards, the stress, workload, and lack of sleep had taken a toll on Dave. He had trouble maintaining his weight, he was always tired, he smoked more pot, and the nights of lovemaking with Sharon became more intense. She understood and did everything she could to help him leave his work at the door, but the denial he used as a defense mechanism, along with the weed he smoked to self-medicate, and the distraction of the sex were barely keeping him functional. He always got six to eight admissions on the days he was on call, so his service was never down to less than ten to twelve patients. There was no respite and no breaks because he was responsible for his service seven days a week. He had trouble sleeping because he constantly worried about his patients, and he was always anxious because he was afraid he had missed something, forgotten something, or failed to do something.

Dave was in the hospital working with very little sleep for thirty-six hours on his day on call and the day after call, and then he was back for another twelve hours on the third day. This went on for two months without a break, and there were times it was even worse.

He admitted a juvenile onset, type-one diabetic in ketoacidosis who was an alcoholic and had been on a bender drinking nonstop for a week. At first, he didn't think she was going to survive because her sugars were off the charts, she was profoundly ketotic, and her renal function, liver functions, and electrolytes were all grossly abnormal. He was up with her all night, reviewing labs every hour and adjusting her treatment. At rounds with the chief, Sheffield look at the chart and simply shook his head without saying a word. Of course, Dave could not sign her out, and he was up with her all the next day and night with labs and treatment orders every hour. Finally, she came under control, but that was a clinic day and Dave was at the hospital until seven that night. He had been at the hospital working with almost no sleep for sixty hours by the time he signed his patients out to the on-call intern and left the hospital. He was on call the next day, so that meant another thirty-six hours after being off for twelve. When it was over, he had been at the hospital working almost the entire time for a hundred hours with only twelve hours off.

Dave was ready to get off the wards by his last day. He said goodbye to Jane, Carol, and the other nurses, thanking them all for their help and support. His first day in the ED was an off day, so he got a one-day break before he had to start. He had not had a break since the weekend of the fourth of July, and it was the last day of August—almost two months of working every day. He had to turn his service over to the oncoming intern, so he got to his apartment around eight.

He was light-hearted because his responsibilities on the wards had ended when he walked out of the hospital. He grabbed Sharon, hugging and kissing her as she put her arms around his neck and her legs around his waist. "I am free, thank God almighty, I am free at last. No more Medicine wards, just stomp-out disease and save lives then come home and make love to my woman. From now on, all I have to do is treat them or admit them, then go on to the next one. I want to go skinny dipping. No, I want to fuck your brains out. No, I want to go skinny dipping then fuck your brains out." He carried her to the bedroom and fell into the bed with her.

Sharon rolled on top of him with her hands on his chest. "Boy, someone is frisky! But you can forget about skinny dipping. I am not going to get naked in a pool, in the middle of a big apartment complex, no matter how dark it is or how unlikely it is someone will see me. As for the other part, I may let you do that. I have to think about it."

Dave rolled on top of her. "Time to think is over." He kissed her, but he did not really want to have sex; he just wanted to play and roll around with her. "We will skinny dip, if not tonight at some time, but believe me, we will skinny dip. If we can't skinny dip, I want to skinny apartment. Tonight, my apartment is clothing optional." Dave pulled her T-shirt over her head, unzipped her jeans and pulled them off by the cuff, and went after her thong.

She rolled away holding her last vestige of clothing. "You are a sexual harasser. You expect me to walk around naked for your viewing pleasure!"

"No, I expect both of us to walk around naked." Dave undressed quickly and stood by the bed. "Now you can take that off, or I will have to take it off for you, your choice." He started toward her.

"Can't I leave it on? It is very sexy, and it leaves something to the imagination." She scooted away from him.

"No, that is not an option. I am naked, and you are about to be naked." He moved to head her off.

"Fine, but how long do you think you will last before the brain fucking out starts if we have no clothes on?" She wiggled out of the thong slowly and seductively, then lay back on the bed with one arm over her head and one leg bent.

Sharon was perfectly groomed and looked incredibly sexy and beautiful lying on the bed. "Now that's what I call some serious viewing pleasure." Dave lay down beside her and snuggled against her. But he was still just interested in playing. "Sharon, I couldn't have made it through the last two months without you. I want to enjoy your beauty tonight. Like you said, we will make love when I can't take it any longer, but until then, I want to bask in your loveliness."

Sharon knew he could not have made it through the last two months without her, and she was basking in that knowledge as he basked in her nude body. She was proud of him for facing his demons and overcoming them, but she was also proud of herself for helping him deal with those demons. "Bask in my loveliness? You really have a hard time keeping that Southern charm in check, don't you? Bask away. I like being basked in." She laughed.

Dave got up and pulled her up with him. "I want a nude beer, a nude smoke, and some nude music. Then I don't want to bask in your beauty—I want to bask in you."

Sharon laughed. "I knew we would get around to that sooner or later." She followed him to the kitchen where Dave got a beer and poured her a glass of white wine. They clinked beer bottle to wine glass and kissed softly. *Helen is right*, Sharon thought, *we are children, adult children playing adult games, but even if the games are X rated, they are innocent and pure, and the rules are based on unconditional love.*

Dave took her hand, led her to one of the beanbags, sat her down, sat down beside her in the other beanbag and rolled a joint from a Jamaican bud. They both took a few hits. Dave went to the stereo, put Etta James on, lit all the candles and incense sticks, turned out all the lights, and returned to join Sharon in the beanbag, enfolding her in his arms. They snuggled together as Etta James's hauntingly distinctive voice took control of their emotions. "At last, my love has come along" prompted a passionate kiss prolonged by Etta James's voice until the song ended. Dave held her in his arms looking into her eyes and feeling her body against his. They were hot and hungry for each other, but they had all night for that.

Dave untangled himself from Sharon and went to the stereo, found a record after some searching, put it on, and placed the needle on one particular song. He walked back to Sharon and held out his hand to pull her up to dance. The strains of Hoagy Carmichael's masterpiece, "Stardust," filled the apartment. "That's all we are, you know—stardust, a miraculous collection of stardust." He whispered in her ear as they slow danced around the front room of his apartment, their nude bodies pressed together, enveloped in the scent of the candles and incenses.

Etta James had surprised Sharon, even though she knew Dave loved jazz and the blues, but "Stardust" was totally unexpected. From the outside, Dave seemed like such a hard rocker. But the candles, the incense, the dancing, and the music revealed the soft, vulnerable, romantic side of him that Sharon loved and never wanted to give up. She knew that part of him was being encased in a hard shell at the hospital. Sharon didn't care what the shell shut out, as long as it never shut her out, and he never lost his soft, vulnerable, romantic side.

The slow dancing turned into fondling, the fondling led kissing, and the kissing ended the dancing as the song ended. They were very high, it had turned into a very romantic evening, they were very much in love, and they were feeling an overwhelming sense of joy. They made love on the floor where they had been dancing, they made love in one of the beanbags, and they moved to the bedroom and made love in the bed well into the night. Dave put the Four Tops on the stereo, and they lost themselves in each other, the physical act of love, and the romance of the music of the night. When their passion was spent, they lay in each other's arms adrift on fulfillment. Sharon went to sleep in Dave's arms, but Dave became lost in thought as he lay holding her close.

First and foremost, Dave was a scientist and an intellectual who patterned himself after his role model, Aldous Huxley. He observed and absorbed everything, evaluating, thinking, reading, questioning, learning, listening, and formulating new ideas constantly. He prided himself in the fact that he learned something new every day. He loved Sheffield's exercise of describing himself in one sentence and had worked on the task since Sheffield had proposed it at orientation. Now, as he lay in bed next to Sharon, he questioned the very roots of his existence.

In Dave's mind, all the unanswerable, complex, perplexing questions mankind faced could be distilled down into one simple question, expressed in the vernacular: what the hell is going on, or in more vernacular terms, what the fuck is going on? You could not ask how or why it was going on, because you did not know what was going on in the first place. Dave knew the universe came from the big bang. What banged? You could not address how it banged or why it banged until you knew what banged. Dave told Sharon they were just stardust, and he knew that was true. All the elements that made up the universe, including them, came from the nuclear furnaces of stars that exploded in spectacular supernovas or neutron stars that had cataclysmic collisions with each other, scattering their elements out into the cosmos. But what was life? You could not ask how life started or why it started until you knew what life was.

Dave boiled the questions down to Sharon. He had spent the evening with a woman with the perfect body of a goddess, the beautiful face of an angel, the eyes of some ethereal being, the mind of a philosopher, the soul of an artist, and the heart of a poet who was as pure and innocent as a child. He loved her so much he burned and ached for her constantly. What the hell was that? What the hell was love?

There probably was an answer to the question, what the fuck is going on, but humans didn't have the intelligence or brains to grasp and understand the complexity of the question, much less the answer. Homo sapiens weren't evolved enough to have the capability to deal with the universe and everything in it, including themselves. It would take a more advanced, higher being. Therefore, humans had to have a philosophy of life to allow them to cope with the vastness that surrounded them and their very existence. They had to have a framework to hang the fabric of their life on in order to function amidst the uncertainties and unknowns they faced every day. Without a philosophy of life, the individual would be overwhelmed and lost.

For some, it was religion. Faith and belief replace understanding and knowledge. Predestination and God's will determined, guided, controlled, and explained everything. All they had to do was believe and put their faith in God. For others, it was cultism. They followed a leader or a set of rules that relieved them of any cognitive participation or involvement. They found safety in turning themselves over to an individual, group of individuals, or set of rules for behavior.

Dave hung the fabric of his life on science and math. Deductive reasoning, the search for understanding and knowledge, the quest for solid empirical answers, and curiosity drove his philosophy of life. That didn't mean he denied other explanations, it meant he only accepted proven facts. Dave's philosophy of life was very complex. It was based on what he didn't know as much as it was based on what he knew. He was a true agnostic, admitting there was much he didn't understand so he dismissed nothing.

One's philosophy of life determines one's behavior, actions, and is the guide for one's belief system. The core of Dave's belief system was Judeo Christianity. He followed those teachings in his behavior and interactions with others. But he also followed the Tao and believed you must do the right thing because it is the right thing to do and to do otherwise is illogical. He had read and absorbed the teachings of Siddhartha Gautama the Buddha as well as the Bhagavad Gita. Life, nature, the flow of the universe and everything in it were sacred to him.

Dave did not believe in organized religion. Organized religions were created by men not by God, and they had all the faults, foibles, fallacies, and problems of men built into them. He tried to model his behavior on the teachings of the Tao, Jesus, the Buddha, the Bhagavad Gita, and the writings of the philosophers he had read from the ancient Greeks to the Age of Enlightenment and the advent of Humanism. He rejected Nihilism and Existentialism. He firmly believed education and knowledge were the keys to a balanced functional society. If everyone behaved accordingly, not adhering to organized religion's interpretations, life could be a paradise on earth. It never failed to amaze Dave how religion could twist, spin, and distort the original teachings to come up with outlandish doctrines and positions that were diametrically opposed to those teachings.

Oh well, he thought, *what the fuck*, and he fell asleep.

They slept late. Dave took her in his arms when they woke up. She looked straight into his eyes and said, "I want to keep our love fresh and vibrant with wonderful romantic nights like last night. I love that tender side of you, and I never want to stop holding your stardust in my arms and swaying to the melody of loves sweet refrain." Sharon sat up and looked at him seriously. "Don't let them take that away from you, no matter what. Do whatever it takes, but protect that vulnerable, tender, romantic side of yourself I love so much. Build a wall around it to keep it safe. Nothing is worth losing the best part of yourself, and that is the best part of the man I love."

"God, I love you!" Dave pulled her to him, and they made sweet, tender love in the soft light of the late morning. It was noon before they got out of bed. Sharon started looking for her clothes. She found her jeans and T-shirt, but not the thong, so she was bending over look for it under the bed, when Dave took the T-shirt and jeans from her. "The rules of the apartment have not changed. No clothes allowed." Sharon stood up with the thong and reached for her clothes, but Dave held them back from her and took the thong.

Sharon glared at him with her hands on her hips. "I am hungry, and I am not going to eat with no clothes on. I pour my heart out to you, then I find out you are a perverted sexual harasser. I take back everything I said about you being tender and romantic; you are a misogynistic, perverted sexual harasser. You want me to parade around with nothing on objectifying myself for you to look at, like your own living center fold. Well that's not going to happen. Give me my clothes." Sharon made a grab for her clothes, but Dave held her off easily. "Big strong man, what next? Do you want me to dance for you like a harem girl?"

Dave laughed. "I hadn't thought of that, but now that you mention it, it is not such a bad idea. You are supposed to objectify yourself. The female, you, has all the secondary sex characteristics and is supposed to display them to demonstrate her attractiveness and fertility to the visual male, me."

She relented. "You are so full of BS. I will make us some sandwiches, but I am not going to do it unless my lady part is covered. At least give me my thong."

Dave held the thong out for her, but when she tried to take it, her grabbed her and pulled her into his arms. "I absolutely adore you." He kissed her. At first, she tried to turn away from his kiss and hit him in the chest, but then she kissed him back, getting her thong in the process.

She put the thong on. "You are such an asshole sometimes. How can you be so sweet, tender, and romantic one minute, and then turn onto such an asshole the next minute? If you want to have lunch with me, you need to cover that thing, so it doesn't get in the food. Wrap a towel around it or something."

Dave got a towel and wrapped it around his waist. He came up behind her in the kitchen as she was making the sandwiches and cupped her breast. "Can I hold the girls for you while you make the sandwiches?"

She turned around to face him. "You are incorrigible. See, this is why I wanted to get dressed. I knew you would get distracted. Behave and leave the girls alone." She turned back and finished the sandwiches.

They ate at the counter and discussed their plans. "I am on every other day in the ED, but every other shift is in Minor Medicine, and I get off between seven and nine with the next day off, so we can go out on those nights. I spend every fourth night in the hospital instead of every third, which means only one night in four that we can't be together. A whole month of relative normalcy."

Sharon started cleaning up with Dave's help. "I tried to make sure on my bid sheet that I was not flying when you are not spending the night at the hospital. I want to go dancing; I had forgotten how much I loved to dance, plus dancing with you last night was magical. We can get everyone together and go to a club."

Dave frowned. "A club? You mean like a disco? I love almost all types of music, but I hate disco. I hate everything about disco—the superficial, fake, phony, narcissistic bullshit clothes; the fake, phony, narcissistic, bullshit people; but most of all, I hate the music. I am with Bob Seger—don't try to take me to a disco, you will never even get out on the floor. No disco clubs."

Sharon laughed. "I have never seen you so worked up—not about civil rights, the war, or the plight of humanity. You make it sound like disco is the root of all evil in the world."

Dave responded. "It is the root of everything that is wrong with our society."

Sharon smiled at him. "You put disco at the top of the list of everything that is wrong today?"

Dave was adamant. "Yes, art reflects life and life mimics art. Take music in America. First came the blues, and the blues is the foundation of American music, then came rag time and jazz; jazz incorporated classical and European music in a mix with the blues and other ethnic music. Jazz became swing, then rhythm and blues mixed with folk music and country music to eventually morph into rock and roll. Everything this country has produced in music since rock and roll is garbage, especially disco. Look at what has happened to our society since disco. And don't even get me started on pop music, which is nothing but hype and promotion."

Sharon was enjoying Dave being illogical and emotional about something rather than his usual pragmatic analytic self. "You are saying disco is a reflection of all that is evil? Art reflects life. Right?"

"Yes, but life mimics art, too. Our society is suffering from an epidemic of character disorders like sociopathy and narcissism because life is mimicking disco music, disco values, and the disco lifestyle. The Disco Generation has been named the Me Generation. They are all a bunch of sociopathic narcissists." Dave was sure he was right.

Sharon stopped laughing at him because oddly enough, what he was saying began to make a little sense to her. "Boy, you really hate disco. Then why don't we try the club the black couple told us about at the concert?"

Dave would do anything for Sharon except go to a disco club. "We can check it out. If it looks dangerous or sketchy, we can leave. Some of us will have to dress down a bit, in order not to attract too much attention."

Sharon stood in front of him in nothing on but the thong, with her hands on her hips, her head up, and her feet planted apart. "You expect me to go clubbing with all this covered up?" She swept one hand down the front of her body. "When you go dancing, you dress to go dancing. I plan to get a new outfit that will bring you to your knees. I am not going clubbing in a burka."

Dave looked at her standing in front of him. "Until we check the place out, it might not be a bad idea, but dammit, Sharon, you go all modest on me with 'I have to cover my lady-part' stuff, and then you tease me by standing in front of me like this. God, look at you, and I am not supposed to want to look at you like this all the time? I will take you dancing, you can dress any way you want, but when you are with me, can you just stay undressed?"

Sharon walked over to Dave and put her arms around his neck. She kissed him. "Now, what are we going to do today, or with what is left of today? We can go to the pool. It is the first of September and a week day, so there is probably no one there, and I have a new bathing suit, or we can go shopping for a new outfit for me to go clubbing in. What do you want to do? It is your first day off in two months. And no—staying in the apartment and fucking all day is not an option." Sharon looked into his eyes and smiled.

He put his arms around her. "I like that option best, but you know what I want to do? I want to take a drive. I am a car guy, and I have this fantastic new car I have only driven to and from the hospital. I want to hit the open road and go zoom, zoom. We can find a little place to have dinner out in the boonies, and get back in time for a little wu chang lang and a good night's sleep before my shift and your trip."

Sharon cocked her head to one side. "Are you trying to schedule our intimate time again? Get it through your head—our wu chang lang episodes happen when they happen and not on a schedule. Don't be such a controlling asshole."

"Why you always call Dave asshole? Dave no asshole. You should not call Dave asshole." Dave looked down.

She hugged him. "Sharon only call Dave asshole when Dave act like asshole. Dave no act like asshole, Sharon no call Dave asshole. Let's shower and get going. I really like your idea of taking a drive outside the city. Let's get away from it all for a while. I should wash my hair since I am flying tomorrow, but that will take too long, and I don't know why I bother any way. I come off each trip with my hair smelling like cigarette smoke. Why don't they ban smoking on airplanes? After a long trip, I feel like I have smoked a whole pack of cigarettes just from breathing the air on the plane."

They showered together with the usual activity that almost led to them not leaving the apartment. They dressed in jeans and sandals, with Dave wearing a T-shirt and Sharon wearing a tube top. The tube top led to more delay, but eventually they made it to Dave's car with Sharon's tube top in place. They took a bottle of chardonnay on ice in the little cooler they used for the pool, two glasses, a joint, and a blanket. Dave put a Steely Dan eight-track cassette in the player, and they were off, driving north on the expressway past the airport exit out into the surrounding countryside. The rural South is never far from the urban areas, so they were on a long straight stretch of freeway in the open country in no time. There was no traffic, so Dave let the 240 Z out, hitting a hundred and twenty, then flooring it for a short time, reaching a hundred and thirty-five.

The Datsun was rock steady at a hundred and thirty-five with perfect control. Dave took his foot off the accelerator and started looking for a pretty country lane to drive on. "God, I needed that. I feel like I left the last two months somewhere on that stretch of road. Now for some real driving."

Sharon looked at him thinking, *Boys and their toys*.

Dave took an exit from the freeway on to a quintessential Southern country lane, a curvy road that led into the forest with open fields and orchards interspersed among the trees. The children were in school, and the adults were working, so Dave drove as if he were driving at Le Mans. Sharon continued to sit quietly watching him drive. The 240 Z handled the curves beautifully. After a few miles, he began to look for a place to stop, relax in the afternoon sun, smoke the joint, and have some wine. He saw a quaint farmhouse surrounded by fields and orchards with a man at the mailbox in front of it getting his mail. Dave pulled over to talk to him. "Would you mind if we sat in your apple orchard to have some wine? We want to put a blanket down and enjoy the afternoon."

The man looked hard at Dave through the window, then bent down to look at Sharon in the passenger's seat, taking a long look at her before saying, "Sure, help yourself, just don't help yourself to any of my apples. They ain't ripe, anyway. You drive up from the city to get away from all them people and that smog?"

"You got it. Say, do you know any place near here we can get a bite later?" Dave said while the man continued looking at Sharon as she smiled at him.

"There is, if you like German food. You go back to the freeway and head back toward the city. Take the third exit on the right and drive toward town. There is a German place on this side of town called the Chalet. You can't miss it, because it looks like a chalet."

Sharon leaned across Dave toward the man still smiling and said, "Thanks, we will leave your apples alone, I promise."

He smiled back at her. "You enjoy the afternoon." He waved and stood watching as Dave drove to the apple orchard and pulled onto the gravel path that led to the orchard gate. They left the car and walked into the orchard far enough to be out of sight of the road and spread their blanket on a nice piece of grass between the trees. The trees were full of green apples that looked like green Christmas ornaments hanging among their leaves, and the grass was soft and full. The air was warm and fragrant with the smell of growing things, and they were in an atmosphere of varying shades of green. They sat on the blanket, poured two glasses of wine, clinked their glasses, and kissed. "I want to come back here in the spring when the apple trees are in bloom and make love on this very spot, surrounded by the scent of apple blossoms with their white petals raining down on us."

Sharon moved against him, and he put his arm around her. "OK, but it has to be after sunset, and we have to ask permission again. This was such a good idea, and I love this spot. I feel protected and sheltered here."

Dave looked at her. "You want to ask permission? 'Say Mister Farmer, we want to spread a blanket in your orchard again, only this time we don't want to just drink wine, we want to fornicate. Is that alright?'"

They laughed and sipped their wine enjoying being out of the city and insulated from the stress and worry of the hospital. "I want to practice in a rural area but not just any rural area; I want to practice in the mountains in a small town near or at a ski area. I checked out Colorado, but Colorado is about as far from the ocean as you can get. The only place that fits my dream is Northern California. The ocean with great sailing and the mountains with great skiing are close enough to have access to both."

"What are you going to do next year for a residency, and where do you want to do it?" Sharon's voice was soft and low. "What about us? Am I included in your dream?"

"You are the most important part of my dream. Whatever I do and wherever I do it, we will be together. I want to spend the rest of my life with you. Right now, in this perfect spot, on this perfect day, I would ask you to marry me, but I know you don't want to get married, so I will ask you to spend the rest of your life with me instead. Sharon, will you spend the rest of your life with me?"

Sharon was quiet for a moment asking herself if she should marry Dave. If she were going to marry anyone, it would be Dave. Two of her roommates were about to be engaged; Harven and Connie were already engaged. Was getting married to Dave what she should do? Then the old fear and anger welled up inside her, causing a knot to form in her stomach. "Yes, I will spend the rest of my life with you. I love you, and I want to be with you." She put her arms around his neck and kissed him.

Dave lay back on the blanket and pulled her with him. "It is starting to come together for me. I know I don't want to do Pedi, that is an easy decision because I'm simply not the Pedi Pod type. I don't want to do

OB/GYN because I don't want to be a midwife. Everyone always tells me I have good hands, and I like doing things with my hands." He rolled toward her, slid his hand under her tube top and cupped her breast.

She put her hand on his hand. "Soft hands."

"And I like Surgery, but the residency is too long. I don't want to spend four or five more years in training, so it's Medicine. That was sort of my plan with this rotating internship all along, to work my way into a better Medicine residency. It would be ideal if I could do that here. You could keep flying and things would go on just as they are for another two years, only I would want us to move in together. Then I will look for a place to practice in Northern California."

"I would have seven years of seniority by then. The only base we have in Northern California is San Francisco, and it is a very senior base. I am not sure even seven years would be enough seniority to transfer there." Sharon frowned.

"Do you want to be a flying waitress all your life? What is your degree in? You are smart enough to do anything you want. What do you want to do?" Dave pulled his hand out from under her tube top and touched her face with his fingertips.

"You are right. When I started four years ago, it was a glamor profession. We used to be air hostesses. We served steak and lobster, and made Caesar salad from scratch in first class. Now, I finish a trip dead on my feet and smelling like cigarette smoke. My degree is in business, and I thought about going back part time to get my MBA while I was flying." Sharon sat up and looked down at Dave. "I could get my MBA while you are doing your residency. I have a lot of money saved, and I could support myself and pay for school, plus we would have your residence salary. Then I wouldn't have to worry about transferring. I could work anyplace you wanted to practice." She smiled. "I have been worried about what was going to become of us. I have tried to put it out of my mind, to enjoy what we have, and to live in the moment. But now I think there is a way for us to have a future together." She lay back down. "Oh, what a wonderful day, following a wonderful night. We do have it all."

Dave stood up and pulled her with him. "Let's take a walk through the orchard." He poured two more glasses of wine; they took the wine in one hand, held hands with the other hand, and strolled through the trees. They were in a dense green arbor with the trees arching over them and the afternoon sunlight filtering through to make bright patches on the grass. "You know we are engaged now. We are engaged to be in love and together for the rest of our lives. I could not be happier."

Sharon looked at Dave walking beside her and thought, is this really what I want, to be Dave's mistress and not his wife? She was happy, but something was nagging at her. Was it because something was missing? Was she denying herself what she really wanted because of her demons she had never faced or dealt with? Was she letting what happened to her parents' marriage keep her from experiencing what her heart told her she wanted and needed to achieve true happiness, or was she succumbing to the myth that a woman had to be married to be fulfilled?

Her generation had started to reject the notion that a woman had to marry to be happy, and she had seen the unhappy side of marriage up close and personal. No, she was doing the right thing. She loved Dave and Dave loved her; that was all they needed. They did not need a contract forcing her to give up her name and her rights.

When they came to the back fence of the orchard, there was a field overgrown with wild blackberry bushes. Some of the vines protruded through the fence into the orchard with rich ripe berries dangling from the vines. They picked some of the blackberries to eat with their wine. They stood at the back fence of the orchard, alternating between feeding each other wild blackberries, taking sips of wine, and kissing.

When they finished their wine, Sharon left Dave behind, skipping and twirling through the trees humming to herself. When Dave caught up with her at the blanket, she pulled him down on top of her and kissed him. When the kiss was over, Dave raised himself up on his hands. "Does this mean what I think it means?"

Sharon rolled him over, so she was on top him. "No, it means I love you. You have to wait until spring for what you think it means."

Sharon sat up straddling him with her hands on his chest. "If I have to wait until spring? I will have the worst reltney any man has ever had."

Sharon asked, "What is a reltney?"

Dave took her hands and pulled her back down on top of him and whispered in her ear, "It is when I guy gets so horny, the horns grow so big they pull all the guy's skin with them as they grow, distorting his appearance."

Sharon sat back up. "Well I don't want that to happen. Will you get a reltney if you have to wait until we get back to your apartment?"

Dave rolled her back over, so he was on top of her again. "If I do, you will have to rid me of it."

She wrapped her arms around his neck and her legs around his waist and smiled. "I have no problem with that."

They finished the bottle of wine and Dave lit the joint. They spent the afternoon laying on the blanket high on wine and weed, planning their future and cuddling. When they drove back toward the farmhouse, Sharon saw the man sitting on the front porch. "Stop. I want to thank him again."

Dave pulled over in front of the house as the man's wife came out with two glasses of ice tea. Sharon got out and walked toward the house as Dave stood next to the car looking over the roof. "I want to thank you for letting us stop in your orchard. It is lovely, and we had a wonderful afternoon. I also wanted to ask you if we could come back some time. You see, it is very special place for us now."

The couple looked at each other in amazement. Here was a beautiful woman and a guy with long hair in a fancy sports car wanting to come all the way up from the city to sit in their orchard. The woman answered, "Well, of course, you can come back. Would you like some ice tea?" She looked at her husband confused and unsure of what to do or say next.

"No, but thank you again." Sharon got back in the car, and they drove off.

"I just don't understand city folks. Why would they drive all the way up here to sit in our apple orchard? I think being crammed up together with all those other people in the city makes them a little crazy." The woman shook her head.

"I think they are some kind of entertainers, or musicians, or something. Did you see that feller's hair? And that's the prettiest woman I ever seen. She has to be an actress or something. I bet they're famous. Did you see that car? That woman can sit in our orchard any time she wants. It's worth it just get a look at her." The man looked sideways at his wife as she frowned at him.

Dave followed the man's directions to a restaurant on the outskirts of a small dusty country town with one main street. The building was a perfect replica of an alpine chalet with a parking lot in front of the two-story structure and a beer garden with tables on one side. The building and the garden were immaculately maintained with a painted sign above the door of the building that read *The Chalet*. The whole thing looked completely out of place in the tired-looking country town.

They parked and walked through the front door. A pleasant, trim, blond woman dressed in an alpine costume greeted them. "I am sorry, we are not open yet. You can wait in the beer garden if you'd like, but the kids have to finish their homework before we can open. Our daughter is the waitress, and our son is the busboy. Their schoolwork comes first. Did you drive up from the city? Are you celebrating something special? Is that why you drove all the way up here from the city?"

"Yes, today we committed ourselves to each other." Sharon looked down and blushed a little as she spoke.

"Oh my God, you got engaged today. That makes today a very special occasion. Come take this table by the window. Don't worry, my husband and I will make a special engagement dinner for you. We were about your age when we met almost twenty years ago. We worked in the same restaurant together. I was the bookkeeper, and he was the cook. We fell in love and married. After we married, we wanted to have our own place. He knew cook and I knew book—that's what we tell people. So, we saved our money, bought this house, and fixed it up. He is from Austria and came over with his parents after the war. Our food is all authentic Austrian dishes. Let me suggest his specialties for this special dinner. His schnitzel is beyond comparison, and his toffle spits melts in your mouth. Let me bring you a nice fresh salad from our own garden, a wiener schnitzel, and a toffle spits. You can share the main dishes so you both get a little of each one. For dessert, we have fresh strudel with homemade ice cream. Now, for the lady, a nice Riesling and for the gentleman a good Austrian beer. The perfect engagement meal for such a handsome couple." She was so excited, she didn't wait for an answer or conformation, but rushed off to the kitchen. "Werner, we have an early guest!"

Sharon giggled. "She is so cute! I just want to hug her. Oh Dave, I want to go to Europe so bad, and I don't mean a one-night layover, but to travel and experience the people and places like you did. Promise me that when we can afford one, our first vacation will be to Europe."

The woman returned with a glass of wine, a big stein of beer, and two waters on a tray. "The children are doing their homework and will not be finished for a while. So, I am going to lock the door and serve the two of you a private engagement dinner."

"You don't have to do that. We don't want to interfere." Dave was worried that such a small place this far out in the country couldn't afford to lose any income.

"No, we want to do it. We don't open until around six on most week nights and by six thirty we are full, and we stay full until nine or nine thirty. On weekends, we open at five thirty and are full until around ten thirty. It is only five o'clock. You are not interfering. Of course, we are closed on Sundays. We don't work on the Lord's day. On Sundays, we go to church and thank the Lord for all our blessings." She beamed at Dave and Sharon.

Sharon stood up. "Can I hug you? I need to hug you. We have had such a wonderful day, and this is like the icing on the cake. Do you mind?"

"Call me Mama. Everyone calls me Mama, and Werner is Papa." The woman held out her arms and Sharon hugged her. "You are so beautiful. I want my daughter to see you. She and my son will be down after they finish their homework. We live on the second floor above the restaurant." She turned to Dave. "You are a lucky young man to have such a beautiful lady. But look at you with your blond hair and bright blue eyes, just like my Warner. He will come out and say hello after he finishes cooking for you." She bustled off to lock the door and return to the kitchen.

Sharon sat down and put her hands out to Dave, and they held hands across the table. "I love this place. What a perfect way to end a perfect day."

They were holding hands when a pretty blond teenage girl in an Austrian peasant's dress appeared at their table. "I will be your waitress now. Congratulations." She smiled and did a little curtsy.

She was followed by a blond boy two or three years younger in lederhosen, with a basket of black bread and a tub of butter. "Fresh bread and butter. Congratulations." His eyes never left Sharon as he sat the basket of bread and tub of butter down on the table and did a little bow. They trundled off back to the kitchen with the boy looking over his shoulder at Sharon.

"Oh my God, they are adorable! Dave, I feel like I am in a fairy tale. This place is not real, and these people are not real. We have crossed over some threshold into a fantasy world right out of the pages of a fairy tale. It is magical and was put here just for us today." Sharon could not contain herself.

The teenage girl brought their food, one course at a time accompanied by the boy with a pitcher of water to refill the water glasses. The boy eyes never left Sharon as he cleared the plates. The food was excellent, far beyond their expectations.

When they finished, the woman reappeared with six glasses of schnapps on a tray, followed by the teenage girl, the boy, and a large man in chefs' garb. Two of the glasses had only a small amount of schnapps in them. She put two full glasses on the table, handed the partially filled glasses to the children, took one herself and handed the last one to the large man. "You have met my children, and this is my Werner."

Dave stood and took the large man's hand. "I am Dave, and this is Sharon. I have been in Austria, Germany, and Switzerland, but this is some of the finest food I have ever tasted. The schnitzel was so light, so flavorful, and I could not believe the toffle spits. You must be a master chef."

Werner beamed. "Thank you. Mama, you tell them why is so good. Is not all my cooking."

"We use only home-grown ingredients from our own garden and from the farmers around here. Everything is fresh, and we choose only the best. I do the baking and my Werner does the cooking, but he is being modest. He is a master chef. But enough about us. Now to you. Sit, please, sit."

"When you drink schnapps, it is all in one drink; you finish the glass in one swallow." She held up her glass and they all did the same. "To you Sharon and Dave, may you have a long life filled with love, happiness, and children to bring you the comfort and contentment that comes from a family." She held her glass to each of them. "Prost!" They all repeated, "Prost!" holding their glasses to each other and downing their contents in one swallow.

Sharon felt something stir deep inside her, a feeling she had never felt before. She looked at the two children, and some instinct she never knew she possessed rose to the surface. It was totally alien to her but very powerful and completely familiar. To be a mother, to have her own family—the thing inside her yearned for it. This place had cast a spell over her. It was the toast that wove the spell. Love, happiness, and family to bring you comfort and contentment; nothing else, only love, happiness, and family. They were left alone as the little family went back to the kitchen chattering among themselves.

"I know why they are out here in the country; it is because of those two kids. They are wholesome, sweet, and innocent, and it is because they are not exposed to the negative influences of the city. They put their restaurant out here for their children. They could have a top spot in the city and make a lot more money, but they put their children first and sacrificed for their children's wellbeing. That's the love of a mother and father." Sharon sat listening to Dave lost in her own thoughts.

What had happened to her today? If there was anything she was sure about, it was that she did not want to marry and have children. Now she was confused and in conflict. Things she had never felt before or knew existed in her, were in conflict with her intellect. She sat quietly looking at Dave. She did love him and in reality, she did not completely understand that either. He was her lover, her best friend, her companion, her soul mate, and they were incomplete without each other. How had that happened? She honestly had not thought she could ever feel that way about anyone until she met Dave, and she knew he felt the same way about her. Is that what happened? Had love allowed those buried instincts to rise to the surface? Was Henry right? Was it all biology, psychology, and genetic memory? Did having a mate cause feelings to formulate that gave rise to natural instincts? Was this a conflict between a Darwinian creation of natural selection and adaptation driven by survival of the species operating on instinct and genetic memory, versus an intelligent thinking being, aware she did not have to respond to those base drives and instincts? Or, as Etta James had put it, at last her love had come along, and she wanted everything that went along with that love. She was frightened because she had been the victim of a bad marriage and a divorce that left her damaged. Until now, she had things the way she wanted them. She felt fulfilled, happy, and content, wanting things to go on just the way they were, but now....

It started when Dave asked her to marry him, by not asking her to marry him. Now, after meeting the family at the restaurant and Mama's toast, it had grown into a conflict deep inside her. Should she listen to her heart and the very core of her being, marry Dave and have a family, or should she listen to her head, reject what she was feeling as biologic instincts originating in her genetic memory and keep things the way they were? And what about children? Did she want to bring children into a world filled with hate, bigotry, racism, hypocrisy, war, conflict, pain, and suffering? Sharon reverted back to her happy, content, self. No, they had it all, and she did not need anything else. She was the happiest she had ever been in her life, and she intended to remain that way.

Mama reappeared and unlocked the door to let in some people who had gathered in the parking lot. "Please have save a safe drive back to the city, and may an angel rest on your bedpost tonight to bless your love." She smiled mischievously.

Sharon stood up and hugged her again. "Thank you so much for the wonderful food and for the wonderful evening."

Dave thanked her and looked at her for the bill. She put her hands in her pockets of her apron and smiled. "There is no bill. Your engagement dinner is our gift to you. You remind us of ourselves, Werner and me, when we were your age—so happy and so much in love. We are still very much in love and very happy. This is our way of sharing our love and happiness with you."

"Oh, we can't let you do that," Dave protested.

"You have no choice. We are blessed, and we never forget to share our blessings. I think you are blessed too, and I think that even though you are happy now, you will be even happier in the future. If you want to thank us, never forget to share your blessings with others." She took Sharon by the shoulders and kissed her on the cheek, and then did the same thing to Dave. "Now go, it's getting late and we have real work to do." She laughed.

Dave and Sharon walked out to the car with their arms around each other. "I feel like I have had a mystical experience. What lovely people and what a wonderful family," Dave said as he opened the car door for Sharon.

Sharon sat quietly in the car as they drove back to the city. She was engulfed in a warm glow that was coming from deep within her. Dave drove sixty-five all the way back, letting the whole day soak in as the Datsun hummed along the road just as quietly as its two occupants as if it sensed their mood and was providing the proper background for it.

When they reached the apartment, Dave put Dvorak on the stereo; they shed their clothes and cuddled in one of the beanbags. They had shaken off the last two months at a hundred and thirty-five miles an hour on the open road, solidified their relationship and future plans in an apple orchard, and reinvigorated themselves with a magical dinner. Now all they had to do was enjoy each other.

They made love that night with a sense of purpose. Their day had been special, and they wanted their lovemaking that night to be special, so they focused on each other. By each of them giving to the other, they reached heights of ecstasy unlike those they had achieved in the torrid nights of passion they had experienced. Their lovemaking was no longer only a union of their bodies; it was a union of their hearts, minds, and their souls to a point where they became one in all aspects of their being, not only locked together physically, but locked together on all levels.

Later, as they lay cradled in each other's arms, Dave knew he would never forget the night they met, nor his first day as a doctor, and he knew he would never forget this day—the day they committed their lives to each other.

Tomorrow, Dave would start a twenty-four-hour shift in the Major Medicine ER at University Hospital, and Sharon would fly off on a long trip with a layover in New York City, but tonight, they would sleep in each other's arms.

7
The ED

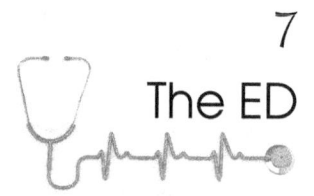

A hospital is a living organism, and the Emergency Department is its beating heart, always pulsating with activity and filled with lights, smells, and sounds. Dave's adrenaline was flowing because it was his first day in the middle of the chaos a large metropolitan area creates for a city/county hospital ED twenty-four hours a day, seven days a week. The security guard checked his ID, nodded him into the ED itself, and the energy of the ED exploded in his face as he walked through the automatic doors.

The security guards of the hospital were an interesting story. They were big, tough black men who never smiled and seldom spoke. They carried a side arm, mace, a night stick, and restraints in the form of zip ties. Their uniforms were gray with black piping and trim, and they wore black jump boots. Most were ex-military, and some were ex-military police. To say they were no nonsense was an understatement. Shit happens, and when shit happened at University Hospital, they handled it quickly and as quietly as possible, with startling efficiency. Every member of the hospital staff knew these men were all that stood between them and the mayhem that could break out in one form or another at any time in the hospital. The staff treated the security guards with respect, and the guards were always professional and courteous in their interactions with the staff. If a new doctor or staff member had a negative interaction with one of the security guards, another doctor or staff member would quickly pull them aside and educate them in no uncertain terms.

Dave wondered how they felt about their job, because the majority of the staff were white, and the majority of the patients were black. Black security guards were protecting mainly white doctors and staff from mainly black people in the South with the turbulence of the civil rights movement swirling around them. Dave thought that was the reason they never smiled or talked. Their job wasn't only physically dangerous; it was emotionally and mentally taxing as well.

The Emergency Department was a long hall with doors on each side labeled, Major Medicine, Minor Medicine, Surgery, OB/GYN, and Pediatrics. The first two sets of double doors were labeled Trauma 1 and Trauma 2. The individual emergency rooms, with the exception of the Trauma Units, were long rooms with the doctors and nurse's stations behind the ward clerk's desk just inside the entry doors. The exam rooms were not rooms, but sections divided by curtains with a third curtain to close them off. The walls between the curtains contained monitoring equipment, oxygen, suction, BP cuff, ophthalmoscope, otoscope, and other things necessary to examine and treat the patient.

Dave entered Major Medicine to find four fresh-faced studs lounging around in the doctors' station. He heard Henry before he saw him. "Hey, Poncho! We back in it, man. We be the emergency doctors. Can you dig it?"

"Hey, Cisco," Dave responded.

Jay walked in. "You guys need to act like professionals so you don't taint the students."

Jay gave the students their instructions. "You two are going to work with Dave, and you two are going to work with Henry. You will take patients in rotation. After you finish your work-up and are ready, present your case to your intern. He will review your work, see the patient, sign off on the case, and make any necessary corrections. Henry and Dave, I know when things get rolling, we will all be pressed for time, but try to spend some time teaching. I talked to the resident going off, and there are only two holdovers: a COPDer finishing his treatment and an OD waiting for Psych. One last thing: don't leave the ED. If you get a chance to sleep, do it in one of the last exam areas in the back. Any questions? Good, I suggest you spend your time reading until we start getting patients."

Dave and Henry walked out into the hall to talk as the students opened their Harrisons. "Now that we have a little free time, let's get together."

Dave smiled. "Sharon and I talked about the same thing. How are things going with Sherry?"

Henry answered. "Sherry is fine. I told her yesterday I was going to continue to pay rent on the Park house. She was fine with it. Mike's team is the one that didn't rotate out of the ED, and he is on the same schedule we are. He is in Minor Medicine today. He is dating the physical therapist that was at the 4th party, but he has some kind of thing for Sharon. It will be awkward to have him around when we all get together."

Jay came out into the hall. "God, they look so young, but that was us only a couple of years ago. I feel so old when I look at their faces, all full of enthusiasm and zeal."

Things improved for Jay once he started dressing better and taking care of his appearance.

Dave answered, "Jay, I can't take another month of your hangdog attitude. I have never seen a man more in need of a woman—any woman, but preferably a very bad woman who will bang your brains out. Are there any prospects?"

"I admit what you guys did with my clothes made a difference for me, and I have thanked you repeatedly, but I refuse to let you alter anything else in my life." Jay was resolute. The three of them had become close over the last two months and were completely comfortable with each other.

Dave didn't keep his politics to himself. "Our internship class has only about a half-dozen women in it and no one of color. My medical school class had ten women out of a hundred, and again, no one of color. Is this junior class all white males or are there any women or non-whites in it?"

"The residents in Medicine are all white males and so are the Surgery residents. There are some women residents in Pedi and OB/GYN, but all of them are white. I don't know about this junior class, but my class was like yours, Dave. About a tenth of them were women, and everyone was white. What's your point?" Jay looked puzzled.

"No point. I was thinking about you needing a woman." Dave kept his politics to himself.

Surprisingly, Henry stepped up when Dave least expected it. "Jay, I hate to admit it, but I think Dave is right about you needing someone in your life. It pains me to have to admit it when he is right, but he was right about the clothes, and he is right about this. You are a really good guy, you have a lot to offer, and there are a lot of women working in this hospital who would be lucky to be with a guy like you. We don't want to interfere with your life, but let us help you meet someone." Henry looked at Dave.

Jay looked frightened. "Do I have any choice?"

"No!" Dave and Henry said at the same time.

The overhead came to life. "One ambulance coming in Code 3 for Major Medicine."

Jay looked relieved. "Cisco, Poncho, time to go to work." Jay would much rather handle a Code 3 ambulance than meet a girl.

There are codes in hospitals and codes for ambulances. Different hospitals and different ambulance districts have different codes. In this city's ambulance district, Code 3 meant lights, siren, and maximum speed; Code 2 meant lights, siren, but reasonable speed; and Code 1 meant just by ambulance. In the hospital, Code Red was fire, Code Blue was a cardiac or respiratory arrest, Code Gray was a call for security, and Code Purple was a major disaster with all available personal reporting to the ED to handle a massive influx of patients. The Code 3 ambulance was probably a cardiac arrest. "Dave, you tube them and take control of the airway with RT. Henry, you get a central line in. RT is already here, and nursing will handle the EKG and IVs. The crash cart is ready, so I think we are set."

Overhead they heard, "Code 3 ambulance three minutes out."

The four students did not seem to know what to do. "You guys stay out of the way and observe."

Overhead again, this time from the triage desk. "Here they come."

The doors slid open and the paramedics ran into the room with a patient on a gurney under CPR with mask, bag, and chest compressions. They stopped just inside the doors, and Jay checked the patient's pupils. "He is responsive." He ordered a nurse to take over the chest compressions and for Dave and Henry to go to work. The code team sprang into action like a well-drilled sports team or the pit crew of a race car, each preforming their task quickly, efficiently, and expertly.

"Strip." Jay looked at the strip. "V tack, stand clear." He pushed the buttons. As soon as the patient settled from the jerk of the shock, they all went back to what they were doing. "Strip." Jay looked at the second strip. "Still in V tach. Dave, check his pupillary response."

Dave pulled the eyelid up and shined a light straight into the patient's eye. "Still responsive."

"Are we at 300 jowls? Good, stand clear." Jay shocked him again. "Strip. Sinus brady. Has he had any bicarb? Atropine one milligram."

"Bicarb is in. Atropine is in," the charge nurse replied.

"Strip. Sinus. Call the CCU and Cardiology. How about his

vitals?" Jay stepped back. "Let's get him off the ambulance gurney and onto one of ours."

"His vitals are good, and his oxygen saturation is good. He is breathing on his own." The charge nurse and the ambulance crew moved the patient.

"Give me a post-resuscitation EKG. Henry and Dave, take over. OK guys, gather around and let's see what the EKG tells us. Someone call psych again and tell them the OD is cleared medically, and they need to come get her, now. Henry and Dave, once you get this guy to the CCU, one of you discharge the COPDer. What a way to start the shift."

The CCU nurse gave report to the nurse, and Dave presented the patient to the resident. The resident and nurse took the patient to the CCU. Henry discharged the COPDer while Jay went over the EKG with the students. It was obvious Jay loved to teach. He was like a different person when he was teaching, calm and confident. The ambulance crew finished their paperwork, Jay signed their forms, and they left. Psych took the OD upstairs. It was only eight o'clock, and they still had twenty-three hours to go on their shift.

"God, I haven't even had any coffee yet. I can't function without coffee." Henry sat down in the doctor's station.

The rest of the shift went by with them treating the typical issues seen in a city/county hospital's Medicine ED. They admitted twelve patients with the usual: CHF, diabetes, DTs, liver failure, kidney failure, COPD, a GI bleed, sepsis, chest pain, DVT, a "we can't take care of him anymore," and a stroke. The three of them treated and released at least another ten, with Dave and Henry supervising the students on another dozen. Dave was involved in the diagnosis and treatment of two dozen seriously ill patients in a twenty-four-hour period. They got a break in the early morning hours that allowed them to crash on the gurneys in the back for a while, and then it was over.

When seven o'clock rolled around, they were totally drained and exhausted. Henry didn't even leave; he went to sleep in the Medicine call room in the basement. Dave drove home in a stupor; he was determined to be home when Sharon got there. He was home before eight and slept until four when Sharon woke him up. She found him sprawled on top of the bed in his scrubs and OR shoes.

"Dave, are you OK?" Sharon came to the bed.

"Don't touch me. I am covered with every type of bodily fluid known to man. What time is it? I meant to set my alarm for two." Dave sat up and looked around still half asleep.

"It's four. Was it that bad?" Sharon looked worried.

"No, I just didn't want to mess up the bed." He grinned. "I understand it was pretty typical for a weekday shift. After a weekend shift, you will probably find me on the floor just inside the door unable to make it to the bed."

"Don't joke; you look terrible, and you didn't even take your shoes off." Sharon wanted to hug him, but he held his hand up.

"I am too funky; I don't even want to shower in my own bathroom. Let's go to the pool. Did you bring your bathing suit?" Dave got up.

"Haven't you noticed there is a little Sharon shelf in your closet and some unfamiliar products in your bathroom? I have left a set of my essentials here, some clothes, and my bathing suits." She went to the closet and got their bathing suits.

They put their suits on and for the first time ever, Dave left Sharon alone when she was undressed. "Are you sure you are alright?"

"No, I am far from alright, but I will be alright, once I get the blood, piss, shit, vomit, and some stuff I don't even know what is off me. Until I am sterilized in chlorine, I don't want you anywhere near me. But understand, it is only my deep affection for you and your well-being that keeps me from grabbing your naked body." Dave grinned maliciously at Sharon. "Beer, I need beer, but I am afraid I will contaminate it. Can you get a beer and pour it down my throat?"

He is fine, just tired, but I have never seen him look so bad. He has lost so much weight, and this is just the first of many shifts to come in the ED, Sharon thought as she went to the kitchen for the beer. "Have you eaten anything? Are you hungry?"

Dave answered, "I had breakfast yesterday and a sandwich last night. I am not hungry, and I smell too bad to eat. I need to get clean, so let's go wash the big chunks off, then I can take a hot soapy soak in the tub. I'll scrub your back and you can scrub mine. I don't want to touch the beer, just pour it down my throat."

"Dave, you have to eat; you have been losing weight. I don't want my big, strong pair bond to waste away. How will you be able to protect me and my nest?" She loved his arms and shoulders. For months, he had not eaten properly, not to mention the toll the lack of sleep and constant unrelenting stress had taken on him. It was starting to show in his body. She looked at him standing there, and her heart ached for him. If she could see the effects on his body, what else was it doing to him? She got two beers from the fridge and handed him one over his mock protest, pointing to his mouth for her to pour it in.

Sharon put on a new black bathing suit made of thicker material that covered more, but it made her flawless body look even hotter and sexier. They were almost out the door before Dave noticed. "Wow, I love your new suit. It makes you look incredible"

"I won't look incredible if I have worry about you not eating, not sleeping, stressing, and not taking care of yourself. Dave, you have to eat, find some way to get more sleep, and take care of yourself while you are going through this. I don't want this to change you inside, but I don't want it to change you outside either." She reached for his hand, but he waved her off.

"Let's go." And he was out the door. They did not have any sunblock, towels, or anything other than the beers they were carrying. Dave slammed down his beer and dove in the pool. Sharon stood on the side of the pool and watched him as he repeatedly went under water, shook out his hair, and rubbed his body.

When he finally finished his ritual bathing, he stood in the shallow end of the pool and looked around for her. She was standing on the side of the pool with her hands on her hips. "We don't have any towels, I need sunblock, and we need more to drink. I will go get the sunblock, towels, more beer, and some water."

"I am sorry, Baby, I had to get the ER off of me. I didn't mean to ignore you, especially the way you look in that suit. I will get out and get the sunblock, towels, and more drinks. I didn't leave the ED at the door this morning when I came in; it was stuck all over me." Dave grinned.

"Don't get out; I will get the stuff. I want to make sure you have the ER off you and the pool has had time to filter it out of the water before I get in." She smiled back at him.

She started back to the apartment before Dave could protest, so he went back to his cleansing ritual in the pool. He was swimming laps when she reappeared with towels, the sunblock, and the little cooler.

It was four thirty in the afternoon and the first week of September, and no one was at the pool. Sharon did not see where the guy came from as he stepped in front of her. "Let me help you with that stuff." He held out his hands.

"It's OK. I got it." Sharon tried to go around him.

"Where do you want to sit?" He stepped in front of her again and tried to take the cooler.

"I am with someone." Sharon held on to the cooler and tried to go around him again.

The man looked over his shoulder at Dave in the pool. "The guy swimming laps?" He moved closer to her. "I think you can do better than that."

"Let me pass. I am flattered, and I am sure there are girls who would like for you to approach them, but not me."

She tried to walk around him again, but he blocked her way. "I live right there." He pointed to a ground-floor apartment. "Come on. Let's go in, have a drink and get acquainted. You know you want to." He smiled at her and took her arm to lead her to his apartment.

Dave was out of the pool in a single bound, and Sharon got a sinking feeling in the pit of her stomach when she saw the look on his face as he came striding toward them. She stepped between them. "It's fine Dave. Let's go sit down."

The man realized the only thing keeping him from being punched by someone bigger and stronger was the woman standing between them.

"Dave, it's over. Let's go sit down," Sharon pleaded and tried to maneuver Dave away from the man. Dave looked at her and saw how frightened she was, and then he looked at the man standing behind her.

Dave had a choice: to go ahead and punch the guy or to let it go. Dave uncoiled his arm. "Y'all want to come sit with us?" But Dave's eyes didn't change as he put his left arm around Sharon to pull her to him and out of the way. Sharon looked at him in disbelief, because Dave had spoken in a deep Southern drawl.

"No. I'm on my way back in."

Dave stood with his feet planted squarely in front of the man with his left arm around Sharon, his right arm hanging down, but his right hand was in a fist. She started to pull him toward the pool, but Dave pulled her back. The man had no choice; he had to walk around Dave, but Dave moved to his right blocking the man's path again and now Sharon was not between them protecting him.

The man looked at Dave's face; Dave was grinning, but his eyes were flat and menacing. The man dropped his gaze and moved to walk around Dave once more, but Dave moved to block him again. He was still grinning, but his features were set in steel. The man tried to walk around Dave again, and when Sharon felt Dave move to block him, she pulled away from him. "That's enough." Dave let the man walk around him.

Dave turned and watched him walk away with malice in his eyes.

"Dave, I deal with that kind of BS from narcissistic assholes like him all the time, and I know how to deal with them. It is better for me to reject them on my own, so they know it's coming from me. That way, they give up and go away."

"That guy wouldn't take no for an answer. You gave him a chance; in fact, you gave him several chances. Sharon, he put his hands on you. You are not going to deal with stuff like that from jerks like him when I am around. He wasn't just hitting on you; he was harassing you. You think I am going to let some asshole harass you and put his hands on you? I only wish I could be there every time something like that happens to you."

"You are such a macho alpha dog. You had to make him walk around you, didn't you? I was so afraid you were going to hit him before I could stop you, and don't tell me you weren't going to." She looked directly into his eyes.

"Yes, I was going to clock him, but you got in the way and I realized it was you who was important, not him. If I hit him, it would have really upset you, so I became a good old boy and defused the situation. But you are right, he had to know if he pushed back, I was going to hit him, so I made him walk around me. I think he got the message, and I don't think he will bother you again." He smiled at her. "You may have been able to handle the situation, but you got a little help from that good old boy."

"Like I said, you had to show him you were the alpha dog." Sharon had to admit the man was pushier than most, and she wondered what would have happened if she had been alone. He actually tried to pull her into his apartment. That thought made her feel vulnerable. "I want to know who that good old boy was? That accent cracked me up."

"His name is Sunshine Billy Peaches, and that's the way people talk where he's from. All I did was lapse back to my roots." Dave hugged her with the arm he had around her. "He can reappear any time you need him." They both laughed. Dave took advantage of her hands being full, crushed her to him, and nuzzled and kissed her neck. She put her head back and kept laughing.

"Sunshine Billy Peaches protected me by using his intelligence, not that coiled fist I saw when you walked up, and that means a lot to me, as well as the fact you honored my feelings above your own." She put the stuff she was holding on a table with an umbrella.

Dave put his hands on her waist and held her away from him so he could look at her. She ran her hands over his shoulders and arms and smiled. "What?"

"What makes you so wonderful?" Dave stood there with his hands on her waist, looking at her.

She smiled at him. "Maybe it is the elixir this cute doctor keeps injecting into me every chance he gets. But not tonight; tonight, I belong to Sunshine Billy Peaches. Does it make you jealous I am going to fuck someone else tonight?"

Dave scooped her up, walked to the pool, and tossed her so high, she had time to yell, "You are such an asshole," before she hit the water.

She came up spitting water and trying to get her hair out of her face.

"Little girls who are not prepared to be thrown in the pool should not make fun of the way Sunshine Billy Peaches talks." Dave jumped in after her.

They played in the pool a while, then got out and toweled off. As usual, Dave took great pleasure in helping Sharon dry off before taking even more pleasure in covering her body with sunblock. The sunblock application resulted in a lot of fondling and caressing, so they ended up intertwined on one lounge chair. "I will be able to leave the hospital sometime between seven and nine tomorrow night, and I have the next day off, so we can do something. I talked to Henry about getting together. When is Labor Day? I imagine the gang will get together for some kind of picnic, party, or something."

Sharon looked at him closely. "Do you want to keep burning the candle at both ends? Shouldn't you take it easy?"

Dave hugged her closer. "Stop worrying about me. I will eat a whole pizza tonight, then we can have a nice quite evening at home listening to music. I am trapped in the hospital so much of the time, I feel like I am missing most of my life. I need to get out and live every chance I get."

Dave checked into Minor Medicine a few minutes before seven. The four studs were already on the station, and Henry and Jay were not far behind, so by seven, they were all ready for their day.

"We can get breakfast in shifts. Henry's team can go first, then Dave's team, and I will go last. If it were cold and flu season, they would be lined up out the door by six waiting for us to open at seven, and we would be shipping a lot of them to Major Medicine at nine tonight. We are lucky it is still summer. We will see all patients in a rotation, not the selective rotation we did in Major Medicine, with the studs getting fewer patients. You guys will see the same number and types of cases as we will. Henry and Dave, you will have to sign off on a lot more patients, but you will be seeing fewer yourselves." Jay the teacher was calm and confident.

Before Henry and his two studs left for breakfast, Dave took him aside. "Do you and Sherry want to meet us for dinner at one of our little neighborhood restaurants after we clear the last patient tonight?"

"Sure. I will check with Harven and Connie to see if they want to go." Henry left with his studs.

Minor Medicine was configured like Major Medicine only in a bigger room with more exam areas and less support items on the walls of the exam areas. Dave sat down in the doctor's station and waited for the nurses to start bringing patients back. It wasn't long before the patients began appearing in the exam areas with their paperwork in the rack at the front of the doctor's station with a number on the rack's slot that coincided with an exam area number. Dave, Jay, and the two students saw them as quickly as possible. On the wards, the goal was to stabilize the patient so they could be followed and treated in the clinic. The goal in Major Medicine was to get the patient admitted as soon as possible if it was determined they needed admission or to stabilize them in the ED so they could continue their treatment as outpatients. In Minor Medicine, the goal was rapid turnover.

Dave waded through URIs, allergic reactions, gastroenteritis, diarrhea, asthma, rashes, headaches, anxiety attacks, depression, unwarranted fears, and drug seekers. The nonmedical psychosocial problems took a lot of time and often created a backlog in the flow of patients. Unlike the wards and Major Medicine, where the work was difficult, stressful, and intense, the work in Minor Medicine was tedious, repetitious, and mind-numbing.

The flow was slow but steady until after lunch when it began to pick up. It accelerated after five when people got off work, and peaked just before seven when Minor Medicine closed. Dave called Sharon at his apartment and told her they were going to dinner at the Italian place. Henry called Sherry first, paged Harven, and called Connie in the ICU. It was Friday night, they had not seen each other for a while, so everyone was excited. Dave and Henry worked through dinner and got help from the senior resident, so they were finished a little after seven.

Sharon was ready and waiting for him when he got to the apartment. Again, he could smell the Chanel #5 before he saw her. He loved the way she smelled in either Chanel or Ambush almost as much as he loved the way she looked. Tonight, she was in a dress that clung to every curve of her body and heels. She had curled her hair, and the curls hung around her face, over her shoulders, and down her back. She had on very little makeup, but it accentuated her eyes and mouth, making them stand out. Dave was so distracted by the way she looked, she had to push him to the shower so they wouldn't be late. Since she had on a dress, he pulled his hair back in a ponytail and put on a dress shirt, pants, and shoes.

They drove to the restaurant and met everyone in the parking lot. All three women had on dresses, and the men were dressed accordingly. The restaurant was crowded, mainly with families out to eat on Friday night after the work week. The dining room was decorated with old-world charm and a distinct *Lady and the Tramp* feel to it. Like the Mexican restaurant, it was family owned and operated with the mama doing the cooking using her family's recipes to produce home-style comfort food.

Once everyone was settled and all the small talk was over, Harven said, "Connie and I have set a date, and we have made an important decision. First, we have decided we don't want to stay here. Even though our parents are opposed to it, we want to go to California. I am applying for a straight Medicine internship at UCSF, Stanford, USC, and UCLA—two in northern California and two in Southern California. Of course, I will apply here as a backup, but we really want to go to California. I graduate in May, and we are getting married the first week in June. Even though my parents are unhappy about us moving to California, they are paying for the wedding and a honeymoon. The wedding is at the Municipal Methodist Church in the city with the reception at the Four Seasons. Then we leave for a week in Paris followed by a week on the Riviera. We will get back in time to move and get settled before I start my internship. With her credentials, Connie can get a job at the hospital where I am training. So next year, hopefully we will be in either LA or San Francisco."

When the waiter arrived, Henry ordered three bottles of Chianti. The wine was poured, they clinked glasses, and congratulated Harven and Connie. Dave looked at Sharon and squeezed her knee under the table. She gave a short nod to Dave. "We will be right behind you. Sharon and I have decided to go to California too. I am applying for a Medicine residency at those same places. Sharon is going back to school to get her MBA while I am doing my residency."

Connie was excited. "We could end up in California together!"

Sherry asked, "Sharon, are you sure you can get into those MBA programs? Cal and Stanford are two of the top programs in the country"

Sharon looked down. "I have a degree in business and my major was economics, but I did get two B's. "

Sherry's eyes widened. "The university you went to has a very good business school and you only got two B's?"

Sharon blushed at bit. "I made two B's, but they weren't in the Business School or in my major. One was in PE, if you can believe that. I didn't like some of the stupid things we had to do, so I didn't do them. The other was in an elective. The TA hit on me, and I turned him down, so he made sure I didn't make an A."

Sherry could not control her reaction. "You are tall and gorgeous, that should be enough, but you are smart too!" Sherry was jealous of Sharon's looks and height, but her solace had always been she had an MBA from Duke.

Dave couldn't help himself. "She was a top dancer in high school and is an excellent diver. She is beautiful, smart, and a good athlete. She is the complete package, and I am going to spend the rest of my life with her." He smiled at Sharon, but she was blushing and looking down. Sharon was proud of her looks, her intellect, and her physical abilities, yet she was always humble and kind.

Connie got more excited. "Does that mean what I think it means?"

Sharon looked up. "Yes. We are committed to each other and to a future together."

A love story and social commentary

This was another blow to Sherry, but she was a lady, cultured and well brought up. She raised her glass. "Congratulations you two. To all four of you. All the best." They clinked glasses.

The waiter reappeared, but Henry told him he should wait until they called for him. "Has another California migration started like the Gold Rush and the Dust Bowl?"

"I have friends from prep school and college out there. I have spent time with them, and I get why they love it—the weather, there is so much to do, plus the attitude of the people in California. It's a haven for the counter culture, tolerance, and change. I think you are right; a third California migration has started, driven by our generation's search of a place to express ourselves, our views, and values. A place where we can live the way we want and not be constrained. The coast is the most." Harven's enthusiasm was infectious.

"In Northern California, the ocean and mountains are only a few hours apart. It is possible, at certain times of the year, to sail or surf in the morning, water ski around noon, and snow ski in the afternoon. There is beautiful scenery, and the Pacific Ocean and the parks are right there. San Francisco is a great city with everything you could want: theater, art, food, and culture. So, we are headed for the coast too." Dave matched Harven's enthusiasm. Then he added. "I would be dishonest if I didn't say I want to get out of the South. I want to get away from the racism and Jim Crow. In California, there is hope for the future that you can feel it in the air. It's almost electric. Here, you feel the toxicity of the past, and the taint of slavery permeates everything."

"I know you two guys; don't try to tell me the drugs, entertainment, and concerts have nothing to do with it and it's all about social change, culture, and outdoor activities. What about you, Sharon and Connie? Are you on board with this? Is this your dream, or are you just following your men?" Henry was skeptical.

Sharon thought for a moment. "I have layovers in both LA and San Francisco, so I have spent time in both places. They are different, but each has a lot to offer. I can think of a lot of worse places, and to tell you the truth, not many better places to live. I am completely on board with it, and I am California dreaming." She took Dave's arm. "I don't want to fly for the rest of my life. It used to be glamorous, but not anymore, and I have done it long enough. There is tremendous opportunity in California, and with an MBA from any of those four schools, my potential is unlimited. Plus, I want to get away from the racism, bigotry, and hatred too. It doesn't only affect black people; it affects women as well. I am tired of the misogyny and sexual harassment. I couldn't even walk to the pool by myself yesterday without a guy blocking my way and trying to get me to go to his apartment with him. Dave's alter ego, Sunshine Billy Peaches, had to fend him off. The guy wouldn't take no for an answer, and I am not sure what would have happened if Dave, I mean Sunshine Billy Peaches, hadn't been there." She smiled at Dave.

Henry laughed. "Really Dave, you brought out Sunshine Billy Peaches?"

"It was either Sunshine Billy Peaches or I punch the guy, and I promised Sharon I was over that sort of thing." Dave looked at Sharon.

"Harven and I have discussed where we wanted to live a lot. With Harven's trust fund, we can go anywhere we want, and we decided on California." Connie looked at Sharon and smiled. "I get the woman thing too, believe me, and the South thing."

It was all a bit awkward for Sherry, but she held her composure. They looked at their menus in silence until Henry called the waiter over. After they ordered, Connie said, "What about you, Henry? What are your plans after your internship? What are you guys going to do?"

Henry was feeling guilty. He knew he could not and should not keep things from Sherry any longer. He needed to be honest and truthful with her. "Until now, it has been all a matter of course: get my degree, chose a specialty, then get a good internship, but I never thought past that. I never thought about what I wanted to do with my degree and my training or what I wanted to do with my life. It didn't become clear to me until I took acid the night of the concert. I know that sounds like a cliché, but it is true. Lying in the park, looking up at the night sky and the full moon, it all unfolded for me. Like Harven, because of my trust fund, I can do anything I want, anywhere I want. I have advantages far beyond most people, and I feel I should use those advantages to do something significant. Again, it sounds like another cliché, but I believe in noblesse oblige.

"I think humanity will continue to face epidemics and pandemics like the ones we have seen in the past; plus, I believe they will get worse and worse. I want to help deal with those upcoming catastrophes. I am going to do an infectious disease fellowship, hopefully at Hopkins, then do research at the CDC and possibly move on to the World CDC in Europe at some time in the future. I think the front line of our defense against the plagues that are coming will be there, and I want to make a significant contribution to the fight." Henry looked at Sherry. "I am sorry I didn't tell you sooner, but I know what you want. I didn't tell you before because I was afraid you would leave me, and I am not ready for it to end. " Henry unburdened himself.

Sherry was overwhelmed and confused. How could she be disappointed that she was not going to be a New York socialite because the man who was going to make her one was going to be saving humanity instead? She could not deal with her mixed emotions and had to excuse herself. Sharon and Connie went after her.

Dave looked at Henry and said,. "You did the right thing, man. It is too bad you didn't do it in private, but you did the right thing. Phi Kai Phi, brother." Dave knew Henry was different. Henry could live for himself, like his cousins and sister, but he chose a life of purpose instead. He was a world-class swimmer who could have won Olympic medals, but he gave that up to pursue his education and go to medical school. He could be a Park Avenue internist, mingle with the rich and powerful; celebrities, actors, politicians, and business leaders, but instead, he was going to confine himself to a lab to do research in order to prevent the deaths of thousands, if not millions.

Sherry walked outside. She felt betrayed, yet knowing what Henry wanted to do made it hard for her to justify her feelings. Sherry was a product of her class, raised in wealth and privilege, but she was not a bad person. She was smart, educated, and aware; that side of her saw Henry as noble, but the other side of her was spoiled and focused on her own desires. She was torn between the two, unable to embrace either.

Sharon and Connie followed her outside. They had no idea Sherry was upset because Henry was no longer her means of becoming a socialite and a leading lady in the most exclusive set in the county. Neither of them thought in those terms or had those types of aspirations, so Sherry's issue was completely alien to them. Sherry was embarrassed to tell them what the issue really was, so she went along with their idea that it had to do with the nature of her relationship with Henry.

Connie started, "He said he didn't want to lose you, and he didn't want things to end. I know you have been dating for about a year, but give it more time."

"How do you know if you love someone?" Sherry asked. She was fond of Henry, but she had seen him mainly as a means to an end, and she didn't actually know if there was more to it than that.

Connie answered. "I can't answer that; I don't know. I just knew with Harven. How about you, Sharon. How did you know?"

Sharon laughed. "You are asking me? Remember, I am the one who took her clothes off and tried to fuck Dave in front of a room full of people right after I met him. I know it sounds hokey, but I think I knew from the first moment I saw him, and he tells me he felt the same way. Of course, we felt like we knew each other because Henry had told us so much about each other. I can tell you this, after I did fuck him, I never wanted to be with anyone else, but it wasn't all physical. We touched on multiple levels. He awakened feelings and sensations in me I never knew existed. We can't keep our hands off each other, but we also have a hard time just not being together, like when I have a layover or when he spends the night at the hospital. Neither of us can sleep well if we don't sleep together, and I don't mean having sex, although that too, but actually knowing the other person is sleeping beside you. It is like the two of us became one entity. We are a pair rather than two separate people."

Connie continued, "It happened immediately for her; it took time for me. I think love is different for different people, but the common factor is the interpersonal connection between two people on multiple levels. Look, let's go back in; you and Henry can talk it out later. I think both of you want your relationship to continue."

Sherry would never lose herself in another person, she was too self-focused and self-possessed, and there was nothing she could do about Henry's career plans, so she decided to let it go. "OK, I think you are right. I am fine now." They went back in.

While they were gone, Henry brought up the fact he was probably going to have to move back to the Park house. Harven told him he would be living alone most of the time because he, Mike, and George spent a lot of nights away, either on call or with the women they were dating.

The women came back, and they ate dinner with very little conversation. After dinner, Dave offered, "Why don't we go back to our place and listen to some music?"

Sharon looked at him thinking, *Our place?* She had moved more and more of her stuff into Dave's apartment, and the only time she spent at her house was when Dave was at the hospital. After this year, they would have their own place, either here or in California. She liked the sound of "our place."

Henry looked at Sherry. "I think we better pass. Maybe next time." *If there is a next time*, he thought. Henry and Sherry left.

Harven looked at Connie. "Sure."

The four of them drove to Dave's apartment. They didn't drink the third bottle of wine at dinner, so they took it back to the apartment with them. Dave rolled a number while Sharon poured four glasses of wine. Dave and Sharon sat in one beanbag with Harven and Connie in the other one, as they listened to Janis Joplin, drank wine, and smoked the number.

The girls talked about Henry and Sherry until Dave interrupted. "I think Henry is using Sherry, and Sherry wants to use Henry. Sherry is like every girl Henry dated in college: pretty, wealthy, refined, sophisticated, and self-absorbed. And they all took care of Henry. Henry needs a woman to take care of him, and he needs them to be cut from the same cloth. He has never been serious about a girl or in love with anyone, and if Sherry dumps him, he will find another one out of the same mold as soon as he can. That's what he did in college. I think his only concern is that it will be harder to find someone because he is tied up with his internship, so he wants Sherry to stick around. Sherry will probably stick around until she is sure she can't ride Henry to some kind of elevated social position. Henry doesn't believe in love; he is too pragmatic and too unemotional, plus he protects himself from any drama, emotion, or physiological entanglements. He is my best friend and I love him like a brother, but I know him. Someday, when he is ready, he will look for a permanent mate, his term not mine, and when he does, he will base his selection on a whole host of criteria and areas of compatibility, not love."

Sharon looked at Dave. "Do you really believe that?"

Dave held her gaze. "I don't just believe it, I know it. Henry and I know each other. How accurate was he when he told you about me?"

Sharon smiled at Dave. "He was very accurate, except he never told me what an asshole you can be sometimes."

Connie sat up and looked at Sharon. "I think that is a given. The asshole part, I mean. If he is a man, he is an asshole to some degree. It is only a matter of degrees." Connie looked down at Harven and laughed. "We women know we have to put up with some degree of assholeishness. It goes with the turf. So, as long as the asshole is cute and the assholeishness is manageable, it's OK."

Sharon sat up. "You men are lucky we women put up with as much assholeishness as we do. We love you; we nurture you; we take care of you; we literally take you inside our bodies to satisfy your desires. Understand, we are very tolerant, but also understand, like Connie said, we will stay only if you are a manageable asshole. If you become unmanageable, we will find some other asshole to lavish our womanliness on and take inside our body."

Dave looked at Harven. "What did we do?"

"You are men, that is what you did." Sharon lay back. "But you are a cute, manageable asshole, so I guess I will keep letting you inside my body."

Harven pulled Connie back down beside him. "How about me? Am I cute and manageable enough?"

"Well, I have been letting you inside my body nearly every night for almost a year now, and I am going to marry you, so I guess you are good to go." They all laughed. "It would be so much fun if we were together in California."

"Except for a couple things like residency and internship. But we wouldn't let little things like that get in our way and spoil our fun, would we?" Dave responded.

They were enjoying themselves so much, they didn't want the night to end, but finally Connie said, "I think we had better go. I can tell by Sharon's body language it's time." They got up and said good night. Dave and Sharon went to bed, shedding their clothes as they went with Fleetwood Mac providing the music to accompany their lovemaking.

They slept late and stayed in bed deciding what to do with their day off. "I don't want to go to the pool and deal with another guy hitting on me. I have an idea of what to do, but first I am going to make us breakfast."

A love story and social commentary

Sharon got up, found her thong, pulled a pair of shorts out of Dave's closet, and threw them at him. "No pants, no service." Sharon made bacon and eggs while Dave made coffee and toast, caressing her every chance he got, then they sat down to eat. "I want to go to the park for a picnic. On the way, we can stop for a bottle of wine and some picnic stuff." They finished eating and cleaned up the kitchen. When he wouldn't leave her alone, she turned on him, and put her arms around his neck. "Am I going to have a problem with you? Didn't you get enough last night?"

Dave hugged her. "I can never get enough of you, and I am not going to get any of you for a while." Dave started backing her toward the bedroom.

Sharon stopped him and frowned. "Is there something wrong with us? I mean, do we have too much sex? I don't think other people do it as much as we do."

"That's their problem." Dave started to push her backwards again.

"Wait. I mean it." Sharon stopped again.

Dave laughed and started them for the bedroom again. "Really?"

Sharon stopped them again. "We are at each other every chance we get. Is that normal?"

"As far as I can see." Dave once more had them headed for the bedroom.

Afterwards, as they lay in bed, Dave said, "I don't think there is something wrong with us. I think there is something right with us."

Sharon raised up on her elbow to look at Dave. "I know. I think it is physical. I don't mean a physical attraction, although that too, but I mean actually physical. We fit together physically; our bodies are a perfect fit; when we hold each other, when we dance, when we make love, we are the perfect size for each other." She blushed a little. "Our parts fit together perfectly too."

"What?" Dave raised up on his elbow to face her.

She blushed more. "You fit perfectly inside me. You are just the right size for me." She smiled through the blush. "It's a three bears thing. It is not too big, it is not too small, but it is just right. Like Goldilocks, or Goldie Cock." She laughed. "You are a bad man."

Dave laughed with her. "What did I do? You are the one talking about Goldie Cock and parts fitting together."

"I never, ever even thought about anything remotely like that before I met you. If I had in some fashion or form, I would have never, ever said anything about it. Now, after you seduced and corrupted me, I am laying here talking about how your boy part fits in my girl part perfectly and calling you Goldie Cock. You did that to me. I had heard about men like you, and now I am the victim of one." Sharon continued laughing.

Dave reached for her and pulled her back down with him. "I seem to remember a beautiful woman evaluating me very closely for some time, before taking me to a dark room, giving me very potent drugs, and exposing her body to me. Then she took me to her room and had mind-blowing sex with me. So, who seduced whom?"

Sharon snuggled against him. "You seduced me, then you corrupted me. You seduced me with your shoulders, long blond hair, vivid blue eyes, and confident manner, but most of all, you seduced me with your knowledge of art, literature, and your sense of adventure. You were at Woodstock, you travelled Europe with a back pack and a Eurail Pass. And don't tell me you didn't know I would find all that seductive and that you didn't work as hard as you could to make sure you presented it all to me."

Dave hugged her. "You bet; I have never wanted anything more in my life than I wanted you. I was so afraid you were out of my league and that you would reject me. But you seduced me. You know very well how great your body is, those long, slender perfectly shaped legs and firm rear, your insanely incredible breasts, and all of it part of a tall, graceful, lithe package. So, what do you do? You wear a short skirt and come-fuck-me shoes that display your legs to their best advantage, and just to make sure I get the whole picture; you undo your blouse to show me just how amazing your breasts are. If that is not seduction at its highest level, I don't know what is."

"Maybe a little bit. But don't tell me you weren't trying to seduce me just as hard, if not harder. No pun intended with the hard and harder." Sharon laughed. "So maybe we seduced each other, but you corrupted me with your wanton sexual ways that made me lose control and scream. I had never felt anything like that and never dreamed it was even possible to feel anything like that. We may have seduced each other, but you corrupted me with sex."

Dave looked at her. "Do you think I had ever felt anything like that? I can't keep my hands off you. I want you constantly."

"I guess there are worse things than wanting to make love all the time. God, Dave, are we always going to be like this and be this happy?" Sharon held him close.

Finally, they got out of bed, showered and dressed, and drove to Sharon's house.

On the way, they bought a bottle of Pinot Noir, a baguette, two different types of cheese, a salami, an apple, a pear and some chocolates. When they got to the house, she added two plates, two wine glasses, and a knife to the stuff they bought, then she ran upstairs for a blanket. Dave carried the bag, she carried the blanket, and they walked to a nice spot in the park to set up their picnic.

When she unwrapped the blanket, there was a kite in it. "It is the symbol of my sorority, and no sister would ever be without one to fly on a perfect late summer day like today. Come on, let's get it up, and I don't mean you, I mean the kite." Sharon was as happy as a child. Dave put the kite together and held it up for Sharon to catch the wind. She let the string out until the kite was high enough then came back to the blanket and sat down with Dave. He staked the kite out, and they set up their picnic, like two children off on a kite-flying lark on a sunny, balmy, summer day. They were very much in love, so the sky looked bluer, the grass appeared greener, and the air bathed them in its warm soft caress.

Dave poured the wine and cut up the fruit, cheeses, baguette, and salami. They lay back on one elbow facing each other while they sipped wine and nibbled the picnic. Sharon wanted to talk about "our place."

"Next year, when your internship is over, we will have our own place, our first home, and I want to talk to you about it. I want it to have two bedrooms. One will be our bedroom, the other will be our library with book shelves and desks where we read, study, and do our work. I want a big front room, big enough to have a dining area. I want lots of flowers all the time and plants. I guess it has to have a kitchen, but I don't intend to use it." Sharon was animated as she told Dave her plans for their first home. "I want nice things. I want a warm, inviting, sophisticated look that reflects our personalities and our values." She sat up.

Her eyes were bright and shining, and her face seemed to glow as she gazed off into the distance across the expanse of the open field, picturing her first home. Dave saying "our place" had triggered something in her that filled her with a domestic urge. Making plans and picturing their home was more pleasant than she had ever dreamed something like that would be. She lay back down. "I can't wait to have our place."

Dave loved to see her so excited. "You don't have to wait. You can move into my apartment now. I know it's not perfect or what you are picturing, but you can make it ours."

Sharon came back from the happy place she had created in her mind. "I thought about that, but there is Helen to consider. Helen is my best friend, and if I move out, it will leave her alone. Audrey and Caroline spend most of their time away. At least I am there when you are at the hospital on call."

She became serious. "There is another factor; the way the guy acted at the pool. I think it is best to leave things the way they are for now." She smiled, the serious look left her face and it lit up again. "I know we will have to move into an apartment because you will want a pool. You are such a water guy. No singles apartment though. I don't want that kind of thing happening again. I have to put up with unwanted advances, but I am not going to put up with them where I live." She looked dreamy again.

Dave laughed. "Do you think guys will stop hitting on you just because they are married? How many married guys hit on you on the airplane or at work?"

Sharon moved toward him. "Well, I can tell you one thing, I better not catch you hitting on anyone. You better be completely and totally committed to me, or I will make of you a eunuch." She smiled and made a snipping sign with her first two fingers.

Dave frowned. "There you go again, threatening my manhood. Every time the subject of infidelity comes up, you threaten my manhood. Sharon, why would I hit on anyone when I have you? Stop threatening my manhood. That is a scary thing to do to a guy."

Sharon took the wine glasses and plates of food and set them aside, then turned on Dave with a malevolent look in her eyes. "Oh, is the big man afraid?" She came at him making snipping signs with the first two fingers of both hands.

"You are not funny." Dave laughed, grabbed her, and they rolled around on the blanket until he was able to stay on top of her, pinning her arms above her head. "You know you are doing this because you are a terrible tease." He held her down. "You threaten my manhood, then you get physical with me." He kissed her again and she kissed him back passionately. He let her hands go, and she put her arms around his neck then rolled on top of him.

Sharon broke the kiss and moved her mouth to his ear. "I want a home with you. I want to live with you in our home. I want us to spend the evenings reading, talking, listening to music, and our nights in wild unfettered lust and passion in our own bed in our own home."

Sharon sat up straddling Dave with her hands on his chest. She looked up and saw Bob and Phil standing over them with a bottle of wine and a blanket. "When we saw you, we thought we would join you, but before we could get a blanket and wine, you were wrapped up in each other, literally wrapped up in each other. Do you have no shame?" Phil was smiling at them.

"Can you uncouple, or should we leave you to continue what you started?" Bob raised his eyebrow still smiling.

Sharon blushed and stood up. "Please join us. We haven't seen you guys for so long." Phil spread their blanket, and they sat down with Dave and Sharon.

Sharon had done a modeling job for Bob and Phil at the Apparel Mart for their fall line. "The photographer from Nieman Marcus has been pestering me about you since the Apparel Mart show. He wants to know who you are, who your agent is, and how to book you for work."

"You must be kidding!" Sharon couldn't believe it.

"No, I am not. It could mean a lot of money, but it would also mean you have to travel."

"I am not a model." Sharon was overwhelmed.

"Sharon, you are one of the most beautiful women I have ever seen, and your body is perfection," Bob added. "Everything you wear looks great on you. That is why they want you, to sell clothes, because if it looks good on you, people will think it will look good on them."

"Look, I am happier than I have ever been. I have everything just the way I want it, and I don't want anything to jeopardize it." She looked at Dave.

"Sharon, if you want to do this, do it. We will find a way to work around it. The one thing I don't want you to do is not do it and then regret it later. You have my support one hundred percent either way." Dave put his arms around her.

Sharon thought for a minute. "Everything in my life is perfect, and I don't want to change it, but I will do it if I can do it on my terms." Sharon looked satisfied with herself. "One more thing, and I want to make this very clear, I will not tolerate any unwanted advances or inappropriate behavior from anyone. If anyone hits on me, I will leave, and I will be paid for the entire time I was booked." Sharon smiled and put her head on Dave's shoulder. "I will use the money to decorate our place."

Phil said, "I will give them your number."

"No, you won't. You got me into this; as of now, you are my unpaid agent, so you set it up. Give them my terms and let them know they are not negotiable. I want a contract that gives me exactly what I want." Sharon smiled sweetly at Phil and cuddled with Dave. "Give them my address, have them mail my contract, the bookings, and details to me."

Phil changed the subject. "OK, are you guys going to make it to our Labor Day Happening? We are having the gang over for brunch, then wine and cheese in the afternoon. Everyone has to work the next day, so we won't go late."

Dave answered, "I will be coming off a twenty-four-hour shift in the ER, so I won't even be up until late afternoon."

Bob pleaded, "Come by anyway. We never see you two anymore. It is the same way with Henry and Sherry. It used to be great with everyone getting together all the time and the parties. I miss the parties."

Bob and Phil looked at each other and smiled. "Halloween is coming up, and that is the biggest party night on the Park. Let's throw the biggest, wildest, most outrageous Halloween party the Park has ever seen."

When they got back to the apartment, they were mellow from the wine, refreshed from being outside, and warm from the late-summer sunshine. They both kicked off their sandals, snuggled in one of the beanbags, and Dave put Canned Heat on the turntable.

"I am not going to be the hot young stewardess who everyone thinks should be a model, and you are not going to be the handsome, dedicated, young intern forever. This time of our life is precious. We need to savor and enjoy every second of it, because when it's gone, it will be gone forever. We need to live every moment to the fullest and enjoy every minute of our time together, because we are young, and our lives are perfect right now." Sharon cuddled closer to Dave and hugged him tighter as they listened to Canned Heat's "Going Up the Country."

After Canned Heat, they listened to Quick Silver Messenger Service and Sharon ordered a pizza for their dinner. While they waited for the pizza, they continued to listen to San Francisco groups, like The Grateful Dead and Jefferson Airplane. After they had more wine with dinner, they were more than mellow. They were slightly buzzed and feeling very amorous. The San Francisco music had them California dreaming as they cuddled in a beanbag after dinner.

Sharon's top and Dave's shirt came off in the beanbag. Both their shorts came off and Date put Steve Winwood on. Sharon's thong came off just before they got in bed. Their wine-fueled lovemaking left both of them asleep in no time. Sharon dreamed of their first home and how she would decorate it. She even accepted the fact it had to have a kitchen and dreamed about how to decorate it. Dave dreamed about Sharon.

—⚡—

Dave had come to love the smell of the ED; it was a clean sharp antiseptic odor. It caused an excitement and adrenaline rush in him similar to the feeling he got from the smell of a locker room in a stadium before a game. When he arrived the next morning, the smell hit him along with the total chaos in the ED.

Patients were on gurneys in the main hall and every exam area in the Major Medicine occupied. The senior resident, the junior resident, both interns, and all four studs from the previous shift were still seeing patients, and in Minor Medicine because people were already lined up out the door at the triage desk. Dave was not surprised having worked three-day holiday weekends in the ED as a student. With the seven of them and the seven from the previous shift working, they cleared the patients from the hall of Major Medicine and freed up a couple of exam areas. The previous shift left after nine o'clock with some semblance of order restored to Major Medicine. Minor Medicine never caught up or cleared the entire shift.

The uncontrollable, bizarre acting, or unconscious drunks, the overdoses caused by suicide attempts or attempts to get higher, the GI bleeds and intractable vomiting caused by alcohol or drugs, the psych cases from schizophrenia to catatonic and delusional states mixed in with patients with pulmonary issues, cardiac problems, diabetes, organ failure, strokes and other medical problems to produce an unmanageable toxic mixture of smells, noises, and visual horrors. The ambulance bay was full for the entire twenty four hours with ambulances coming and going constantly, hauling the broken, battered, shattered, convulsing tide of humanity in extremis to the overwhelmed, stressed-out, and overworked staff of University Hospital. For the doctors, students, and nurses, it was a fight against insurmountable odds. They were able to win battles, but they could never win the war, yet they fought on until they were physically exhausted and emotionally drained.

There were cases and situations that occurred during Dave's internship that he was never able to talk about or think about for the rest of his life. He repressed them because they affected him so deeply. There were others he could never forget. They were always as vivid in his mind and psyche as if they had just occurred. One of those happened later that morning.

At one point, Dave was running a code on an ambulance patient who had just arrived, Henry was running a code on a patient in the hall who had coded while waiting for an exam area to open up. Jay was lavaging and pushing blood on a GI bleeder as he bled out in an exam area, and all four studs were over their heads with patients beyond their capabilities.

A biker was brought in unconscious from drugs and alcohol. His blood alcohol was off the charts and his toxicology screen was pending, so the nurses started an IV, put a Foley catheter in him, and gave him Narcan on Jay's orders. Then he was forgotten in the ensuing chaos.

Dave had just finished putting a chest tube in a COPD patient with a spontaneous pneumothorax in the last exam area in the back of the ER, when he heard the crash of a Mayo stand going over and the sound of broken glass. One of the nurses rushed toward the exam area the sounds had come from as the biker emerged with a broken IV bottle in one hand and his Foley catheter in the other.

"Get this mother-fucking tube out of my dick, you cock suckers!" he screamed as he waved his broken IV bottle like a broken beer bottle in a bar fight. The nurse backed off. Dave was trapped at the back of the ER with the biker blocking his way. "I am going to cut you mother fucker for sticking this tube in my cock!" He advanced on Dave with the broken bottle at the ready.

Dave was standing beside the Mayo stand with the chest tube packet on it. He grabbed the chest trocar, held it in his right hand and pointed it at the biker's chest and picked up the Mayo stand tray to use as a shield in his left hand. "I am a doctor, and I know exactly where your heart is. It is right there at your fourth rib." Dave thrust the trocar at the biker's chest. "You may cut me, but this is designed to penetrate the chest wall." Dave waved the trocar. "And I will drive it into your heart, and you will bleed out and die immediately. So, come cut me and die."

The biker had been in a lot of bar fights, and he realized the trocar was a much better weapon than the broken IV bottle. Plus, Dave was not intimidated and looked capable of doing just what he said. He lowered the broken IV bottle and looked around. "I am getting the fuck out of here. I want this fucking tube out of my cock." He turned back to Dave who still had the trocar leveled at his chest, and he never saw the two security guards coming. The night stick made a "tonk" sound on the back of his head like a ripe melon breaking open, and he went down with the two guards on him immediately. One put his knee in the middle of the biker's back and held up his hands for the other to zip tie. Then they rolled him over and zip tied his feet together. They jerked him up and slammed him down on the gurney in the exam area he had come from and had him in four-point restraints in no time. Dave heard a sound like a butcher hitting meat with a cleaver, and then the two security guards came out.

They looked at Dave then looked at each other. "You alright, Doc?" Dave was still holding the trocar, but the shaking in his hand was nothing compared to the quivering going on inside him. His whole core felt like a bowl of jelly slopping around. "If you mean, am I hurt, no, he didn't hurt me. If you mean am I alright, hell no. I have never been so scared in my life, and I am still shaking. Thanks, guys. I don't know what would have happened if you had not gotten here when you did."

The two security guards looked at each other again. "We saw you stand him down as we came through the doors. You had him under control. We just put him down. He is going to need stitches in his head, and his nose is not where it is supposed to be. He must have hit his face when we took him down." They looked at each other with the faint hint of a smile showing at the corners of their mouths. "He won't give you any more trouble. We will notify the police, and they will pick him up when you are through with him."

Dave put the trocar and Mayo tray down so he could put out his right hand. "Thank you again. I don't know what we would do without you guys." They both shook his hand.

The other security guard spoke. "Don't worry, Doc, we've got your back. We will never let anything happen to any of our people if we can help it. But I want to tell you something; you are the one who kept him from hurting someone. I know you were scared, but give yourself some of the credit. What you did took guts, and you protected the rest of your staff."

"It was not like I had a choice. I was the someone who was going to get hurt."

The two guards actually smiled. Everyone was standing around listening and watching. The other doctors, the nurses, and the students all said something to him, patted him on the back or touched him in some way.

"I need to sit down for a minute. Give me a minute before I pick up the next patient." Dave went to the doctors' station and sat down still shaking.

The rest of the shift went on unabated until Dave and Henry left on Monday morning, Labor Day. Dave mentioned the gathering at Bob and Phil's, but Henry declined stating he was going to sleep until he woke up, then go back to sleep, and sleep some more.

Dave got home around nine, fell on the bed and was asleep in no time. He woke up at four and stumbled into the front room to find Sharon dressed for the party sitting in a beanbag reading. "Dave, you look terrible. I am afraid the ER is going to kill you. Let's skip the party. When did you eat last?"

Dave smiled at her. As always, she looked incredible, and seeing her lifted Dave out of the hole he was in. "It almost did," he said under his breath.

"What?" Sharon stood up. She had dressed for Dave, making sure she didn't cross the line beyond European allure while giving him what he liked. Her hair was down and curled just the way he liked it, and her makeup accentuated her eyes and mouth perfectly. She had on a halter top with a square neck in periwinkle blue that exposed just the right amount of swell of her breast and midriff, with dark blue shiny jeans that were tight but not too tight. She never wore a bra because she did not need one with her breasts, so the halter top hinted at what was under it in a tantalizing way. She always wore heels to enhance her long legs.

Driving to Bob and Phil's, Dave brought up something he thought they needed to clarify with their friends. "I think we need tell people we are engaged. For us, there is no change. We never have to get married; we will simply remain permanently engaged. What do you think?"

Sharon thought for a minute. "You mean I won't be your mistress anymore? I will be your fiancée? I like being your mistress. It sounds sexy and forbidden." She ran her hand along his thigh and smiled.

"Where we are concerned, you will still be my mistress." Dave looked at her. "But to everyone else, you will be my fiancée. They already think we are engaged. I can't introduce you to everyone as my mistress; we have to be more conventional."

"I think you are right. I always fumble around trying to explain that we are in a committed relationship, so I will become your permanent fiancée for the public, but I will still be your mistress where it counts." She ran her hand higher up his thigh and laughed.

Dave looked down at her hand. "Really."

They parked near Bob and Phil's house and went in. It was after five, and some of the gang had already left. Connie and Harven, Audrey and Jake, Janice and Mike, George and the grad student, Sam and Rachael, and of course Bob and Phil were still drinking wine and talking when they arrived.

Phil greeted them. "Gorgeous, there is wine and cheese on the little table by the wall. Help yourself, then come sit beside me. Dave, you find your own place to sit. You have had her," Phil paused, "all to yourself and now you have to share." Phil sat down and patted a place beside him on the couch smiling.

Sharon and Dave got some wine and cheese then Sharon sat down with Phil. "I talked to the photographer, and he mailed the proposal to Nieman's along with shots he took of you at the Apparel Mart. He is sure they will accept it. If they could see the way you look today, they would jump at it."

"What!" Connie and Audrey said at the same time.

Phil answered, "You are looking at Neiman Marcus's newest model."

Janice interjected, "I thought you said you weren't a model."

"I am not. I am a flight attendant who some delusional people think could be a model." Sharon looked at Janice and smiled.

Phil continued. "Maybe Bob and I are delusional, we certainly smoke enough weed to be, but the fashion photographer at Neiman Marcus certainly isn't. He thinks you are perfect for their catalogues and print ads. He also said you can do that on the terms you outlined."

Dave sat down beside Mike and waited until the modeling conversation was over. "I want to let everyone know that Sharon and I are officially engaged."

Phil offered a toast. "To two of the nicest people I know." The way Jake looked at Audrey told Dave it was just a matter of time before they announced their engagement.

Bob followed Phil's toast. "Wow, first Connie and Harven, now Sharon and Dave, and I have a hunch others are going to follow soon. To those engaged and those about to be engaged. Best wishes to you all." As they drank, Bob and Phil looked at each other with a slightly sad expression.

Mike didn't drink to the toast, and his dark clouded brow told volumes about how he felt about Dave being engaged to Sharon.

The rest of the month in the Medicine ED ground on just as the first two months on the Medicine wards had ground on, with no let up or respite. Twenty-four hours in the Major Medicine ER every fourth day was taking more of a toll on Dave than every third night on call on the Medicine wards. He was lucky to get some breakfast and maybe a sandwich during the whole shift. Then he went home the next day and fell asleep until afternoon, so he went for over twenty-four hours with very little to eat and hardly any sleep. Not eating much on those days coupled with the stress and lack of sleep was causing Dave to lose more weight. He looked in the mirror and realized he was getting thin. Dave had never been thin. He had an athlete's body: trim, muscular and balanced, with broad shoulders, well defined arms and legs, and a deep chest. He had always been proud of his body. It had taken him his whole life to hone and sculpt it. He started water skiing when he was twelve, sailing when he was sixteen, and snow skiing when he was eighteen. He had built his body through years of workouts, training, games, practices, and drills then maintained it through recreation. He was starting to look like the interns he had met when he went through orientation.

Sharon made sure he ate when he was not at the hospital and she enticed him to bed early with lovemaking so that he got enough sleep, but nothing she did seemed to help. The weight kept melting off him with each passing week. The weed use was escalating too. They smoked a number every night. Sharon knew the herb smoking was self-medication, and she realized he needed it to cope, but like the weight loss, it worried her. The thing that worried her most was what the stress and pressure were doing to him inside. What kind of unseen and undetected damage was he suffering? She loved the man she had met that first night at the party, and she didn't want that man to change.

It is odd, she thought, *now I am worried about the same thing he was worried about when I first met him. I helped him get over his fear, but who is going to help me get over mine?* The epiphany that really shook her was the realization that her worry for him was affecting her health. She was drinking more and smoking as much weed as Dave. All she wanted was to get through the year with both of them and their relationship intact.

There was another incident in the Medicine ED that Dave never forgot. Dave was sitting in Major Medicine one evening feeling down because he had run several codes that day, none of which had been successful. When a patient was down for a long time, was a homeless derelict or a wino with no family, Dave could cope with losing them. But if CPR had been started quickly, there was a chance of reviving them and if they had family, he had a hard time coping with the failure of a resuscitation. The worst part was telling the family he had not been able to save their loved one. He was in the doctors' station, lamenting his last failed attempt, when they brought the patient in.

He was a small mixed-race man in four-point restraints on a gurney with straps across his knees, his waist, and his chest and one across his forehead. There were two large city police officers at the foot of the gurney and two big burly firemen, instead of paramedics, at the head of the gurney.

Jay walked over to the patient, looked at the extreme measures taken to immobilize him and said, "OK. We will take it from here. Take the restraints off."

One of the firemen responded. "I don't think you want to do that, Doc."

Jay bristled. "Of course, I do. I want him unrestrained. How can I examine him tied down like this?"

The fireman tried to tell Jay the man had trashed the inside of the ambulance and injured a paramedic, and that it took all four of them to get him restrained in the first place, but Jay cut him off. "I said take the restraints off."

The fireman looked concerned. "If we untie him, do you take full responsibility for him?"

Jay frowned. "I am the resident in charge here; of course I take full responsibility. Now, take the restraints off."

The man waited until the last restraint was off, and then he opened his eyes and went after the two policemen at the end of the gurney, tipping it up and over as he went off the end. He took the two policemen down, kicking and punching them. The two firemen looked at each other then jumped into the fray. A Code Gray was called. Two big security guards responded and jumped into the fight. They all crashed into the supply shelves on the wall, bringing them down to the sound of shattering glass. It looked like a cartoon with one of the six men flying out of the pile backwards from time to time only to get up and jump back in. At one point, the little man was up and all six of the men, who were twice his size, were down. They finally subdued him and got him on the gurney restrained again.

All six of the big men were bruised and bloodied, but the little man was fairly unscathed. The big fireman who had spoken before had an innocent look on his face as he said, "Do you want us to untie him again, Doc, or did you get all your examining done that time?"

Even though everyone in the ER was horrified, they could not help laughing. That comment broke the tension and allowed them to overcome their stress and anxiety with laughter.

The man was on PCP. The staff was seeing more and more patients on PCP, meth, cocaine, heroin, and hallucinogens every day. The drug problems were adding to the already heavy traffic through the ED, causing more violent outbursts and behavior problems, putting the staff at risk and keeping the security guards busy.

Dave rotated off the Medicine service in survival mode. He had taken damage but was still fairly sound. Now, he had to focus on getting through Surgery.

A love story and social commentary

Dave left the Minor Medicine ER on his last day, went to his apartment, and got dressed for dinner with Sharon. She had a turnaround, so they were going out to dinner to celebrate the fact he was still standing after his Medicine rotation. She wanted to go to a small, exclusive French restaurant in the Park Area.

Dave knew Sharon wanted to dress for their night out, so he wore gray slacks, a dress shirt, tie, and a dark blue blazer. Helen came to the door when he got to the Park house. "I know, you are here for Sharon." She laughed. "I didn't know at the time you were literally here for Sharon to take her away. I will miss her, but I want you to know how much it means to me that my best friend is happier than I have ever seen her."

Sharon came down the stairs while Helen was talking to Dave. Dave said, "Jesus Christ!"

Helen turned to look at Sharon. "Damn, girl, you are letting this modeling thing go to your head."

Sharon had on a shimmering green, sleeveless, low-cut, cocktail dress that matched the green rings around her irises, a green gauzy shawl draped over her shoulders and arms, and green heels. As always, her hair and makeup were perfect.

"Where are you guys going?" Helen asked.

"To Paris," Sharon said as she swept out the door. Outside, she said, "I wish we were in Paris tonight. We would have drinks at the Ritz on the Place Verdun, dinner on the Eiffel Tower, and then go to a little Bohemian jazz club on the Left Bank, before we went back to the First Arrondissement to dance in the moonlight on the steps of the Louvre. Then we would walk to our hotel on the Rue Rivoli and make love as the sun came up over Montmartre."

Dave stopped and turned to her. "I promise you that night in Paris someday." Dave looked at her in the low glow of the street lights and felt something stir inside him that was painful in its intensity. What he felt wasn't motivated by her beauty and his passion for her physically; it was a gut-wrenching emotion emanating from the very core of his being caused by his overwhelming deep love for her, not for her physical beauty, but for her, her goodness, her almost childlike purity, her sweetness, kindness, and her gentleness. He wanted to hold her, to protect her, to shield her from the world and everything in it that wasn't as good and pure as she was. She had no idea what the real world was like. She was far too soft for the hard, harsh, cruel realities he dealt with every day. His constant ache for her physically was now coupled with a desperate demanding need to protect her and to keep her safe.

They walked on to the restaurant pretending they were walking to a cafe in Paris. It was a perfect early autumn night, and they felt like they had the world all to themselves as they walked along the sidewalk in the soft light of the street lamps, not wanting to break the spell of the evening by talking.

The restaurant was not crowded, and they got a nice table by a window looking across the street at the lake. Dave ordered two champagne cocktails to celebrate rotating off Medicine. He took both Sharon's hands across the table. "I know you are worried about me, but I am OK. I have lost some weight, and I have a few dings, but overall, I am intact. I don't see or feel things the same way, but I am still me. I haven't undergone any fundamental changes. I am going to get through this; we are going to get through this. I am going to be fine; we are going to be fine. There is only one more hard rotation, not that the other two were easy, but the OB/GYN and Pedi rotations are not like Medicine and Surgery." Dave looked into her eyes. "I can do this; we can do this. There are some things I will never forget, and there are some things I have to forget. I have to repress them, so I bury them deep inside me someplace, and I never go there. That may not be healthy, but it works, and I know how to do it now. I have been through the fire, and I may be singed, but I am not burned. I have grown up and matured some, that's all. Surgery is going to be tough, and I may come out of that rotation battered and bruised, but I will still be me. After the Medicine rotation, I know that. Remember *Invictus* by Henley. My head is bloody but unbowed. I may come out of this bloody, but I will be unbowed. I will still be me, maybe a leaner, more mature, grown-up me, but still me." He dropped her hands and raised his glass to her. "One down and three to go. I, *we*, are halfway through the worst of it." They clinked glasses.

Sharon smiled as she thought how she had helped Dave get over his fear of what his training was going to do to him, and now he was helping her get over the same fear. She relaxed for the first time in weeks. He was right, it was a learning curve, and like all learning curves, it had taken time and experience for him to master it. She felt relieved, but that did not mean she would not continue to feed him, make sure he got enough sleep, and the other things he needed to combat the stress, including as much of her as he needed. Her smile widened as she thought, *I like fulfilling his need for me best.*

They finished dinner and walked back to Sharon's house to spend the night. When they got to her room, Sharon let Dave take his clothes off while she stood just inside the door. She waited until he looked at her, and then she reached back to slowly unzip the dress and slide it off while he watched. She stood by the door in the green heels, thigh-high nylons, and a green thong that matched the dress.

"It is fashion week in Paris, and I am a runway model you met at an exclusive club. You have invited me back to your hotel room, because you want me to become your mistress and travel the Cote d'Azur with you." She walked to the bed and put one knee on the bed beside him and leaned over to put her hands on the bed with her arms straight. "I have agreed to be your mistress on one condition. You have to satisfy all my sexual desires in one night." She crawled on to the bed and lay on her back with her hair spread out and her arms above her head, looking at him with a smoldering expression on her face. "Do you think you can do that?"

"You bet." Dave fumbled trying to finish undressing because he could not take his eyes off her laying there. When he finally managed to get the rest of his clothes off, she let him slip her thong off. Their lovemaking was passionate and intense because of the sense of relief they felt.

Sharon and Dave had eggs, bacon, fruit, cereal, and toast for brunch before driving to Dave's to spend the afternoon at the pool. Summer was over, and it was a weekday, so they had the pool all to themselves. Sharon had to fly the next day, and Dave was starting the Surgery Wards at seven AM, so they ordered a pizza and went to bed early. They both slept soundly, secure in the cocoon of Dave's apartment.

Part 3: Surgery

8
The Wards

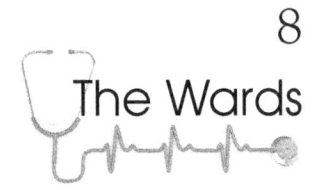

Dave drove to the hospital on the first day of his Surgery rotation knowing Henry wouldn't be there to greet him with "Hey, Poncho." Dave and Jay talked for some time about the last three months on Dave's last day in the Medicine ER. Changing the way Jay dressed had made a difference in the way he was treated by others, and his confidence surged. When Dave and Henry thought Jay was ready, after they did some coaching, Dave approached Carol about finding Jay a date. Carol showed up one morning in Minor Medicine after the shift change with a pretty nurse from Medicine 1 to ask Jay if he had time for coffee. Jay had a minor meltdown but recovered quickly and said he would like to go to coffee with them.

As they were leaving, Jay looked over his shoulder at Dave and Henry with his worried expression, but they smiled and waved him on. Once Jay and the two nurses were gone, Dave and Henry laughed and high-fived each other.

"I would be delighted to take coffee with you." Dave bowed to Henry as Henry fell into his chair laughing.

Jay returned from coffee with a smile on his face and just a slight amount of cockiness in his walk. "She is a new hire who finished nursing school this year. We like the same things, and she even wears the same kind of glasses I do with no rims. Carol is going to have us over for dinner as soon as our schedules line up where we all three have a night off." Jay looked down. "Thanks, guys."

By the time they finished their ED rotation, Jay and the nurse from Medicine 1 were kissing goodbye in the parking lot in the morning. Jay had come out; he was a better man, and because he was a better man, he became an outstanding doctor and teacher.

Dave replaced an intern on a Surgery team that had been together for three months, so Dave knew he would have to go through a period of adjustment with his new team and prove himself in order to be accepted. He also knew the milieu of Surgery was different from Medicine with a more aggressive competitive atmosphere.

There was an unhealthy relationship between Surgery residents and Medicine residents in a lot of teaching hospitals, and University Hospital was no exception. The Surgery residents called the Medicine residents "fleas" who were too cerebral, jumping around being a nuisance, never making a decision or getting anything done. The Medicine residents called the Surgery residents "cowboys" or "gun slingers," who shot from the hip without thinking and were simply carpenters or plumbers. The two actually came to blows on occasion, fighting over a patient's diagnosis or whether the patient belonged on the Medicine service or Surgery service.

Dave found the Surgery chief resident waiting for him when he reported to the nurse's station on the Surgery floor. The chief resident gave him a quick orientation and introduced him to his team. The orientation was short, and the introductions were clipped so his team could get on with morning rounds and their elective surgeries.

Surgery teams were made up of one student, one intern (straight Surgery or rotating), one junior resident (first or second year), and one senior resident (third or fourth year), and just like the Medicine teams, they stayed together for a three-month rotation in order to provide continuity. They were on call every third day and made rounds every morning. They did elective surgeries in the morning and clinic in the afternoon the day before call. They did follow-up rounds the morning after call but no clinic so they could leave after morning rounds, but they could not sign out an unstable patient. The whole team had to stay until all the patients on their service were stable, and they left together.

Unlike the two studs Dave had worked with for a month in the Medicine ED, he would be with this student for three months. His name was Jason, and he was a typical kiss-ass gunner concerned only about his grades and rank in class. The junior resident was Richard, a second-year resident from a good school and a good internship, who had spent two years in Vietnam as a GMO (general medical officer) in a combat zone with I Corps. He was calm, steady, unassuming, and quiet with a military haircut and a decidedly conservative outlook. The senior resident was Tom, a third-year resident from Texas who attended an Ivy League school, did a straight Surgery internship at University Hospital, and was the exact opposite of Richard. He was big, loud, brash, and cocky with a personality that filled the room, overshadowing anyone and everyone around him. Although not a military cut, his hair was short, like his temper, but he was long on intolerance and more conservative than Richard.

Richard and Tom had been together for three months and got along amazingly well, mainly because Richard never said anything, and Tom never shut up. They both took one look at Dave and immediately decided they had been saddled with a worthless lazy hippie who would not be able to pull his own weight, much less make any contributions to the team. They dealt with Dave by ignoring him. Dave had been down this road before. He knew the best way to handle them was to do his job, prove his worth, and ignore their attitude toward him. The stud was worthless, the residents knew that, but Dave was not, and he would soon have an opportunity to demonstrate his value.

Tom told Dave they did everything as a team; they made rounds as a team, and they operated as a team. Dave would operate with Richard, and the stud would operate with Tom. They ate breakfast, lunch, and dinner together. They hung out in the doctors' lounge during downtime together, and they left the hospital together. They were a unit, they functioned as a unit, and they did everything as a unit.

They never saw their attending, and there were no rounds with the chief. The only time they saw the chief of Surgery was at Grand Rounds on Saturday, and the attending only operated with the senior resident on the most difficult cases. The stud went to class from eleven to twelve on weekdays. Rounds and elective surgeries started at seven on the day before call, with clinic in the afternoon. They were out of the hospital by seven on those days. The day after call, they were usually out of the hospital by noon.

They wore scrubs and OR shoes all day, every day, so Dave wore his trader beads and tied his hair back with the bead on the leather thong, which did not win him any points. Tom called him Goldilocks, Richard did not talk to him at all, and the stud acted like contact with Dave would contaminate him in some way. Dave had little contact with any of them other than supervising the stud during clinic. Their team was on call the next day, and their service was fairly small, so they got out of the hospital before seven, and Dave drove to his apartment to meet Sharon. They had a relaxing evening and went to bed early. Dave needed to overcome the rest of the team's preconceived notions about him, and as he slept soundly beside Sharon that night, he didn't know he would do just that the next day.

They finished rounds, ate breakfast, and were in the lounge when they got the first page from the ER. It was after noon, and Jason had returned from class, so all four of them went down to see the patient. When they got to the ER, they smelled the patient before they saw him. As the ER resident led them to the exam area, he handed each of them a mask and put one on himself. The smell got stronger as they got closer to the patient. The ER resident opened the curtain of the exam area, and the smell was over-powering, causing Jason to start gagging.

"I hope you have strong stomachs. I have seen some gross things, but this is as gross as it gets." The resident pulled the sheet back from the legs of a small Latino man in his sixties, and the smell overwhelmed them. Jason threw up in his mask and started to faint.

Dave caught him and called for ammonia capsules. Dave popped an ammonia capsule and stuck it under Jason's nose. He started to revive, but as soon as he was up, he saw the man's leg and went down again. Dave laid him down on the ER floor, turned him over to a nurse to get him out of the area, and stuck the remaining ammonia capsules in his pocket.

The smell was so bad it made their eyes water, but the sight of the man's leg was even worse. His leg was rotten from the knee down with maggots in the rotting flesh of his leg, foot, and between his toes. He was a diabetic with peripheral vascular disease, and he had lost the blood supply to his leg, causing necrosis. The maggots had probably saved his life by eating away the dead flesh before gangrene could set in. The ER resident said his family had been afraid to bring him in because he was an illegal immigrant, so they let his leg rot until they couldn't stand the smell anymore. "We typed and crossed him for four units, cultured his leg and blood, drew all his labs, and started a big bore IV with normal saline. He is all yours. Oh, don't try to kill the smell with air freshener; it only makes it worse, not better."

"Fuck!" Tom said, followed by, "Call the OR and tell them to get ready for an AK amputation and to notify anesthesia. Richard, you and Goldilocks take this one. That little shit, Jason, is worthless." Then again he said, "Fuck!"

Dave and Richard looked at each other as Tom left to take care of Jason; they both knew Tom should be doing this case. Tom was using Jason as an excuse to get out of an unpleasant task, but Richard had

A love story and social commentary

learned the way to get along with Tom was to never question anything he did or said. Richard went to the doctors' station to write an admit note and pre-op orders.

Dave swallowed hard trying not to vomit and dove right in. "I want a lot of saline, two suture sets, some plastic bags, a really big bowl, a gallon of betadine, and a nurse who can handle herself. Also, see if any of the nurses have any perfume with them; if they do, put some on two masks."

In no time the charge nurse showed up with everything Dave had asked for and laid it all out in the exam area. "I'm not going to ask one of my girls to do this." The charge nurse handed Dave one of the perfumed masks and put the other one on herself.

Dave and the charge nurse put the big bowl under the man's leg. "Put a tight tourniquet above his knee. It may help prevent a shower of bacteria."

Dave open the two suture sets, took out the tweezers and scissors, and handed the other set to the charge nurse. Then he started pouring saline over the leg, wiping off the dead tissue and maggots, using the tweezers to pick out the embedded maggots and the suture set scissors to cut away the hanging flesh. It took them about an hour to debride the leg because they had to stop from time to time to get away from the smell. When they finished, Dave poured betadine over the leg, then put the leg in a plastic bag, and taped it to the man's thigh above the tourniquet. He and the nurse dumped the contents of the big bowl into another plastic bag and tied it shut.

"Someone take this out and dump it in the proper place." Dave took off his mask because the smell was finally clearing. He thanked the charge nurse and walked back to the doctors' station where Richard was waiting. "He is ready to go when the OR is ready for us. He needs a Medicine consult. I will page them." Richard did not say anything, but Dave could tell from the way he looked at him that his opinion of Dave was changing.

The amputation went smoothly with Dave demonstrating he could cut, tie, and use both hands with dexterity, so by the end of the surgery, he was doing his side and Richard was doing his. Richard looked at Dave, their eyes met, and from the look of respect he got, Dave knew he had proven himself.

"Go ahead and close. I will go dedicate the op note." Richard left Dave to close the stump with the scrub nurse.

One down and one to go, Dave thought as he sutured the stump.

It took Dave a while to close because they had taken the leg very high in order to get viable tissue, so the stump wound was large and required a drain, all of which took extra time. Dave knew if he survived, the man would be on crutches the rest of his life, because he was illegal and there was no way he could afford a prosthesis.

When Dave got back to the lounge, and Tom greeted him with a snide comment. "Did you take a little siesta in there?" Dave realized he would probably never win Tom's respect no matter what he did, so he decided to stop trying and ignore him. He would be working mainly with Richard anyway, and he had established himself with Richard, so Tom became irrelevant to Dave, just as Jason was irrelevant to him.

Tom continued to trash-talk Dave, and Jason tried to imitate Tom's behavior. Dave was able to ignore Tom's comments, but eventually Jason's got on his nerves because Jason was just a junior student and Dave was a doctor. When Jason chimed in with Tom's teasing of Dave about having to wear a bonnet in the OR, like the nurses because of his long hair, Dave had heard enough from Jason.

"You know you're going to hurt yourself fainting like that every time you see a few maggots eating someone's rotten leg." Dave still had some of the ammonia capsules in his pocket from the ER, so he walked up to Jason, put them in Jason's breast pocket, then hit Jason with an open hand breaking them all at once, while he made a gagging sound. The excessive ammonia smell hit Jason in the face like a brick, and that coupled with Dave's sound effects, plus the memory of the maggots, drove Jason to the bathroom vomiting again.

Tom almost fell off the couch laughing. "That was great!" Tom stopped laughing and looked at Dave. "Perfect."

Dave shook his head and thought, *I don't get any respect from Tom for doing my job, but I get it for bullying someone.* Dave understood that tormenting Jason had made him one of them in Tom's eyes—a tough, take no prisoners, hard-ass surgeon. Dave thought, *Is that all I have to do to keep him off my back, be an asshole like him?* Then he remembered how Sharon was always calling him an asshole, and he smiled. Tom thought he was smiling about belittling Jason and smiled back.

The rest of Dave's first shift on call went by in typical fashion. Dave and Richard did an appendectomy, Tom and Jason did a small bowel resection for an acute obstruction due to adhesions and a gall bladder. They also did several consults but were able to rest and even get some sleep, sprawling out on the couches in the doctors' lounge between cases.

Dave had learned how to sleep in any position, any place, at any time when he was a student. He could sleep sitting up, standing up if he had something to lean against, and had once fallen asleep holding a retractor in surgery. No one knew he was asleep, even when he woke up with a start, causing him to move the retractor. The only comment from the resident doing the surgery was to tell him not to move the retractor.

The next morning, they made rounds and were out of the hospital by noon. Dave had rested and slept some, but he was fatigued from the physical effort of standing and operating. He drove home to get some sleep before Sharon got back from her trip. She was on a layover and scheduled to be back by early afternoon.

He was sitting in a beanbag drinking a beer and listening to Steely Dan when she unlocked the door and came in. "Wow, you're not in bed after a night on call."

"I can go back to bed and you can join me, if you want." Dave got up and kissed her. "Or we can go out for an early dinner."

"Or we have a third option. Connie called about the Halloween party. She said everyone is getting together tonight at the Park house to plan it, so we can have an early dinner then drop by for a while." Dave could see Sharon was dressed for option three in a nice blouse, pants, and heels.

"We are good for Halloween. The day before Halloween is my last call on the Surgery wards, so I should get out of the hospital on Halloween no later than early afternoon, and I am off the next day. My first day in the Surgery ER is an off day like when I started the Medicine ER. Let's have an early dinner, meet everyone at the Park house to help plan the party, come back here, go to bed early, and fornicate." Dave got handsy with Sharon's rear.

Sharon took his hands off her backside. "I noticed how you put fornicate in there as if you needed to make sure it was on the list of things we were going to do tonight."

"You better believe I want to make sure it is on the list." Dave got a glass of wine for Sharon and rolled a number; they smoked while listening to Steely Dan. "I have been thinking about residency. I'm putting the places in California first on my match list because I am ready for a change. I have lived in the South my whole life, and I am tired of the BS." Dave had been thinking about the residents he was working with, and he knew if he stayed here, he would continue to encounter the same narrow, conservative, judgmental people. "I want to get the hell out."

Sharon took a sip of wine and thought for a minute. "I can get behind that."

"You need to look into the MBA programs at Berkeley, Stanford, UCLA, USC and here, in case I end up here." Dave went to the fridge for another beer and brought the bottle of wine to pour Sharon some more, and then he put another album on.

Sharon got up to join Dave in one beanbag. "So, we are going to California next year unless we have to stay here." Sharon slid under his arm in the beanbag and put her hand on his chest. "You never told me about Woodstock. We have time this afternoon, so tell me."

The smell of her Ambush and the touch of her body acted on him like another drug, adding to the high from the weed and beer. He pulled her to him and kissed her, letting his hands roam over her body and losing himself in her. "Do you really want to hear about Woodstock?" Dave nuzzled her neck and cupped her breast in his hand.

"Yes, I do. It had such an influence on you, and I want to hear about it." Sharon pulled away, sat up, and looked at him. Whenever she turned those eyes on him, he had no choice but to do whatever she wanted.

Dave pulled her back down. "Only if you stay right here." He put his arms around her again.

She snuggled against him. "I have no problem with that."

Dave began. "We left Providence Town on the Cape around ten in the morning that Friday. When we exited the freeway, we started down the two-lane road to Bethel. It wasn't long before the traffic piled up, and we were just creeping along, and then the traffic stopped. We sat there for a while, then got out, and stood around talking, waiting for the traffic to start moving again. We got to know the people in the cars in front of us and behind us. Two guys brought out guitars, and we sang along with them while we waited.

"The traffic started to move, we drove a little further, and it stopped again. We got out, sat on the cars, and sang folk songs with the two guys with guitars again. This happened over and over all morning and into the afternoon. The best way I can describe the drive is the line from the song, 'Everywhere there was the sound and the song of celebration.' When we got to the little towns along the way, it was like a parade with all the people lining the road waving. Some of them came out with fruit, drinks, ice tea, pieces of pie, cake, and other stuff to eat, handing it out to us while we waited for the traffic to start moving again.

Finally, late in the afternoon, we reached a place where the highway patrol was stopping all the cars and having everyone park on the side of the road; we parked, got our stuff, and started walking down the road in a long line of people. We walked for quite a while before the crowd thinned out, and we saw painted buses coming and going on the road. They would stop, people would fill the bus and get on top until absolutely no one else could get on or in the bus, and they would drive back down the road. They were from the communes, like the Hog Farm, Morning Star, and even the Pranksters were there. We got in a bus painted in day-glow colors, and it drove us the rest of the way. The driver pointed us toward the trees on the side of the road and said to follow the crowd. It was almost sunset when we started toward the faint sound of music.

"There is no way to describe the scene that unfolded below us when we walked over the hill and looked down. There was a large natural bowl filled with a sea of people sitting on the ground. The stage, which was massive, looked like a postage stamp—it was so far away, and there was nothing but people between us and it. The sun was going down, and Ravi Shankar was playing to the sunset creating a magical setting. As long as I live, I will never forget standing there looking out over all those people, listening to the Indian music and watching the sun go down. Even now, it gives me chills to think about it.

"The guy I was with took off through the crowd, stepping over and around people and heading for the stage. I had no choice, so I followed him down through thousands of people sitting on the ground, and I must have said excuse me a hundred times as I chased him. Remarkably, we found an open spot, center stage about thirty yards back, right between the speaker towers. It was perfect, so we spread our stuff out and sat down to listen to the most incredible music I have ever heard.

"I'm not going to go down the lineup of groups, but I will tell you about the performances that blew me away. Understand, everything I heard was great, but there were moments that were totally over the top.

"We had our sleeping bags, some food, beer, water, and a half tent, so we spread our sleeping bags out to sit on, and arranged everything else around us to make sure we had enough room to set up the half tent that night. As soon as we sat down someone passed me a joint. I had never smoked weed, so I passed it on, but it kept happening. Joints were passed to us from the right and left. After I had passed them on two or three times, I took my first hit of herb. By the time Arlo Guthrie came on, I was pretty high, but he was more fucked-up than any of us. Arlo looked out at us and said, 'Wow, do you fuckers know what you look like? There's half a million people here. The New York State Freeway is closed, man.' I heard music stoned for the first time. But it was Joan Baez that transported me to another magical, mystical world. She sang in the most amazing voice I had ever heard in front of half a million people accompanied only by her guitar. A light misty rain began to fall, so she pushed the guitar behind her back and sang a cappella. It was freaking amazing. The night, her voice, and the light rain all combined to produce a fantasy that was literally out of this world. In the pauses in her singing, there was absolute silence; half a million people were dead quiet. I can't tell you the affect that moment had on me, and I will always carry that night with me.

"After she finished, we set up the half tent on our spot and didn't move again until Monday morning, except to go to the port-a-potty and try to find something to eat during the day. The groups that tore it up were Santana; Ten Years After; The Who; Crosby, Stills, Nash, and Young; Canned Heat; Blood, Sweat, and Tears; Creedence; the Dead; Jefferson Airplane, and the Band. Then there was Joe Cocker and Janice Joplin, one right after the other, all afternoon, all night, and into the morning. It was ongoing, unbelievable, almost-nonstop music. Country Joe and the Fish played after the big storm Sunday when everyone else was afraid of getting electrocuted. They plugged in and Joe said, 'Fuck it, we'll play.' At one point they had the whole crowd on its feet singing, 'Whoopy, we are all going to die.' But the highlight of the whole thing was Saturday night when Sly sang, 'I

Want to Take You Higher' with half a million people on their feet dancing and screaming, 'Higher,' as huge spotlights swept across the crowd in the early morning hours.

"By Monday morning, we were tired, muddy, and hungry, so we started walking over the hill while Jimmy Hendrix was playing. Just as we got to the top of the hill, he stopped us in our tracks. He played the National Anthem in feedback, making the sound of bombs bursting and rockets whooshing through the air with his guitar. It made our blood run cold. It reminded us that while we were there, enjoying three days of peace and music, guys just like us were losing their lives, limbs, and their minds in a war that could not be won and was being fought for no valid reason. The tired old men who occupied the White House couldn't find a way out. Nixon was afraid of being known as the first American president to lose a war, so the people in Washington continued to sacrifice the lives of young men, causing others to be maimed and crippled or to have their lives ruined by PTSD. It was a fitting end to the fantasy and brought us back to the reality of the world. We found the car and drove back to Providence Town. End of story."

Sharon sat up and looked at Dave. "I guess it was more than the music you experienced. You looked through a window into the kind of world we could live in if peace and love were priorities. It was an experiment in the philosophies of Buddha, Jesus, Gandhi, Dr. King and others who have tried to show humanity a better way."

Dave sat up beside her. "Humanity doesn't want a better way. Look at what humanity did to those men you just mentioned and the countless others who tried to point to a correct path for mankind to follow. If you try to fix what is wrong with mankind, mankind will kill you for your effort. Starting with Socrates, then Buddha and Jesus, to Gandhi and Dr. King—all of them were destroyed for showing mankind the way to a more perfect society. I like the line from 'Symphony for the Devil,' 'They shouted out, who killed the Kennedys, when after all, it was you and me.' It is the same old never-ending story. There is evil in the world, good has to confront evil, but good is destroyed in the process. How many writers that we both love and admire have hammered that theme home over and over again in their works?"

"I get it and you get it, but the vast majority don't. Just look at the right wing, the holy-roller Christians, the televangelists, and the megachurch preachers. What Bible are they reading, and what teachings of Jesus are they following? Jesus wants me to be rich! Throw in the politicians who call on God to justify what they are doing, plus the racists, the bigots, and the misogynists who use the Bible to justify their acts, and you have evil hiding behind God or using God to justify itself. More people have been killed, tortured, and maimed in the name of God than anything else in the history of man. Your God, my God, the best God, the right God—you name it. In reality, they are using God to justify their greed and horrendous acts. Look at the history of Christianity. The Pope duped poor people into giving money to build a huge cathedral, and when Martin Luther spoke out against what he was doing, it triggered the reformation and a hundred years of war among Christians over how to worship the same God. Then the greed of Christian knights caused the crusades—a war between Christians and Islam that is still going on today. Tell me how the Sermon on the Mount or the Beatitudes justify war, much less the Spanish Inquisition, which was used to take the possessions of Christians and non-Christians for the church. And don't even get me started on Islam, the peaceful religion that is spread by the sword and jihad— 'convert or die.' Not to mention the way women are treated, that anyone not a Muslim is an infidel, and the whole religion was started over control of trade routes. How many people died as that peaceful religion was spread throughout Africa, the Middle East, India, the Caucuses, and Europe? Oh, and don't forget the Jews and their never-ending wars with the Arabs over which one of them is the chosen people of the God of Abraham and gets to live in the Promised Land. I almost forgot the witch burnings, another way of taking people's possessions over religious beliefs. Jesus said it was OK to burn women, didn't he? Follow the money, and you will always find the answer. Money and power, not peace and love, rule the world. At Woodstock, you got a chance to see a world where peace and love did rule for three days." Sharon sighed, obviously agitated.

Dave hugged her. "Love and hope are the only things we humans really have to hold onto in this world. That is what pulls us through in the face of everything else." He pulled away from the hug to look into her eyes. "One of the reasons we love each other is that we see things the same way. We are more than lovers; we are friends, companions, and soul mates." Dave kissed her and she kissed him back passionately, clinging to him as the music ended.

A love story and social commentary

Dave and Sharon lay back in the beanbag holding each other in the silence that followed, lost in their own thoughts. Then Sharon whispered softly in his ear, "I never want to be without you."

Dave whispered back, "And I never want to be without you." They lay there for some time just holding each other and feeling the comfort and security of being together in the face of all the turmoil in the world swirling around them. They had no control over what was happening, but they had each other to hold onto in the face of it all.

They went to dinner early at the little Mexican place. After, they drove to the Park house to meet the others and to plan Halloween. The whole gang was there when they arrived. Phil started by reminding everyone that Halloween is the biggest party night on the Park, and sometimes, things get out of hand, so it was important they didn't lose control. Connie talked about the potential problems of underage drinkers and smoking weed in the house because of the police presence. "If you see anyone who looks young, show them out, and if you see someone smoking in the house, show them the zoom room."

Sherry went over what they were going to provide and how they were going to pay for it. "We are going to have a keg in the dining room at one end of the table with wine at the other end and food in between, like at the Bar party. I will collect thirty dollars per couple to pay for everything." She glared at Mike.

Harven talked about the music and dancing. "There is a guy in my class who worked as a DJ in college, and he is going to provide the music and sound system. He will work for wine, beer, weed, and food for himself and his girlfriend. We will push all the chairs and couches in the dining room and front room against the walls to make room to dance like the 4th party. He will set up in the dining room with speakers in the dining room and front room."

Bob talked about costumes. "We are going to give gift certificates from our store as prizes for the best costumes. The categories are Best Costume, fifty-dollars; Best Couple's Costumes, a hundred dollars; Sexiest Costume, fifty dollars; Sexiest Couple's Costumes, a hundred dollars. You can only enter in one category. If you go for the sexiest costume categories, my advice is to show more skin than costume. We will take a vote on each category to get the party started."

Everyone agreed to start at seven. Phil told them that if past experience counted, the cops would shut everything down around midnight, and everyone should plan to sleep at one of the three houses on the Park that night. "I am sending out thirty invitations, but we know everyone who lives in the Park area will be going from party to party and from house to house all night, so who knows how many people we will have here at any one time. It might be raining, so we are going to bring a rolling clothes rack and put it at the front door for coats and raincoats. I would advise you not to bring anything you like, because with all the people in and out, it might disappear." Phil went on, "Halloween on the Park is an adult affair, so if you are offended by nudity, it is not the place for you." Everyone laughed. "Last year, there were nude statues, people nude covered with thick white powder, nudes in body paint, and people nude for the hell of it. We will not get any trick-or-treaters. No sane parent would let their child trick-or-treat around the Park. But like Connie said, we will get teenagers, so we need to keep them out because giving alcohol to a minor is against the law, and I assure you the law will be out in full force."

Connie finished up by saying, "Please tell anyone who was not here tonight what we went over. Also, anyone who wants to decorate should do it the day before the party."

The meeting broke up into small groups. Harven brought out a couple of six-packs of beer and opened two bottles of white wine. Connie, Harven, Mike, Janice, Sharon, Dave, Henry, and Sherry sat down together in the front room.

Mike jumped right in. "Are we going to take the acid you guys have?"

Dave said, "I am down with it if you guys want to do it. I am off the next day, but I would advise anyone working the next day not to do it. Does everyone have a day to recover?" Everyone said they did, so Dave went on, "There are eight of us, and I have eight tabs, but Cousin Jane said to split the tabs. This is righteous stuff made by Owsley, so a half-tab should be enough to get us off. We need to meet here early to do it."

Janice said, "I am not going to do it."

Dave looked at her thinking, *Good, the last thing we need is someone who's never taken anything flipping out.*

Dave and Sharon mingled and talked with their friends before they left to drive to Dave's apartment. Dave put Fleetwood Mac on the stereo to accompany their lovemaking. Tomorrow, Dave would be back with Jason, Richard, and Tom, but tonight, he was with Sharon, so he made the best of it, letting their passion insulate him from that world.

Dave found the Surgery wards less taxing than the Medicine wards. There was more down time while he was at the hospital, a half-day off after call, more opportunities to sleep during call, and a lot less stress because of the team approach with a senior resident making the decisions and taking all the responsibility. He was able to eat breakfast, lunch, and dinner almost every day either at the hospital or out, so he was no longer losing weight. The only down side was the physical fatigue from standing in the OR for long hours and actually using his muscles in the mechanics of doing the surgeries. Even though there was less stress, there was still the emotional duress. The worst cases were the cancer surgeries, especially when they were done only to buy time with no chance of a cure. It was hard enough to deal with someone who knew they were going to die, but it was harder to deal with their families, especially young families where the wife would be left alone with fatherless children or the husband would be left with motherless children. Like on the Medicine wards, the dying mothers were the most difficult cases Dave had to deal with emotionally, and he could never fully come to grips with them.

On the Medicine wards, all the days were pretty much the same with every third day being worse, but the work was the same. On the Surgery wards, all three days were different. On one day, the team did elective surgeries in the morning and clinic in the afternoon. The day started at seven with surgeries and rounds between the cases, then clinic in the afternoon from one to five, followed by rounds again, then out of the hospital usually after seven. It was a long twelve-plus-hour day, and it was tiring because they did the big cases, like cancer surgeries and resections, on that day. The next day when they were on call, they made rounds and admitted patients for emergency surgery, usually doing about four to six surgeries in the twenty-four-hour period; they also did consults. Dave managed to get some sleep at night and some rest during the day on most call days. The day after call, they made rounds, stabilized their patients, and got out of the hospital usually by noon.

Dave was slowly gaining Tom's respect but not Jason's, not that Jason's respect mattered to Dave, but the lack of it caused friction on the team. Dave had embarrassed him that first day on call, so Dave became the target of Jason's resentment. Dave decided to reach out to him to try to defuse the situation and decrease the friction. Tom still called Dave Goldilocks, but it was with a different tone and attitude; he was Tom's Goldilocks now, the team's Goldilocks, and Goldilocks had proven he could hold his own.

They were on call when they admitted an emergency appendectomy. Dave had done several appendectomies with Richard where Dave did the case with Richard assisting him, so Richard told Tom to let Dave take this one with Jason. Tom looked at Jason, shrugged and said, "Sure."

Jason could not believe he might get to do more than hold a retractor for Tom. Dave let Jason tie where it did not matter much under close supervision, making him do it over until it was perfect, and Jason would cut when Dave tied. Then he let Jason close, again under close supervision. He was patient and helpful, teaching Jason how to do things right without being harsh or critical. Jason was walking on air when he left the OR.

Tom greeted them when they got back to the lounge. "How many appendices did the guy have? As long as you guys took, he must have had at least three." Jason took it in stride and followed behind Dave like a puppy.

"I let Jason tie and close. He did fine; I think he can help and make a real contribution to the team now." Dave looked at Tom and Tom smiled. Dave knew they were finally a real team. None of the three would ever be his friend, and frankly, he did not want to be friends with guys like them, but they would be a tight functioning team whose members respected and trusted each other going forward. It took time for Dave to notice one other result of his interaction with Jason—Jason stopped cutting his hair short and let it grow out.

Two things happened near the end of their rotation on the wards that sealed Dave's position on the team and finalized Tom's respect for him. They were on call when a post-op patient in the recovery room coded. Dave got there first, tubed the patient quickly, and ran the code smoothly and efficiently, resulting in the patient's survival. The rest of the team, including Tom, followed Dave's orders during the code. Tom and Richard did not like Dave's hair, the beads, or his liberal attitude, but they respected his work ethic, nerve, and abilities. They began to ignore the hair, beads, and attitude after the code.

A love story and social commentary

The other thing involved Sharon. Dave's 240 Z needed its new-car service. Dave had been postponing it, hoping to find some extra time to get it done, but he never did. He was on call in the middle of the week on a day Sharon had a turnaround and was off the next day. They got up early, and Sharon followed him to the dealership, where he did a key drop for the service, and then Sharon took him to the hospital and drove to the airport for her trip. She picked him up the next day after call to take him to get his car.

Call was light, and when Dave was sure everything was taken care, he called Sharon to pick him up at the entrance to the staff parking lot where she had dropped him the day before. As usual, the team all walked out together. They were walking toward the parking lot when Dave saw Sharon standing beside her car with her ankles crossed, leaning back with her hands on the front of her Volkswagen. She had on tight, skinny jeans, ankle boots with heels, and a fuzzy red sweater with an oversized collar that dropped off one shoulder with its sleeves pushed up to her elbows. She saw Dave and stood up straight with her feet apart and her hands on her waist.

Tom reacted by saying, "Jesus, what a fine piece of ass. Watch the big dog work, and no little dog better get between the big dog and his bone."

Dave started to say something to Tom, but he knew it wouldn't do any good, so he decided to let Sharon handle him. They walked up to her and Tom was about to speak, when Sharon said, "How was your night?"

"It wasn't bad, Baby."

They had all heard Dave on the phone with some hippie chick he called Baby. Tom looked from Sharon to Dave and back to Sharon. "You're Baby?" Tom asked, staring at Sharon.

Dave walked past Tom, put his arm around Sharon's waist, and she leaned into him. "Sharon, this is my Surgery team. This is Tom, Richard, and Jason. Guys, this is my fiancée, Sharon Kelly."

Sharon turned on a huge smile and her eyes lit up as she stepped toward them and put her hand out. Tom looked at her in disbelief as he took her hand. He was actually speechless for once. Then she offered her hand to Richard and Jason in turn, smiling and saying how pleased she was to meet them.

She turned to Dave. "Let's get going. We have half a day and a whole night off. I'm not tan, but I am rested and ready, so let's go." Dave walked around to get in the passenger's side of the car.

The three men continued to look at her as she stood in front of them. Richard, who never said anything to anyone, was the only one who spoke. "I hear Dave on the phone with you when we are on call. It is nice to meet you and to know who he is talking to now."

Sharon beamed at him, told him it was her pleasure, tossed her hair, got in the car, and waved to them as she drove away.

They stood there watching her drive away. Jason said, "Wow."

Richard said, "Who would have thought Baby looked like that? I thought she was some hippie, granola chick."

Tom said, "What a stone-cold fox. I wonder who she is and what she is doing with someone like Dave."

Driving to the Datsun dealership, Sharon asked, "What's with the military haircuts? Are they all ex-military?"

Dave smiled at her. "Only one of them is ex-military, but in their case, you can judge a book by its cover. They are exactly who they appear to be, and there are others just like them in training here, which is another reason I am ready to go to California."

Dave picked up his car and followed Sharon to his apartment where he showered and changed out of his scrubs before they drove to the mall to look for costumes for Halloween. They both found things they liked then walked around the mall window shopping before getting something to eat and driving back to Dave's apartment.

The next morning, Tom pounced on Dave as soon as he arrived. "Who was that incredible hot piece of ass?"

"She is my fiancée, Sharon Kelly," Dave said, acting nonchalant.

"What does she do, and what is she doing with someone like you?" Tom was relentless.

Dave answered patiently, "She is a flight attendant, but she does do some modeling. Check out the Neiman Marcus Christmas catalog. She is in it. Since I am a Southern gentleman, I can't tell you what she does with me." Dave smiled at Tom enjoying having an advantage over him.

Tom looked at Dave and thought, *There must be more to this guy than I thought.* Tom's opinion of Dave went up considerably, not because of Dave's abilities, but because he was with a woman like Sharon. Tom started calling him Dave instead of Goldilocks, but where Dave's stock really went up was with Jason. For Jason, women like Sharon weren't real; they only existed in his imagination. To meet her, touch her hand, have her smile at him, and realize she was real was a pivotal moment for him. His mind exploded with the realization that if an intern he worked with could be with a woman like Sharon, so could he. After he met Sharon, Jason didn't just let his hair grow; he mimicked Dave in every way.

One of Dave's worst nights on call was due to overflow from the Trauma teams. The Trauma rooms in the ED were really Surgery suites, and cases were done in the rooms. The teams did what was necessary to stabilize patients, and then they handed them off to the correct specialty to be taken to the OR. Head injuries went to neurosurgery, chest injuries to thoracic surgery, extremity injuries to orthopedics, back injuries to spine surgery, and so forth. Abdominal injuries were done by the Trauma teams, then admitted to the Surgery team on call. Multiple injuries were handled by multiple teams working in tandem according to the threat to life of the injuries. When both Trauma rooms were occupied, any overflow went to the ER, and if all members of Trauma teams were working, those cases went to the on-call Surgery team.

Dave's team was called to the ER for a patient with multiple gunshot wounds to the abdomen because all the members of both Trauma teams were occupied. The ER resident told them the man had been shot multiple times with a small caliber handgun at close range. They had identified six entry wounds in the abdomen but only four exit wounds. The man had lost a lot of blood and needed to go to the OR right away.

The story the resident got from the police was that the man's wife was the one who shot him, and she was in custody. The man had a habit of getting drunk, coming home, beating her, then having sex with her while he continued to beat her. She got fed up with his behavior, so she bought a small caliber handgun at a pawn shop, and told him if he did it again, she was going to kill him. He came in drunk, so she emptied the gun into him before he could touch her. Tom told Richard and Dave to take this case so he could stay out to cover since all the teams were tied up with cases, but they knew Tom was just dodging another unpleasant case. The ER resident took them to an exam area where a large black man was lying on a gurney with normal saline going in one IV and blood going in another. Dave examined the man while Richard wrote an admit note and pre-op orders.

Richard had started talking to Dave after he met Sharon. "This is an all-night sucker. We are going to find hole after hole in this guy's bowels and organs, and then we have to go fishing for the two missing slugs. I hate little handguns. I think they should be outlawed. People should only be able to buy big handguns so when they shoot somebody, they stay shot. All little handguns do is keep us up all night patching little holes."

Dave thought this was a somewhat novel and unique way of looking at gun control, so he added, "What if all handguns were outlawed?"

The way Richard looked at him made Dave think Richard was going to stop talking to him again. But Richard had accepted him—hair, beads, liberal attitude and all—so he just shook his head and said, "Jesus, Dave, I don't know where your head is sometimes, then I realize it is squarely up your ass. Where do you get these ideas from unless you pull them out of your ass? Have you ever heard of the Second Amendment? Do you know what the Constitution is? You are a good guy, a good doctor, and I think you would probably make a hell of a fine surgeon, but you continue to amaze me with some of the things that come out of your mouth." Dave decided never to say anything political to Richard again, especially not about guns, gays, or God—the three Gs that conservatives went ballistic over.

Richard was right, they were up all night repairing the wounds in the man's bowels and organs. Each time they thought they were finished, they ran the bowels and found more holes. Finally, around dawn, they had finished repairing all the holes and began looking for the missing slugs. They found one embedded in the back muscles, which was easy to remove, but the other one was near the spinal cord. They decided to leave it, irrigate the man's abdomen with a lot of saline, and close. It was well into morning by the time Richard dictated the op note, Dave wrote post-op orders, and they left the man in the recovery room to get breakfast.

When Dave and Richard got to the floor, Tom and Jason had finished rounds on all their patients except the man Dave and Richard had operated on. Thinking he was still in recovery, they all went down to see, but he wasn't in recovery. They checked back with the floor, but he wasn't there either, so Tom sent Jason down to the basement to check Ground East, the morgue, thinking maybe the man had died. He was not in the morgue either. He was not in recovery, not on the floor, and not in the morgue. Tom began to panic, because misplacing a patient was an unacceptable thing for a senior resident to do.

Tom asked Richard if the guy was doing well enough after surgery to have walked out of the hospital on his own. Richard thought it was unlikely, so Tom called the attending to tell him they could not find one of their patients. The attending told Tom to call the city police and report the man missing, which Tom did. He then called the hospital administrator to have him search for the patient. Tom's conversation with the city police left him embarrassed and humiliated. The officer who had arrested the wife was more than a little critical of Tom for losing the victim.

By now, Tom was beyond panicked, so they all went back to the doctors' lounge to try to figure out what happened to the patient. The team was free to leave the hospital if they could find their patient. Tom called the attending again to ask him what they should do. The attending told Tom he could let the rest of the team go, but he had to stay until the patient was found. The attending demanded Tom search the entire hospital, bed by bed if necessary, until the patient was found, and God help Tom if he had let a patient walk out of the hospital status post-op with multiple gunshot wounds.

Tom was already in trouble for an incident that took place before Dave joined the team. Richard told Dave about it while Tom was on the phone with the attending. Tom had punched a Medicine resident. They had argued about whether Medicine or Surgery should admit a patient. The Medicine resident got in Tom's face, so Tom knocked him down with one punch. Tom was almost dismissed from the program and could not afford another incident.

They all volunteered to stay and search with Tom. Richard and Dave had spent the night on their feet in surgery, but they pulled themselves together and joined Tom and Jason in a floor-by-floor, room-by-room, bed-by-bed, station-by-station search of the hospital.

It was early afternoon when Dave walked into the ICU and saw the man. Dave was tired, so he was a little less than cordial when he asked the nurse how the patient got to the ICU and why they had not been notified he was there. The nurse was just as sharp with Dave when she told him she did not know how the patient got to the ICU, and they didn't know who to notify. Someone had deposited him without a chart and left. The man had recovered enough to talk coherently, but he didn't remember how he got to the hospital much less how he got to the ICU.

Dave paged the others overhead, and they made their way to the ICU. Tom and the ICU charge nurse yelled at each other until they both calmed down enough to work together to get the patient transferred to the Surgery floor.

9

The Halloween Party

Dave woke up at four, ate a ham and cheese sandwich, then drove to Sharon's to get into his costume and makeup. Dave was going as a pirate. The costume included a pirate vest, a head scarf, mid-calf duct pants, a wide belt with a sash that went under it, and a realistic-looking toy flintlock pistol to put in the belt. When Dave got to the house, no one came to the door, so he let himself in and went to Sharon's room.

She was waiting to help with his costume. After Dave put on the vest, pants, and belt with the long colorful sash under it, Sharon braided his hair in a Navy pigtail, and tied the scarf around his head so the tails hung down with the pig tail. She used makeup to draw a big anchor on Dave's chest, a heart with the initials SK and DC on one arm, and a skull and cross bones on the other. Then she made his eyes look dark and sinister, adding red scar down one side of his face. Dave jammed the pistol in his belt and was ready to go, so Sharon sent him downstairs to wait for her.

Sharon was going as a black cat. Her costume was a black full-body leotard with a tail that hung down to the ground and curled up at the end. The leotard was shear, tight, and fit her like a second skin, so it looked like she was simply painted black. She wore black pumps with four-inch heels, had a ponytail at the top of her head with a wide black band around its base, and black cat ears sticking up through her hair. She was over six three from the top of her hair and ears to the ground. Her face was even more alluring than her body. She had used black eyeliner to make her eyes look even larger and more cat-like. She used the liner to make whiskers and to put a black spot on the tip of her nose. She had long black false eyelashes, her lipstick was gray, and there was a wide black collar with a bell at its front around her neck. She was a tall walking big black cat.

She walked into the front room where Dave was waiting for her, stopped, and turned around so he could get the full effect. She said, "I think it came out pretty good. What do you think?"

"What do I think? Jesus Christ, Sharon, I am going to have to beat the guys off you with a stick. My God, you look sensational." Dave stood up and walked up to her.

"I wanted to turn you on, and from the look in your eyes, I think I succeeded." She laughed.

It was a mild Indian summer night, so they wore light plastic raincoats over their costumes to walk to the party. The other three couples were sitting in the front room when they got there. Connie and Harven were going to put their costumes on in Harven's room later, but Henry, Sherry, Mike, and Janice were dressed for the party.

Janice was dressed as Dorothy from *The Wizard of Oz*, and since she looked and acted like she was twelve years old, it was the perfect costume. Mike didn't really have a costume on. He was dressed in casual clothes and said he was a college student. Sherry was dressed as a hula dancer in a skimpy bikini top and a small bikini bottom under a grass skirt. She had flowers around her ankles, her wrists, and her head, and she wore several flower leis around her neck. Henry was dressed as a competitive swimmer, with a swim cap and swim goggles on his head, a Speedo bathing suit, and nothing else.

Dave and Sharon hung their coats up at the front door, and there was the audible sound of air being sucked in as the other three couples watched Sharon walk across the room toward them. Janice spoke up, "Do you have something on or are you just painted black?"

Mike blurted out, "You have the greatest body I have ever seen."

Connie laughed and said, "Wow! That's what I call a cat suit. Well, if you've got it, flaunt it. Girl, you sure have got it, and you sure are flaunting it."

Sharon smiled. "I have on a black leotard, or like Connie said, a cat suit, only this one has a tail, see." She ignored Mike and showed them her tail.

Dave waved. "Hi, guys. I am here too. Nice to see everyone. I am a pirate."

Henry answered, "Hey, Poncho, do you think anyone is looking at you or cares that you are a pirate when they can look at Sharon in pretty much nothing but Sharon?" Dave and Sharon sat down on the couch next to Sherry and Henry.

Sherry shook her head. "I thought Henry and I were being risqué wearing a Speedo and a bikini, but even though you're actually covered, it looks like you have nothing on. Mike is right, you have a beautiful body. Jesus Christ, what I wouldn't give for your height. How tall are you with the stilettos, the hair, and everything?"

Sharon crossed her long legs. "I don't know, four inches of heels and several inches of hair."

"Man, that's a lot of, ah...cat." Harven looked at Sharon and laughed. Connie hit him. "I said cat. I didn't say..."

Connie hit him again. "If you say it, I guarantee you won't get any tonight." Everyone laughed.

Dave had cut the four tabs of Owsley Window Pane in half with a razor blade and put them in an envelope at his apartment. He took them out and gave everyone one. When he got to Mike and Janice, Janice took one. "I changed my mind," she said.

Dave knew Mike had changed her mind for her, and he was worried because he knew no one should be coerced into taking a hallucinogen. Everyone put the tabs on their tongue to let them dissolve. Dave and Sharon kissed to start their trip.

Connie and Harven went upstairs to get dressed for the party, and the other three couples settled back to let the acid come on as they waited for everyone to arrive. There was a bowl on the dining room table for everyone to put money in when they got their drinks. People came in, hung their coats up, went to the dining room for beer or wine, put their money in the bowl, then walked into the front room. The costumes were all exceptional, and the partiers acted their parts, staying in character as they entered the front room, providing fantastical images for those in the initial rush of some very potent LSD.

Mike and Janice had never dropped acid before, and Dave could see it was hitting them hard as they watched the exotic stream of costumes flow into the room. Mike had done mescaline, but Janice had never done anything, so she had no idea how to handle it, and the Owsley Window Pane acid was like nothing any of them had done before.

Dave, Henry, Sharon, and Sherry knew to hang on for the initial rush caused by the massive release of neurotransmitters in their brains. Janice had no idea when or if the overload of dopamine was going to stop or if she was ever going to feel normal again. To her, it was an overwhelming experience that tore her consciousness and shattered her brain into fragments like a supernova exploding and scattering its fragments across the universe. It was a terrifying for her. She was literally hanging onto the arms of the chair with white knuckles. Mike jumped up and ran down the hall to the restroom as he felt the shearing of reality and the tearing of his consciousness caused by the initial rush of the drug.

Dave put his arm around Sharon, pulled her to him, and whispered, "Are you alright?"

Sharon whispered back, "Are you fucking kidding me? Of course, I am not alright. Are you alright? I am so glad we only took a half. I can't imagine what a whole one would be like." She pushed her body against him. "But I can tell you one thing, I want to be fucked tonight, and I mean fucked."

"Jesus, Sharon, don't start that. I am turned on enough just looking at you in that cat suit. If you start that, we will miss the whole party." Dave hugged her closer. "Don't you want to dance?"

"I want to dance, and then I want to fuck." She nibbled his ear.

"If you keep that up, there won't be any dancing and we will go straight to the fucking." Dave was really high. "Don't think I don't know what you are doing. You are teasing and tormenting me like you always do, and as fucked up as I am, it is having a major effect on me."

Sharon pulled back and laughed. "Good, that's just what I want. I want you out of your mind and crazy for me."

Mike came back from the restroom. "I just had a psychedelic barf. I barfed rainbows." He sat down in a chair next to Janice.

Sherry sat up. "Really, Mike, we don't want to know about your barfs."

Henry sat up beside her. "Man, I am way fucked up. I am so glad we only took a half."

They were all sitting up now looking around, except Janice, who still had a death grip on the arms of the chair. "How long does this last?"

Dave answered, "Probably about six to eight hours, but it will mellow out."

"Oh shit," was all she said.

Everyone was standing or sitting around drinking and talking, when Harven let out a gorilla roar from the landing at the top of the stairs. Everyone gathered in the hall to watch them as Connie and Harven made their grand entrance.

Connie was dressed in tight khaki short shorts, knee-high lace-up boots, a short-sleeve khaki shirt that was two sizes too small, and an Australian bush hat pinned up on one side. Since Connie's endowments were two sizes too large, she could only get the shirt partially buttoned, so she was showing a lot of Connie above the straining buttons. Her hair was in a long braid down her back and she was holding the leash of a gorilla with a studded collar. One look at her eyes told Dave how high she was, and Harven thought he really was a gorilla. He looked like a real gorilla, and he assumed all the attributes of a gorilla as he shuffled along beside Connie.

Everyone followed Connie and Harven into the front room. "It is time for the costume contest. Everyone find a place, and we will go through the categories." Harven sat on his haunches picking at himself while Connie talked, and then he lay down on his back with his arms out holding his feet.

Connie went on. "OK, first category is sexiest costume. If you want to participate, walk to the center of the room, and we will vote to determine the winner." Connie swung her arm around pointing at everyone as she went, but no one stepped out until she reached Sharon.

Sharon leaned over to Dave "This is for you." She stood up with a huge smile on her face, her legs apart, and her hands on her hips; then she cat walked to the center of the room amid wolf calls, whistles, and lewd comments. She stopped, turned back to face Dave with feet apart and her hands on her hips again, then shifted her weight from one hip to the other, tossing her head from side to side with the hip action, just as she had seen professional models do. The wolf calls, whistles, and comments increased, including Harven scurrying toward her sideways making his gorilla roar again. No one else stepped out as Sharon stood in the middle of the room smiling at Dave with her hands on her hips and her feet apart.

Connie jerked on Harven's leash. "I warned you about that cat before. I won't warn you again." Harven slunk back to sit at Connie's feet with his legs straight out. "It looks like we have a winner by acclamation for sexiest costume. Does everyone agree?" Shouts went up along with more whistles.

Sharon did her runway walk back to Dave. She stood in front of him with her legs apart then knelt on the couch, straddling him. She put her arms around his neck, leaned down and kissed him before whispering in his ear, "I hope that earned me what I asked for."

Dave put his arms around her and whispered back, "You bet." The shouts and lewd comments reached a crescendo as she stood up, turned, put her hands on her hips, tossed her head from side to side in sync with her hips, and posed with one hip out before sitting down beside Dave. Her act had the effect on Dave she intended, but it also had the same effect on every other man in the room.

It had a profound effect on Mike. He was completely mesmerized the whole time and could not stop looking at her, even after she sat down next to Dave. He watched as Dave put his hand on her thigh and she hugged his arm to her breast as they sat there cuddling with their heads together. He was tripping hard, and his imagination went wild as he watched movies, all starring Sharon, in his head.

The shouts, whistles, and yells had shattered Janice. She was tripping hard and trying desperately to keep it together as she clung to the arms of the chair. Henry had stood up yelling and whistling like everyone else during Sharon's walk and posing. "Jesus Christ, Sharon, you just severely messed with every guy in this room and some of the women too. I am way fucked-up and that blew my mind. I am surprised Dave is able to control himself after that."

Dave looked at Henry. "You have no idea how it hard is."

Sharon was flying high after her performance. "How hard is it?" She laughed at her own comment.

Sherry was sitting next to Sharon, and she was as high as the rest of them. "You know, of course, every woman in this room hates you now, and every man here wants you. After that performance, they are all picturing you naked, and believe me you painted quite a picture for them. How can any of us compete with you? You and your six feet whatever of … cat?" They all laughed.

Normally, Sharon would have blushed at the thought of all the men in the room picturing her naked and wanting her, but she was too high and too turned on to register anything that would produce a blush.

Connie was tripping just as hard as the rest of them and enjoying the attention of running the costume contest. "Well, that got the party started. I guess we need to do sexiest couple's costume next, right?" There was a resounding cry of affirmation.

"If you want to participate, walk to the center of the room, one couple at a time." Harven sat up on his haunches to watch.

The first couple was Audrey and Jake. Audrey had on her airline jacket, her airline hat, and nothing else. She had a black lace bra and black bikini panties under the jacket with nylons and heels. The jacket was cut like a suit coat, so it acted like a very short skirt and exposed most of the black lace bra. Jake had on black wing-tip shoes, black knee-high socks, black briefs, his airline jacket, pilot's cap, aviator sunglasses and nothing else. They were the stereotypical pilot and stewardess fantasy. Like Sharon, they were greeted with whistles, wolf calls, and lewd comments.

Phil had invited some of George and Harven's friends from medical school, as well as some of his and Bob's gay friends, and it was one of these couples who stepped out next. The girl was pretty, brunette, curvy, and young, and the guy was tall, dark, and handsome. They were dressed as Indians. The girl was in a short, fringed leather skirt, moccasins, and her small, beaded leather Indian vest was laced together with a single leather thong, so it exposed much more than it covered. The guy was wearing nothing but a piece of leather as a loin cloth with overhanging flaps in front and back, Indian style, and moccasins. They had matching leather headbands with feathers in the back and war paint on their faces and bodies. Once more, the jeers, cheers, and whistles filled the room.

Next, two women wearing nothing but body paint flitted to the middle of the room. They had wings on their backs, curved antennae on their heads, and slippers on their feet with turned up toes. They were both slender and attractive. Their hair was teased up and dyed green. Their bodies were painted in varying shades of green, and covered with glitter. They were fairies. Harven kept jumping up and down, running at them sideways, and roaring. They won the sexiest couple's costume.

Sherry did a very authentic hula dance and won best costume, which went a long way to counter her jealousy of Sharon. The best couple's costume was won by Connie and Harven the same way Sharon won, by acclamation.

Connie wrapped it up. "The music is going to start soon, so eat, drink, visit the zoom room, or whatever. Also, I imagine we will start getting people from other parties as soon as the music starts, so stake out a place for the night." Connie walked over to where they were sitting, leading Harven on his leash. "I assume you are all just as fucked-up as I am, but I don't think anyone is as fucked-up as Harven is; he really thinks he is a gorilla. We did some peyote in Mexico. He has a friend at school who gets us magic mushrooms occasionally, but that is nothing compared to this shit. It came on while we were trying to put our costumes on, and as soon as Harven put on the gorilla suit, he said he realized he had been a gorilla in a man suit all his life, but now he was finally comfortable because he was a gorilla in a gorilla suit. That was the last time he said anything." They all laughed and Harven sat up, shaking his head up and down.

Dave looked at Connie. "Don't stand right in front of me, Connie. If you popped a button with all that force behind it, it would go right through me." Everyone kept laughing.

Henry countered. "Look at Mike. If Connie pops a button, it will put his eye out." More laughter, but Mike was so high, he paid no attention and kept staring at Connie, even when Harven saddled toward him and roared.

"Very funny, guys, but what I am going to do with Harven?" Harven scurried over to Connie and started sniffing up her leg. "Behave, Harven. I told you there was no way we were going to do it with you in that gorilla suit, so put that out of your head. Stand up and act like a man, because that is the only way you are going to get laid tonight." By now, they were all laughing uncontrollably.

Phil walked over dressed as Louis the Sixteenth, complete with a wig, stockings, and pumps. "Here are your gift certificates." He handed one to each of the winners. Harven took his, sniffed it, then gave it to Connie. "I have to find Sam and Rachael's friends to give them theirs." He looked at Sharon, Sherry, and Connie in turn, then walked off shaking his head saying, "You three could drive a gay man straight."

Dave stood up. "We should stay hydrated. Let's get some water." He held his hand out to Sharon, and they all six headed for the dining room with Harven scurrying along beside Connie on his lease. Mike and Janice remained in the front room because Janice was still fighting the acid and Mike was totally out of it. Audrey, Caroline, Jake and Ron were in the dining room.

"I think we would have won if we had worn just our jackets with nothing on under them," Jake said to Audrey.

Audrey laughed at him. "You are so competitive. Really, you wanted us to walk around with nothing on but our jacket just so you could win?"

"They weren't completely naked. I talked to them earlier; up close you could tell they had some kind of tape over the business part of their who-haws," Ron informed everyone. Ron had on a three-piece suit with a wolf mask on his head, wolf gloves on his hands, and wolf's slippers on his feet.

Caroline was in a sexy Little Red Riding Hood outfit. "I bet it is going to hurt when they take the tape off their *who-haws*. What kind of man do I have who says who-haws instead of—"

Connie stopped Caroline. "We are not using that word tonight in deference to Sharon, who is a very tall one. But I agree. Is who-haws some kind of East Coast, Ivy League term, like whiffenpoofs?"

Helen and her date walked up to the group. "Hi roommates, friends, and significant others. This is Jackson. Jackson, these are my roommates, friends, and their significant others. Jackson lives on the other side of the Park and is some kind of consultant, only I don't know what he consults on."

Jackson was a good-looking and well-built man in his late twenties. They were dressed as Helen of Troy and Paris, both of them in lace-up Greek sandals, short white pleated Greek skirts, with garlands in their hair. The guy was bare chested with white briefs under his Greek skirt. Helen's white Greek blouse was sleeveless, very low cut exposing a lot of Helen, and she had white bikini panties on under her skirt. They all shook hands with Jackson and told him their names, except Harven, who sniffed at him.

Jackson looked at all the girls. "God, I have been living in the Park for years, and I never knew so many beautiful women lived in one house just across from me."

Helen responded, "Down, boy. Sherry and Connie don't live in our house, and my roommates are all in relationships. Sherry's boyfriend is the big one with nothing on, and Connie is engaged to the gorilla." Harven scurried at Jackson and roared.

"Well, at least I can look. Wow, I am in a paradise of pulchritude. I feel lucky there was at least one left for me." Jackson smiled oozing charm and looking at Sharon. "What a night it would be if I could dance with each of you."

"You can look, but you can't touch, and if you have designs on the cat, forget it. She is engaged. In fact, I am surprised she and the pirate haven't swum upstream to spawn already after her performance in that cat suit," Helen added.

"Don't be mean, Helen." Sharon took Dave's arm.

Bob and Phil came up to them. "Look at all the pretty people. You guys have no idea what an attractive group you are, and there is so much of you on display. Gay or straight, there is plenty of eye candy in this group either way. We have been standing over there drooling over all of you."

Bob was dressed as a Hobbit, with furry feet and all. "Gorgeous, does the little cat walk you did in that cat suit mean that you will model lingerie?"

"No, that walk was for my guy. I thought I made that obvious. And he is the only one who will ever see me in lingerie. So, forget it." Sharon hugged Dave's arm.

"Pity," Jackson said still looking at Sharon. "I would love to see that."

"Why? I don't know how you could see much more of her than you are already seeing," Helen responded.

The speakers came alive with, "It's time to commence to get ready to rock and roll, people!"

Connie jerked on Harven's leash. "You are not a gorilla, Harven. You are a man, and if you don't stand up and act like a man, you will be sleeping alone tonight."

Harven stood up. "OK, but if I take my gorilla suit off, I will be a naked ape because I don't have anything on under it. It is my true skin."

"It is not your true skin. But keep it on because I am not dancing with you naked either. I hate to break this to you, but you are a man not a gorilla, and your true skin is under that gorilla suit." Harven beat his chest and roared as the music started.

Henry put his head back and gave a wolf howl, and everyone followed with a howl of their own. It went on as they all howled together. Jackson was somewhat taken aback. "What's that all about?" he said to no one in particular.

Henry answered, "That means the pack is on the prowl tonight." Then Henry yelled, "Stones Mother," as the driving beat of "It's Only Rock and Roll" blasted out of the speakers.

About half of the partygoers were in the dining room and about half were in the front room, but no matter where they were, most of them started dancing on the spot. Sharon backed out of the group, curled her index finger at Dave, put her hands close together above her head, closed her eyes, and started shifting her hips back and forth, moving her head in time with her hips as the music took control of her body. Dave was soaring as he danced close to her with their bodies almost touching. He yelled above the music, "It's going to be a hell of a night, Baby!"

Sharon threw her head back and laughed as she moved against Dave, then she turned sideways so they could bump, first one side then the other, before backing off to put on a show for him.

Dave was not the only one watching her. "Jesus Christ," Jackson blurted out as his eyes followed Sharon's body.

"Hey, I am over here. I told you, she is engaged, so forget about her," Helen shouted above the music.

"Take a look around. There isn't a guy here who isn't watching her, and you can tell she likes to be watched. Look at her go," he shouted back.

"Understand there is only one guy she likes watching her and only one guy she is dancing for," Helen reminded him.

By the time the DJ played "Johnny be Good," the house was packed with people in every manner of costume and state of dress or undress one could imagine dancing in the dining room, the front room, the hall, and even on the landing upstairs. More wine and beer had shown up, and the air was heavy with the pungent odor of ganga. All the admonitions about teenage drinking and dope smoking had gone out the window as massive amounts of alcohol, plenty of herb, and various chemicals took control. As the music played on with Iron Butterfly's "In-A-Gadda-Da-Vida," the crowd began to spill out onto the front porch. Dave pulled Sharon to him saying, "That is pure acid-eating music, Baby."

The acid peaked when the DJ played "Shout." The front porch was full, the dining room was full, the front room was full, the hall was full, and the upstairs landing was full of people throwing their hands up and yelling "shout" all together. All the lights were on, the music was loud, and the party was a beacon for anyone in the Park Area that night.

Dave looked to one side to see a gorilla throw its paws up and yell "shout." The gorilla was dancing with Connie who was on the verge of a major wardrobe malfunction, so her considerable endowments were almost completely exposed as she threw her hands up and yelled "shout." Behind Sharon, Henry had lost his swim cap and goggles, so he was down to nothing but his Speedo as he threw his hands up and yelled "shout." Sherry no longer had a grass skirt and most of her flowers were gone as she threw her hands up and yelled "shout" in nothing but a tiny bikini. On the other side was a guy in combat boots and a male G-string with chains crossed over his bare chest like bandoliers and rabbit ears on his head throwing his hands up and yelling "shout." He was dancing with a woman who was also in a G-string, with stiletto heels, smaller chains crossed between her bare breasts, and rabbit ears on her head throwing her hands up and yelling "shout."

Dave looked around, and there was a woman completely nude, except for her high heels, dancing on the card table throwing her hands up and yelling "shout." He looked back at Sharon, who was enraptured in a dancing trance, just as she had been at the Santana concert, throwing her hands up as she yelled "shout." His brain was completely overloaded as he watched the scene around him and threw his hands to yell "shout." The front room looked like a living Hieronymus Bosch painting with the array of exotic costumed and partially dressed dancers shouting and gesticulating with their hands as the music blasted through them.

The music went on song after song without a pause as more people gathered in the yard in front of the house. Dave and Sharon had to dance very close because it was so crowded. Dave reached out, pulled Sharon to him, wrapped his arms around her, and kissed her passionately. He buried his face in her neck as he hugged her. She responded by jumping up, wrapping her legs around his waist, and putting her arms around his neck. They finished the song like that, locked together kissing. Sharon put her feet back on the ground but kept her arms around Dave's neck as he held her, and they stood looking at each other. T Rex's "Bang a Gong" blasted out of the speakers. They didn't dance but began to grind against each other as the song seemed to describe Sharon and Dave's passion for her. Sharon's eyes were liquid pools that engulfed him the same way her body engulfed him when they made love. The next song was "One after 909" followed by "Back in the USSR." Dave and Sharon held each other, swaying in time with the music, but they didn't dance. They were ready to do more than dance.

The song ended but another one didn't start. Instead, Phil's voice came over the speakers. "OK, people, we have to wrap this up. We have to get everyone out of this house by midnight. The house has

A love story and social commentary

to be dark, quiet, and unoccupied except for the people staying here before the police start shutting down the parties. We can't have them come in here with the air reeking of ganga, underage drinking, nudity, and people fucking in the zoom room. If you want to keep going, move the party outside into the street. The music is over, and we are going to turn out the lights so everyone needs to start moving out the door."

There were a lot of boos and grumblings, but with the music gone, there was no reason to stay, so people began to leave. Bob got the couples dressed and out of the zoom room. George and his date, both dressed in roller derby costumes, cleared the landing on their way to George's room. Phil herded everyone out of the front room and dining room. Sam and Rachael moved them off the porch, out of the yard, and on into the street. The DJ and his date packed up his stuff and moved it out to his van.

Connie took Harven's leash to lead him to his room, saying, "I told you I am not going to fuck you in that gorilla suit, so give it up."

Mike and Janice, who had rallied during the dancing, followed Connie and Harven, with Janice chattering away about taking acid. Sherry went to the dining room to find a lot of beer and wine on ice in the wash tub, six-packs of beer with more unopened wine bottles on the table, and the bowl not only full of tens and twenties, but bills overflowing onto the table around it.

Henry stayed with the group. "Jesus fucking Herman Christ, that was some awesome party. We tore it down; I mean, we tore the mother fucker down."

Jake was holding Audrey in his arms. "Henry is right. I have never seen a party like that. Did you see all the people in body paint and bizarre costumes, not to mention those with no costumes at all? Talk about your pagan rights on All Hollow's Eve."

Caroline was holding Ron's hand. "Did you ever go to a party like that back East at your Ivy League school?"

"Are you kidding? I thought this was the Bible Belt, but that was pure debauchery at its finest." They all started for the door to walk home except Henry; he went to the dining room to find Sherry.

Helen and Jackson caught up to them. "Who are you people? I have seen some crazy shit on this Park and have been to some major parties but nothing like this. A bunch of doctors live in this house? Is this the way doctors party?"

When they got outside, they saw a lot of people in the street dancing to the music of a boom box someone had brought out. There were police at both ends of the street and more lining the Park, but they were letting the party go on. The four couples walked arm and arm or hand and hand back to the other house.

It was well after midnight when they planned to meet for breakfast the next day. They said good night and went upstairs to their separate rooms. With the other three couples in the house, Sharon and Dave were confined to Sharon's room for their lovemaking, but they didn't let that constrain them in any way. Their passion, fueled by the LSD, carried them long into the night in an excess of multiple couplings before they fell asleep in each other's arms, spent and exhausted.

They woke up in the late morning. Dave put on his pirate pants, Sharon put on her short terrycloth robe, and they padded downstairs barefoot. They heard voices from the kitchen once they were on the landing, so they knew some of the others were up. When they walked into the kitchen, they were greeted by applause by the other three couples.

"What?" Dave looked around.

"Not for you, for Sharon. She won a well-deserved title, representing our house." Helen held up her coffee cup in salute. "Let's hear it for our tall walking big black cat."

They got some more chairs and moved around so all eight of them could sit at the table. "Have you guys been up long?" Sharon sat down between Dave and Helen.

"Not long. I think Caroline and Ron were up first; we got here right before you guys. We were waiting for you to start breakfast or to go out for brunch, but after last night, I don't think anyone is up for cooking or for getting dressed." Audrey, like all the women, had on a short robe.

"I don't want to do anything," Caroline added.

"So, let's just have coffee, toast, cereal, and hang out. Someone start making toast, and I will get out the cereal, milk, and bowls." Ron got up.

"I will make toast and get the OJ out." Jackson followed Ron.

Jake turned to Dave. "Man, that was one full tilt boogie last night. I am still trying to wrap my head around it."

Dave confessed, "I am not sure everything I saw was real, I was so fucked up."

"It was all real." Ron had only been drinking. "Man, you weren't the only one fucked-up. There were some of the most fucked-up people I have ever seen in my life at that party. And with the costumes or lack of costumes there were a lot of who-haws and ding-a-lings on full display. Did you see the S and M couples in the latex, with collars and leashes, whips and shit?"

Jackson chimed in from the toaster, "Halloween is always wild on the Park, but I have never seen anything like last night."

Once everything was ready and they were all sitting down, Helen looked around the table. "This is so much fun having everyone here. I wonder how many more times like this we will have before everything changes."

Jackson had spent the night with Helen even though he lived right across from their house, and he was being included in the group unlike the other men Helen dated. Sharon, who spent more time at the house than the other two women, had not seen him before, and she wondered how long it had been going on. He was certainly good looking, charming, and bright.

Jake and Audrey looked at each other. "This seems like as good a time as any to let everyone know Audrey and I are getting married in May next year. We don't want to get married in winter, so we are going to wait until spring."

They all congratulated Audrey and Jake but realized this put a punctuation mark on what Helen had said. They spent the rest of the morning talking and enjoying each other's company before splitting up for the rest of the day. Dave and Sharon went back to her room to shower and get ready for tomorrow before driving to Dave's apartment in separate cars. Sharon was flying, and Dave started the Surgery ER at seven the next morning.

10
The ED

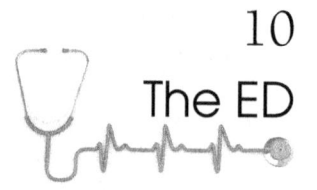

The Surgery ER rotation was twenty-four on and twenty-four off. Dave was back to making the decisions and being responsible for his patients, as well as Jason's patients. The stress level went back up, and time to sleep, down time, and time off went back down. The one positive thing was they were able to eat on a regular bases because Tom liked to eat, so he saw they got breakfast and at least some sandwiches for lunch and dinner.

After a shift in the Surgery ER, Dave usually got to his apartment around eight or nine and slept until Sharon came over in the afternoon; then they would have dinner, smoke a number, listen to music, talk, and be in bed by ten. Sharon saw he got eight hours of sleep every other night, and he slept at least six hours during the day after his shifts. Occasionally, they would meet their friends for an early dinner on a Friday or Saturday night. They never saw Henry and Sherry. Sherry had given Henry an ultimatum: either Henry took their relationship to the next level, or Henry was moving back into the Park house and Sherry was moving on. Henry was not going to marry Sherry, so he was planning to move back to the Park house after the holidays.

Dave struggled through his days in the Surgery ER in a blur of fatigue and sleep deprivation, wading through lacerations, abscesses, surgical abdomens, fractures, crush injuries, avulsed and severed body parts. After twenty-four hours, he was covered with blood, pus, body fluids, excretions, and other things he did not even want to think about, so he showered, washed off his OR shoes, and changed his scrubs before he drove home.

One morning, Dave was sitting in the doctors' station drinking coffee when the nurse walked by with a man with a bloody bandana tied around his head, so Dave thought it was just another scalp laceration. The man told Dave he had been clearing his land with a chainsaw and the saw kicked back, causing a cut on his head. He had not worn any protective gear because he knew how to handle a chainsaw and didn't need any. Dave had the nurse help him as he unwrapped the bandana, parted the man's hair, and washed the area with saline to expose the laceration. He got the site exposed and realized he was looking at the man's brain through a wide groove cut in his scalp and skull by the chainsaw.

"Give me a stack of four by fours and some koban, then page Neurosurgery stat! Sir, you need to lie down right now. Then I need someone in here to start a large bore IV!" Dave got the man down despite his protests that he was OK and that it was just a little cut. He pressed the four by fours over the wound, then secured them with the koban wrapped around his head. The neurosurgery resident showed up, and Dave described the wound to him, then the resident and a nurse whisked the man away to the OR amid protests from him that it was just a little cut and all he needed were some stitches. Dave sat back down in the doctors' station to take some deep breaths, try to get his heart rate down, and finish his coffee. Most mornings weren't too bad, but it picked up in the afternoon, and became untenable at night.

It was the Friday and Saturday night meetings of the city's knife and gun clubs that turned the ER into a hell on earth every weekend and demonstrated the violent destructive nature of humans to the fullest. The true nature of man is on display every weekend in its unvarnished form in the ER of a big city/county hospital, and University Hospital was no exception. First, there are the fights and beatings with facial lacerations, fractured noses, fractured jaws, and fractured facial bones. Then there are the blunt trauma cases with scalp lacerations, skull fractures, rib fractures, subdural and subarachnoid bleeds. Next there are the stabbings and lacerations from knives or broken bottles. Finally, there are the gunshot wounds, either self-inflicted or the results of altercations. Along with all this carnage came the tears, anguish, and grief of the loved ones of the victims.

There were times on a late Saturday night in the Surgery ER when Dave could hardly hear for the cries and screams of pain, suffering, anguish, and grief that filled the entire department. He saw a man who shot himself in the genitals trying to get his gun out to shoot someone else; he was screaming not only in pain but for his lost manhood. He saw people screaming in agony, and then heard the screams of grief of their loved ones when they died. The cacophony of misery recurred every Friday and Saturday night without fail. Dave had one classmate doing his internship at Bellevue Hospital in New York City and another one at Cook County in Chicago. If things were this bad in the city/county hospital of a large Southern city, he could not imagine what it was like in New York, Chicago, or LA. There were rumors that an intern had been stabbed to death in an elevator while taking a patient from the ED to Surgery by gang members going after the patient, who they also killed.

The realization that no one was immune had already been demonstrated to Dave in crystal-clear fashion by his interaction with the biker in the Medicine ER, but the fact was further driven home one night in mid-November in the Surgery ER. He had finished suturing a laceration and was on his way to the doctors' station to write his note when two city policemen came into the ER.

"Close and secure these doors. No one leaves this room. You are to shelter in place." The policemen stationed themselves on each side of the doors with their weapons drawn.

Tom approached the policeman who had spoken. "What's up?"

"A man shot his wife, but she survived and was brought here for surgery. The husband showed up at the triage desk looking for her. The nurse notified your security, who notified us. We think he is armed and is trying to find her to finish her off."

Tom called the charge nurse over to him. "Let's get all the staff and patients as far back as possible and put any empty gurneys, Mayo stands, chairs, or anything else we can find between them and the doors. Once we get everyone relocated, the staff needs to keep taking care of our patients. Richard, try to find out where the wife is and what's going on."

Richard got on the phone with the Trauma charge nurse. She told him the patient had been taken to the OR. The police were guarding the ED and OR while the security guards were searching the hospital for the man.

"OK, everybody, just stay calm and do your job. We are well protected, and we will be fine. Let's get back to taking care of our patients." Richard had been through this kind of thing in Vietnam.

After some time, they heard the policeman on his walkie-talkie, then, "It's all OK. We got him," and the police officers left. Later, they heard there had been a gunfight in the hall outside the OR, and the husband had been killed. The doctors operating on the wife could hear the gunshots, but they kept operating on the wife, trying to save her life.

Richard shook his head. "I never thought I would have to deal with this kind of shit again after I left Vietnam."

What happened on the hill overlooking the ambulance bay was another example of the lack of humanity Dave dealt with every day. There was a road that led into the hospital campus from the main street. On the right side of the road was the ambulance bay and the ED; on the left was the entrance to the staff parking lot. The staff parking lot was on a hill that overlooked the ambulance bay, and every Friday and Saturday night, groups of people gathered on the hillside to watch the ambulances unload. With some trauma cases and patients getting CPR, the doctors and nurses would be waiting on the ambulance dock to begin treatment as soon as the ambulance doors opened so the crowd got a good look at the drama as it unfolded. The fact that the life-and-death struggle of one human being would be considered entertainment by another human being left Dave sickened by the depravity it demonstrated.

But one foggy morning, the hillside revealed the other side of human nature. As November dragged on, the mornings became foggier. On this particular morning, the fog was so dense, Dave could barely see to drive. When he got out of his car, he could only see smudges from the lights of the ambulance bay and dull red blurs from the ambulances themselves. Then he heard a hauntingly beautiful voice floating on the fog, singing "Just a Closer Walk with Thee." He knew the voice was coming from the hillside, but he could not see anyone, and the sunrise added a dull homogenous glow to the fog, so it seemed as if the voice was disembodied, without a source, and emanating from the fog itself. The singer had perfect pitch and the warm melodious voice of a black gospel singer. It was so filled with sorrow and emotion, it tore at Dave's very soul, and when she let her voice soar on the chorus, "Oh Lord let be," it cut through the fog like a knife that also cut through Dave's heart. He stood there engulfed in the pain of the voice and shaken to his core by its effect on him. How could a species that could produce something that beautiful and filled with emotion also produce the death and devastation he was about to deal with in the ED? He knew it was that man-made horror that had produced the beauty and emotion in the voice. That dichotomy left him confused. The fact that man, the most violent and destructive species on the planet, could also produce such beautiful and soulful music was difficult for Dave to reconcile. He walked to the ED asking himself, *What the hell is wrong with people? Why the fuck do they behave the way they do?*

The last case in the Surgery ER that left an indelible impression on Dave occurred before Thanksgiving. The two med students and the other three flight attendants were going home for Thanksgiving, and Henry and Mike were working, so Sharon and Dave were having Thanksgiving with Bob and Phil. Caroline and Ron announced to everyone they were getting married in April, so they were going to Caroline's home to tell her parents. Connie and Harven, Audrey and Jake, and Helen and George were all going home too. Sharon knew her mother would be lonely at Thanksgiving, but if she went home, Dave would be alone since he was off, so she was staying with Dave. Thanksgiving was a family holiday, and Sharon realized she would never have her own family, so the urges she fought so hard to control troubled her again. She couldn't help thinking about marrying Dave and having her own family, especially since she knew Caroline and Audrey were getting married in the Spring. But she pushed those feelings down and told herself she was happy with things the way they were.

Dave had been working steadily all day when he and Jason caught a patient around ten o'clock that night who was brought in by the city police. Dave had worked out a system with Jason that was more efficient. They saw patients together, and if it was something Jason could handle, Dave left him with the patient and moved on to the next one, but if it was beyond Jason's capabilities, Jason helped Dave with the work-up and treatment.

The patient was a black man whose hands and feet were shackled to a gurney; he had been severely beaten. His eyes were swollen almost shut, his nose was crooked, his lips were split, and he had multiple burst wounds and lacerations on his scalp. There were three policemen with him, and one spoke to Dave. "We need him treated and cleared medically as soon as possible, so we can take him to jail."

Dave had seen other injured patients who needed to be treated and cleared so they could be incarcerated, but he had never seen one this badly beaten. "What did he do?" The man reeked of alcohol, urine, and feces.

The policeman responded, "He murdered his wife. Then he killed one of our officers who was responding to the domestic disturbance call." The policeman looked at the other two officers. "He resisted arrest and we had to subdue him."

Dave checked the man neurologically, examined his chest and abdomen, then turned to Jason. "Wash and get some pressure on the scalp wounds to control the bleeding. Get a tech to cut his clothes off and clean him up. Once that is done, call me, and we can check him carefully before we send him to X-ray. Order a skull series, rib series, and facial bones. When he gets back from x-ray, call ENT to take care of his nose and any other facial fractures, then we will suture his wounds. I am going to see the next patient. Be sure to tell the radiologist we need a wet reading on the films right away."

Dave looked at the policemen. "I am very sorry about your officer. I will do everything I can to get this man treated and cleared right away. Is there anything else I can do to help?"

The officers shook their heads. "No, but you can imagine what it does to us when we lose one of our own."

Dave turned back to Jason. "Stay with this patient and ride herd on everyone to get him out of here ASAP. Page me when you have everything done." Dave left and went on to the next patient.

After a thorough exam, the patient returned from x-ray, ENT took care of the man's fractured nose, then Jason and Dave sutured his wounds with one of them working on each side of the man's face and scalp. All the x-rays were negative, so when all the wounds were closed, Dave signed off on the patient and cleared him to be incarcerated.

Dave went back to the patient he had been seeing when Jason paged him and continued where he had left off. He finished and was walking back to the doctors' station when he met the officer who had spoken to him before. "We need you back, Doc." The policeman led Dave back to the man shackled to the gurney. Both the man's eyes were now completely swollen shut, his bandaged nose was smashed again, he had new wounds and some of the sutured ones were split open. He had been beaten again, and there was a new policeman who spoke. "He tried to escape."

Dave looked at the four policemen. "We just spent hours neglecting other patients to take care of this man so you could get him out of here as quickly as possible, now we are going to have to do it all over again, and more patients are going to have to wait. If you are going to do anything more to him, do it now, so we don't have to do our work all over again a third time."

The new policeman stepped up to Dave and pointed his finger at Dave's chest. "This mother fucker killed my partner, and he is getting what he deserves, so you will do what we tell you to do as many times as we tell you to do it."

"No, I won't. Your authority ends at the medical care of this patient, and my authority begins there. He is under my care, in my emergency room." Dave looked with disdain at the finger the policeman was pointing at his chest.

The policeman's face was a vivid red, his eyes were menacing, and the veins in his forehead were bulging as he jabbed his finger into Dave's chest. "Look, you nigger-loving hippie, you want to go to jail for interfering with a police officer in the performance of his duty?"

Tom walked up because he had heard the commotion. "He is not a hippie; he is a doctor, and a damn good one at that, so knock that shit off. This is a hospital ER. I think it would be a good idea for you guys to get this officer out of here for his own good. We will take care of this patient again after we clear the backlog caused by putting his case above our other patients to begin with. If you have a problem with that, give me your captain's name, and I will call him and discuss it with him. I am sure he will be pleased to know how one of his officers is conducting himself in a hospital ER in front of a lot of witnesses, no matter how distraught that officer is." Tom was big, loud, and imposing, so when the policeman confronting Dave turned to respond to Tom with "Fuck you," the other two officers intervened and hustled him out the ER.

The remaining officer who had been talking to Dave apologized to Tom. "I am sorry, but he just lost his partner so give him a break."

"I understand, but Dr. Cameron did not kill his partner, and he is doing everything he can to help. Attacking a physician who is trying to do his job is not going to bring his partner back. We will get your prisoner taken care of, but we have a lot of other people to take care of as well." Tom turned to Dave. "Go ahead with your other patients, Dr. Cameron, then you can take care of this man when you are caught up."

"Jason can take care of him. He knows what to do because it is simply a repeat of the work-up and treatment we just did." Jason nodded. He had been standing by watching the whole exchange.

A love story and social commentary

Tom looked at the officer. "If I were you, I would thank Dr. Cameron profusely for going out of his way to help you, because he is going to have Jason write a follow-up note on this patient and what happened here. The chart and that note will be evidence, so how he writes the note will determine if your friend keeps his badge or not as well as how you and the other two officers involved in this incident are viewed. This is not the streets, and you are not dealing with criminals here. This is the ER in a hospital, and you are dealing with dedicated professionals doing their jobs. How dare one of you treat one of us this way. If any police officer ever insults or threatens one of my doctors again, you will see me on the six o'clock news publicly filing charges against him after the hospital administrator calls the mayor to report the officer. Make sure your captain knows that. And one more thing, don't think you can beat a prisoner in this ER no matter what he has done, and make sure the rest of your colleagues know that too. Is that clear?"

The officer nodded.

Jason sutured all the wounds, ENT put the man's nose back in place, and all the other x-rays were negative, so Dave signed the man out as cleared for incarceration again. The remaining officer took Dave aside. "Look, Doc, he is not a bad guy, none of us are bad guys. He lost control because this guy killed his partner. Don't ruin his career because he was reacting like anyone would under the circumstances."

Dave looked at the officer. "That man is emotionally unstable, and you know it. He was coming after me. What is going to happen to the next black man he arrests? What's going to happen to the next innocent white man, like me, who crosses him? I looked the other way when you brought this man in badly beaten because of the very reasons you just mentioned. But you want me to look the other way when he is beaten while he is shackled to a gurney in the ER of the hospital hours after the shooting? I am having Jason write this up exactly as it happened, and then I am going to cosign it and add my own note. I would advise you and the other officers to get on the right side of this thing while you can. My first note doesn't mention anything but the injuries, so you guys are not implicated in any way with how he presented to the ER, but the second note will outline just what happened here because that officer shouldn't be carrying a badge and a gun."

The officer shrugged. "Have it your way, Doc, but some of our guys just protected some of your guys."

Dave looked the officer straight in the eyes. "And we are grateful. I agree we need to stick together, but that guy is out of control and you know it. Do you want to be responsible for his actions? If I protect him, will you take full responsibility for his actions and any further damage he does? Do you want me to put his protection on your head? I will be happy to sign a note stating you reported to me that a man whose hands and feet were shackled to a gurney needed to be beaten senseless in order to prevent him from escaping, that you were present, and you participated. Is that what you want me to do?"

The officer looked down. "I guess not."

"OK." Dave walked away to find Tom to thank and tell him what a good job he did in handling the situation. Tom was a jerk, but he was an excellent surgeon, and when the chips were down, he always came through, handled things correctly, and did the right thing. Dave finished his shift and drove home to get some sleep before Thanksgiving dinner.

Dave did not sleep well. His two experiences in the ED, coupled with the gun fight outside the OR, had unnerved him considerably. He had been in danger twice, and one of the times he was threatened by someone who was supposed to be protecting him. The news media reports the worst of the violent behavior, but that is only the tip of the iceberg. They ignore a lot of the violence in the non-white communities and some of the less sensational things that occur. The vast majority of violent events go unreported and unnoticed. Only in a big city ED is the complete magnitude of the brutality and its effects on the significant number of people who are its victims evident. There are violent muggings and robberies, domestic violence, fights and beatings, violence associated with alcohol and drug abuse, violence associated with the drug trade, and violence committed by unstable and psychotic individuals. It all adds up to a bleak outlook for mankind in the dawning of an age of peace and love. That gnawed at Dave as he drove to meet Sharon for Thanksgiving.

Dave and Sharon had been raised in good Southern families who dressed for Thanksgiving and Christmas dinners, so Dave wore a suit and Sharon wore a nice conservative dress with heels. They rang the doorbell at Bob's and Phil's house around four o'clock in the afternoon.

Phil answered the door. "My God, Ken and Barbie are here to have Thanksgiving with us."

Sharon sounded annoyed when she responded, "Ken has dark hair and Barbie is blond."

Phil frowned. "Don't tell me you two have had a lover's quarrel?"

Sharon smiled. "No, I am sorry, it's just I usually go home for Thanksgiving to be with my mother. This is the first time I haven't been at home for Thanksgiving, and I feel guilty."

Bob came up to them as they walked in with Phil. "Why didn't you invite her to have Thanksgiving with us?"

"No offense, guys, but I have a big picture of that." They walked into the living room together. "Mom, why don't you have Thanksgiving with me, my new lover I sleep with most of the time even though we are not married and our two gay friends."

Phil motioned them toward the couch. "Mom is old-school I take it."

Sharon laughed. "She is past old-school. Victorian is more like it. She is still upset I didn't marry Bar so he could keep her in the style she deserves. All I have to do to complete the disappointment is tell her I am sleeping with a guy with shoulder-length hair and hanging out with gays."

Bob left the room. "I will be back with some bourbon, and we will wash those blues away."

Phil turned to Dave. "Dave, you don't look happy either. I have never seen you two like this. It's Thanksgiving; let's be thankful."

Dave smiled at Phil and replied, "I am sorry, Phil. I guess the world is too much with me. I have been spending time with the fine citizens of our fair city getting a close-up look at how they treat one another, and it is disheartening." Dave thought about what Phil had said about the police at their lunch before the concert.

Bob returned with four bourbons. "Wrap your lips around these, and I guarantee, it will lift your spirits." When they all had a glass, Bob lifted his. "Happy Thanksgiving." They drank the toast together.

"Wow, is there anything in this, or is it just a big glass of bourbon?" Sharon's voice was hoarse.

Bob smiled back. "Big damn glass of bourbon, and here's to it." He raised his glass again and drank so they took a second drink. After two big shots of bourbon, the mood lightened considerably.

They talked about the three weddings, Dave's and Harven's plans to apply to programs in California, and Sharon's plans to get her MBA.

Dave told Bob and Phil he was sure Henry would be back in the Park house by January, but he had plans to get his own place before his residency.

Bob fixed them all another drink, so by the time they sat down to eat, they had a good buzz going. Dinner was excellent with traditional turkey and dressing, cranberry sauce, gravy, sweet potatoes, mashed potatoes, and pumpkin pie for dessert. They drank a bottle of wine with dinner plus Bob brought out port and brandy after dinner. They thanked Bob and Phil profusely and went back to Sharon's house to go to bed early since they both had to work the next day. They cuddled in bed a long time before they made love and went to sleep. Dave slept better snuggled next to Sharon, but he was still troubled, and Sharon's instinctual yearnings for a traditional family life troubled her, so she didn't sleep well either. All the alcohol helped, but they were still down when they were supposed to be thankful.

Dave was glad to get out of the Surgery ER. His next rotation was Trauma. His Surgery team would become Trauma 2. Again, his last day in the Surgery ER was a day off and his first day on Trauma was off, so Dave and Sharon decided to do something with their friends. Dave had promised to take Sharon dancing at a club, and this seemed like the perfect time. Mother's Blues was the place to go for the hip crowd on Saturday nights, it is was a hangout for the college and grad school crowd on Wednesday nights, Friday nights there were a mix of black and white couples, and the rest of the time it was mainly a black club. They talked to their friends about going, but Henry and Sherry were out because Henry was out, Audrey and Caroline both had trips, Helen and Jackson had become an item, but they opted out, so that left Connie and Harven. They didn't ask Mike and Janice.

The two couples had dinner together and got to the club about eight. It was crowded with college and grad students, so they stood around for a while until some college kids left, opening a table for them. The crowd was mainly white students with some black couples at the tables and black singles at the bar. The house band was hot, playing college tunes, like "Louie Louie" and "Hot Nuts," to please their Wednesday night audience, so it wasn't long before Sharon and Connie were both up to dance. The two women had on quintessential party dresses, short, tight, and low cut; Connie's was red, and Sharon's was black, both with matching heels.

A love story and social commentary

The dance floor was crowded so it was back-to-back and belly-to-belly, but they fell right in with the student crowd, reverting back to their college days. As the night went on, the band got hotter, the dancing got better, and it became less crowded because the students with classes the next day began to leave. Dave noticed those that stayed were more mature and there were more black couples than white couples, yet everyone was getting along and having a good time. There were no fights, no beatings, no stabbings, and no shootings. There were just happy people, black and white, dancing and partying together without any problems. Dave began to think maybe he was seeing a skewed picture of humanity in the ED and there was hope after all.

The night out dancing helped Sharon deal with the things bothering her too. She had Dave, their love, and their future together, which included a possible move to California, her return to school for an MBA, and a career that would let her reach her full potential. She decided again she didn't need anything else.

When they got back to Dave's apartment, their lovemaking was intensified by the music and dancing. They slept soundly until late the next morning because Sharon had shaken off her Thanksgiving blues and Dave once more had hope for the future of the human race. They made love with the same unrestrained desire and passion the next morning, immersing all their emotions in the physical act as they merged their bodies. They spent the rest of the morning lying in bed cuddling and fondling as they talked about their dreams and plans for the future. Dave was almost halfway through his internship, and he was starting to see a light at the end of the tunnel. He saw no reason for them to get dressed because they weren't planning to leave the apartment, so after some negotiation, Sharon agreed to her lingerie and Dave's short silk robe.

Later, as they cuddled on the beanbag, Dave said, "I am going to file my applications for the four residencies in California and the program here after the first of the year, and you should apply to the MBA programs at all five schools soon. It will take some time to get everything together, request recommendations and transcripts, and do all the paperwork, so you should get started this month. With your grades and score on the GMAT, you will have no trouble getting into all five programs."

Sharon snuggled against Dave. The thought that she had a goal and something to work toward that would lead to a fulfilling career was exciting. She drifted on the weed dreaming of her future as Dave talked. Dave would be a doctor, she would have a meaningful career, they would live in a beautiful small Northern California town near or in the mountains, with clean water and clear air, close to skiing and not too far from the water so Dave could have a boat. They would have plenty of money with both their incomes, so they could travel to Europe, drive nice cars and have a nice home that she could decorate the way she wanted with original art and stylish furniture. They would go to the theater and concerts in the Bay Area and spend time on the beaches of Hawaii. She was so lost in her fantasy that she didn't hear what Dave was saying as she dreamed on.

"So, what do we do for the rest of this afternoon and tonight?"

She didn't answer because as she came back from her fantasy, it occurred to her that she had undergone a fundamental change. She had never had plans for the future. She had been a beautiful woman getting by on her looks, running or flying away from her past, but now she was going to go as far as her intelligence and capabilities could take her. That realization awakened a drive and ambition in her she had never felt before. She wanted the dream she had just dreamed and the future she had just fantasized about. She wanted it so badly, she was motivated to achieve it with a longing like nothing she had ever experienced before. These feelings were completely foreign to Sharon, but she embraced them, and it all came together for her as she sat up and looked at Dave. He had done this to her. He had taught her the pleasures of sex, he had brought back the joy of dance to her, he had taught her how to love and be loved, he completed her and showed her how wonderful life could be in a loving relationship, but more importantly, he had helped her find herself and who she wanted to be. She cradled his head to her breast and hung on to him without saying a word. She loved him so much, she did not know how to express it, so she simply clung to him in silence, and then she took his face in her hands and kissed him tenderly and sweetly.

Dave looked into her eyes and melted the way he always did when he lost himself in her eyes. "Is this what you want to do for the rest of the afternoon and tonight?"

She smiled. "Pretty much." They didn't get dressed and they didn't leave the apartment until the next morning when they both went to work.

11
The Trauma Service

None of Dave's rotations were like the Trauma service. The stress level on Trauma goes from zero to maximum instantly then back to zero just as quickly. The physical demands also go from sitting or lying around in the Trauma call room, to doing everything as fast as possible, then back to doing nothing. Tom, Richard, Dave, and Jason had become a tight cohesive unit that functioned extremely well. They each knew their role and place on the team, they communicated well with each other under stress. Jason's transformation was nothing short of miraculous. He no longer got sick or fainted but jumped right in, no matter how gross the situation was, and he was calm, confident, and competent.

They had also developed a camaraderie that permeated their interactions. They were comfortable with each other, so they joked, jibed, and poked fun at one another. Their confidence bordered on cockiness, and they had a certain swagger because they were one of the best, if not the best, Surgery team in the hospital.

The Trauma team shifts went from seven AM to seven AM, like the other ED shifts. Trauma teams never left the ED during a shift, but waited in the call room for announcements alerting them about their next patient or patients. They ate there, sending the stud to the cafeteria for sandwiches and breakfast trays, and slept on the couches. During the down times between patients, they read or napped. There were long periods of boredom interspersed with intense periods of frantic activity and maximum duress.

The overhead in the doctors' lounge gave the particulars of an incoming ambulance. They ran to the Trauma unit to meet the Trauma nurses and to get ready. The doors flew open and the ambulance crew ran in with the patient, shouting the necessary information as they transferred the patient to the trauma table. A choreographed dance began. Dave tubed the patient and handled the airway until the anesthesiologist arrived, and then he put in a central line. Jason put in the peripheral lines. Richard and Tom gowned and gloved and went to each side of the table with one Trauma nurse at Tom's elbow with the instrument tray, while the other Trauma nurse hung blood or fluids and acted as the circulator. Tom assessed the patient then he and Richard would start whatever procedure was necessary. Dave, also gowned and gloved, joined them at Richard's side after the central line was in. When all the peripheral lines were in, Jason stood by for orders and instructions.

They took on car accidents, industrial accidents, gunshot wounds, and the whole meridian of broken, torn, damaged bodies that arrived in the ED daily, from severed or partially severed limbs, to gashed or ripped open abdomens and chests, to smashed heads, and other mangled body parts. It was bloody, ghastly work.

Dave still called Sharon when he was at the hospital to talk and say good night. About halfway through the month on a Saturday night, Dave was on the phone with her when Tom made a comment loud enough for Sharon to hear. "Tell Baby if she ever gets tired of a long-haired hippie like you and wants a real man, I am available."

Dave gave Tom the phone and Sharon responded, "You couldn't handle a woman like me." They all laughed and teased Tom about the put down.

Jason wanted Dave to say hello to Sharon for him. Dave handed the phone to Jason and said, "Say hello yourself."

Sharon used her sexiest, husky voice to say, "Hi, Jason, are you taking good care of Dave? I am depending on you to look after him for me."

Jason responded that he was taking care of Dave for her, then handed the phone back to Dave visibly effected by Sharon's voice. "Jesus, does she always talk that way on the phone?"

Dave answered, "She does it to tease. Did it turn you on?"

Jason blushed.

Even Richard got into the act and took the phone from Dave. "Sharon, can you get this hippie to get a haircut?"

Sharon responded, "Never, he gets his prowess from his long hair." Richard just whistled.

After Dave hung up, he had to deal with lewd comments from them. Tom led with, "You are without a doubt the most pussy-whipped man I have ever seen, but I do have to admit that is some mighty fine pussy to be whipped by."

Jason followed, "I wouldn't mind being whipped by a pussy like that."

Richard countered, "You wouldn't mind being whipped by any pussy."

Dave responded, "Jealousy, pure jealousy from horndog who can't get laid."

Tom responded, "Who said I can't get laid? Women line up and have to take a number to wait to be serviced by two studs like Jason and me."

Richard interjected, "You two are the ones who have to wait in line to get serviced." Everyone laughed.

It had been a quiet day, so they had spent the time sleeping and reading. Jason had made three food runs.

Tom was restless. "It has been too quiet. Something big is going to happen tonight. I can feel it. I am going to crack a chest tonight. I need to crack a chest."

"Trauma 1 and 2, four, repeat four ambulances five minutes out with multiple injuries due to MVA."

They ran to the unit and quickly got the room ready with a second table set up, so everything was duplicated and ready for two patients. The Surgery ER charge nurse joined them to circulate so the two Trauma nurses could assist the doctors and the Trauma charge nurse joined Trauma 1. They had everything ready when the doors burst open and the ambulance crews ran in with two gurneys. They quickly transferred the two patients to the tables, and the ambulance crews gave their reports. The nurses started cutting the patients clothes away. "My God, they are babies!"

Dave turned toward the first patient to tube her and saw she was a very pretty young blond girl not more than sixteen or seventeen. He looked over at the other table and saw another young girl about the same age with dark hair. Dave quickly tubed the blond girl, then moved to the other table to tube the second girl as the anesthesiologist and RT ran into the room. The dark-haired girl's abdomen was grotesquely distended, and they were both very pale. Dave and the anesthesiologist put central lines in the two girls while Jason and the charge nurse started the peripheral lines. After the lines were in, Dave and the anesthesiologist checked the girl's pupils; both girls were reactive, but the nurse reported they had virtually no BP. They got more help in the room and started pushing fluids and untyped blood, as the RT and anesthesiologist got both girls on ventilators with 100% oxygen.

Dave joined Richard as Richard opened the girl's abdomen and blood gushed out. "Suction and retraction. She has a ruptured spleen. I need to isolate the splenic artery and clamp it." Richard and Dave got the splenic artery clamped, but the massive bleeding continued, and more blood was coming out than they could push in. "She has a lacerated liver; we have to clamp the hepatic artery, and then I can get that bleeding controlled. More suction." They clamped the hepatic artery, but the bleeding continued. "More suction and more retraction." Richard continued to search for another source of the bleeding. "Oh my God, she has massive vascular damage. We can't control this, and there is no way to repair it."

The anesthesiologist said in a matter-of-fact voice, "She is fixed and dilated."

The charge nurse added, "She has no pressure or pulse."

Richard looked up at Dave. "She is gone."

Dave and Richard went to the other table to help Tom and Jason. Tom had made an incision in the girl's chest and had his hand inside her chest cavity squeezing her heart rhythmically as blood and fluids were pushed through the IVs.

"She has no pulse or pressure and her CVP (central venous pressure measured through the central line) is zero. Your compressions aren't doing any good because she is not filling between compressions. Let's look. Dave, retract. Tom, take your hand out." Richard and Tom pulled the incision apart and blood poured out. "All of her pulmonary vessels are torn. We are just putting blood in her chest cavity. There is no blood return to her heart."

"She is fixed and dilated," the anesthesiologist added.

Richard looked at Tom. "She is gone." They let the incision go and Dave pulled the retractor out as the wound closed, oozing blood.

Tom exploded, "God damn it! God damn it!" He stormed out of the room.

Richard looked at Dave and Jason. "They both had lethal injuries. There was nothing we could do. Jason, help the nurses get them cleaned up and tagged. I will pronounce them and write the note. I don't think Tom is very functional right now. Dave, check with the desk and see about their families. Come get me when you know what's going on out there."

Dave looked at the scene, and it was burned into his memory for the rest of his life. The endotracheal tubes and lines had been pulled. The beautiful blond girl was lying on the table nude, looking like she was asleep with a calm look on her angelic face; the only sign anything was wrong was a red line under her left breast. But the dark-haired girl's abdomen was gaping open with blood covering her, the table, and the floor. Her head was back with her mouth and eyes open in an expression of horror. Dave could not look away from the two girls as he stood there with emotion welling up in his chest.

He thought about what it meant for these two young girls to have their lives cut off. They would never go to any more proms or homecoming dances, they would never graduate from high school and go to college, and they would never experience love, get married, or have children and a family. The questions exploded in his head as they always did. Why did things like this happen? How did it fit into the overall scheme of things? He didn't ask where a benevolent, caring God was in all this. He had given up on that question. But he did ask, as he did when he was confronted with death, what is life? Was there more to life than complicated electrophysiologic biochemical processes and organic chemical reactions? If there was, what was it? What was the life force? The girls were here one minute and gone the next. Where did they go? Where did their essence go? Did it just drift off into the ether? Was there really a soul? Did all living things have a soul? Death was too much for Dave, and every time he dealt with it, he struggled with trying to get his head around it.

He went to the ED waiting room, and the triage nurse pointed him to two highway patrolmen who told him they had notified the four kids' parents of the accident. One boy was DOA, but they had not told that boy's parents he was dead. The other Trauma team's senior resident told them the second boy was brain dead, on life support, and he needed the parents' consent in order to pull the plug on him. The highway patrolmen had not told the second boy's parents that either. Dave asked the highway patrolman to come get him in the Trauma call room when the girls' parents got to the hospital.

The incident had affected Dave deeply but not as deeply as it affected Tom, who was sitting in the trauma call room covered in blood with his gown and gloves still on. "I had her little heart in my hand. I should have been able to do something. I held her life in my hand, and I let it slip away." He looked at his bloody gloved hand like Lady Macbeth.

Richard tried to console him. "She had lethal wounds, and there was nothing you could have done." Tom kept looking at his hand.

Dave broke the trance. "The parents of both girls are on their way in."

Tom looked at Dave and then looked down at himself. "Dave, can you and Richard handle them? I have to get cleaned up." He headed for the locker room to wash up and change his scrubs. Tom was never the same after what happened, but the change was for the better. He was humbled by the experience and stopped being such a self-centered, arrogant, cocky jerk. He had always been a good surgeon, he had always handled things well and done the right thing, but now he became a good human being and a caring doctor, but a beautiful, young girl had paid a terrible price for his transition.

The highway patrolman appeared at the door. "They are all here."

Richard said to Dave, "You take the dark-haired girl's parents. What was her name? I'll take the blond girl's parents. No details just the facts. They had lethal injuries. That's all. Nothing more. Spare them any details." Dave went out to do one of the most unpleasant tasks he would do during his internship.

Dave and Richard talked to the parents, got the on-call psychiatrist to see them, and Richard contacted the chaplain to come comfort them. The poor parents broke down, shattered and decimated with grief. That was another thing Dave would never forget—their destitute screams and cries of anguish.

Some more highway patrolmen arrived. After talking with them and the parents, Richard and Dave were able to put together what happened. The four kids were juniors in high school. They were good kids, from good families, popular, with good grades, and very bright futures. They had gone to the city to see a movie and were on their way home, when a drunk driver, driving out of control and very fast, careened into them and side-swiped their car, sending it over the median into the oncoming traffic where an eighteen-wheeler, doing over eighty miles an hour according to the skid marks, hit them broadside. The drunk driver did not have a driver's license because it had been suspended for previous DUIs. His car skidded to a stop on the shoulder, and he was unhurt. He was arrested for vehicular manslaughter and for driving under the influence. The driver of the eighteen-wheeler seemed out of it when the highway patrol questioned him, so they searched his cab and found amphetamines; he was arrested for DUI and speeding.

What a waste, Dave thought. *Four kids killed because of drugs and alcohol.* If the man had not been drunk, he would not have sideswiped the kid's car, and if the truck driver had not been loaded, he may not have been going so fast. The highway patrolman said the truck was fully loaded and probably doing close to ninety, so it was like the kid's car was hit by a freight train. That's what burst the girl's internal organs and ruptured their blood vessels; their bodies literally exploded from the impact. The emotion of the whole incident, coupled with the realization of what happened to the girls' bodies in the accident, sickened Dave. His brain cried out, and it was all he could do to keep from throwing up.

Dave went back to the trauma call room and buried the whole incident in the same graveyard he had buried all the other incidents he had experienced during the course of his internship, but the graveyard was getting crowded, and it was becoming harder and harder to keep the ghosts from escaping to haunt him. In truth, his emotions were being turned off in order for him to survive psychologically. The question was, would they turn back on of their own accord, or would he be able to turn them back on when his training was over?

There was one other incident that left an indelible impression on Dave while he was on the Trauma service, but it had nothing to do with medical training; it was about race and racism. Trauma 2 had just cleared their unit of a patient and Trauma One was working on a GSW to the chest, when Dave saw an overweight black woman in scrubs in the hall. He told her, "We need to get Trauma 2 cleaned right away. Trauma 1 is working on a GSW and Trauma 2 is the only unit open, so we need it cleaned ASAP."

The black woman turned slowly to look at Dave. "And who might you be?"

"I am Dr. Cameron." Dave realized from the way she acted and spoke, the woman was not a member of the cleaning crew.

She looked Dave up and down with disdain. "Well, I am the chief resident of thoracic surgery, and I am on my way to see a GSW to the chest, not to clean a room. Do you think every black woman you see is a maid?"

Dave's face colored. "No, I guess, yes, I don't know. I am sorry. The GSW is in Trauma 1."

The black woman scowled at Dave. "You think I don't know that? Are you stupid, or do you think I am stupid, because I am black?"

Oh shit, Dave thought. "No, I am not stupid, and I don't think you are stupid. I am not a racist. It's just that I have never met a black doctor before, especially not a black woman doctor. I am sorry."

"You may think you are not a racist, but you are. You are a white, Southern boy who is the product of his upbringing and his environment, both of which are decidedly racist. You are inherently racist, whether you are aware of it or not; otherwise, you would not have assumed I was the cleaning lady. Have you ever talked to a black woman who was not a maid in your house or some other white person's house? No, I doubt it. Now, I have to get a bullet out of a man's chest, and I don't have any more time to waste educating you on who and what you are. I suggest you do a little self-evaluation and soul searching on your own time." She turned back and continued to Trauma 1.

Dave stood watching her walk away as if he had been struck by a thunderbolt. He realized what she said was true. He only knew a few women doctors or medical students, none of whom were black. He had never talked to a black woman other than his mother's or grandmother's maid or the black women who did their washing and ironing, and then only to say hello. His subconscious mindset was racist because that was all he had ever been exposed to. Racism had been programed into him. No matter how he intellectualized it consciously, or how hard he tried to override it in his behavior and thoughts, it remained rooted in his very being. And if that were true for him, how about the vast majority of other people out there?

No wonder racism was such a problem. If you add man's inherent tribalism, mix in a little xenophobia, stir it with fear, hate, and bigotry, you get a complex problem with no simple solution. Racism was something that would take fundamental changes in the whole milieu of the entire human experience to resolve. That conclusion left Dave with a hollow feeling regarding his support of the civil rights movement and his intellectualization about his own racism. The thoracic surgeon was right, he needed to re-evaluate himself and look deeper into himself in order to correct his inherent racial bias.

A love story and social commentary

Christmas came and went without much fanfare. He and Sharon drove around his neighborhood looking at the decorated houses and Christmas lights one night. They had dinner in the city after walking around looking at the decorations in the store windows another night, and they shopped in the mall near his apartment to enjoy the decorations there. That was it.

All the students and stewardesses went home for Christmas, leaving only the three interns in town, and all three of them were working on Christmas Day. Dave had always gone home for Christmas when he was in college and in medical school. This was his first Christmas away, and he spent it in the hospital. Sharon had left her mother alone at Thanksgiving, but she would not leave her alone for Christmas, Dave was working, so she went home on Christmas Eve and stayed through the day after Christmas. She was flying and Dave was working the day she came back, so they did not see each other for four days—the longest they had been apart since the night they met.

They exchanged gifts before she left. Dave gave her a gold bracelet with a heart locket on it engraved with the word *Forever* on one side and *Love, Dave* on the other. She gave Dave a nice leather case with his initials on the outside and *Love, Sharon* on the inside. Sharon also had a gift for both of them to share. It was a carved wooden wall hanging that read *Our House, Our Home, Where Our Hearts Live*, and she had written on it in gold leaf *Dave and Sharon*.

Bob and Phil had people over for drinks on Christmas Eve, but everyone was gone except Dave, Mike, and Henry. Like the medical students and stewardesses, Connie and Janice had gone home. Henry was back in the Park house, so he and Mike walked over together, and Dave drove in from his apartment. Rachael and Sam also showed up, but no one else.

Bob and Phil's house was decorated, and they had a Christmas tree, so it was very festive. They stood around talking and drinking Champagne for a few hours then Dave went home to get a good night's sleep before his shift on Christmas Day. Sharon called later that night to wish him a Merry Christmas, but they didn't talk long.

The ED was busy on Christmas, but there was only one trauma case and it went to Trauma 1, so Dave's team hung around in the trauma call room listening to Christmas music playing on the overhead and watching TV. They slept through the night on the couches, and Dave went home to spend the next day without Sharon. He was lonely and missed her terribly. He smoked weed, listened to music, and watched football on TV. Sharon called that night, but again, they didn't talk long. Hearing her sexy, husky voice on the phone made Dave ache for her. It was absolutely the worst Christmas in his life.

Dave's last day on the Trauma service was also the last day of his Surgery rotation so he said his good byes. Tom told Dave he could be on his team any time, even though he was a long-haired, liberal, panty-waist hippie.

Tom took his hand firmly and said, "Take care of yourself, Goldilocks, and take care of Baby. I wish you both all the best. I am proud to have had you on my team, and I will miss you." It was high praise from the "new" Tom.

Richard said goodbye and added, "You are going to start your applications for residency soon. Think about doing Surgery and think about doing it here. I think you would make a fine surgeon. You have nerve, you handle tough situations well, you have excellent hands, and you can perform under stress. Tom and I will support your application." He shook Dave's hand and patted his shoulder. Dave valued Richard's respect more than anyone he had worked with during his internship.

Jason thanked Dave for all he had done for him and all he had taught him. "I will never forget how you helped me." Dave thought about the kid who fainted and threw up at the sight of blood when he first met him and what a solid steady man he was now.

Dave drove home thinking about the last six months. His weight was way down, he was pale, and hollow-eyed. His Surgery rotation had been tough on him. He had suffered emotionally and physically, yet a part of him would miss the drama and intensity. He had always been a bit of an adrenaline junky, but he knew it was not something he wanted to do for the rest of his life. He shifted his thoughts to the New Year's Eve party that night and Sharon. He would start in OB/GYN ER next, but first there was the party and a night with the woman he loved, then a whole day and night to spend with her after that. He buried the bodies deeper, pushed the ghosts back into the graveyard with them, and his mood brightened thinking about Sharon—her beauty, her warmth, her intellect, everything about her including her amazing body. Thinking about Sharon not only made him smile; it made him laugh and say, "Wow!"

It was New Year's Eve, and he was halfway through his internship. The poem "Invictus" came to him again. "My head is bloody but unbowed."

Part 4: OB/GYN

12
New Year's Eve

Dave wanted to get as much sleep as possible before the New Year's Eve party. Jake, Audrey, Dave, Sharon, Harven, Connie, Henry and a date were going to a party at a downtown hotel. Henry had reserved a table for eight at a party billed as a New Year's Eve Ball with a no-host bar, a Champagne greeting, a midnight Champagne toast, and a live band. The dress was formal or semiformal with attendance limited to fifty couples. It was expensive, so Sharon paid half. Dave said he had about five thousand dollars saved from his summer jobs and the monetary gifts from his family for his graduations, so he could afford a special night out, but Sharon insisted.

Dave attended an expensive private university that his grandparents had paid for and a state medical school where there was plenty of financial aid in the form of scholarships. His parents picked up the rest of his medical school cost. Sharon had attended a state university with the help of academic scholarships, and her mother paid for everything the scholarships didn't cover. Sharon had been living on half of what she made as a flight attendant, saving the rest, and she had signed a contract with Neiman Marcus.

Dave and Sharon decided to split a half-tab of acid and give the other half-tab to Connie and Harven to split. After what Dave had seen on the Trauma service, he did not want to drive on New Year's Eve with all the drunks, so they booked a room at the hotel. Sharon was excited about staying at the hotel, saying it made her feel naughty, like she was a real mistress. She had bought a sexy negligee and a new dress in New York for the occasion.

Dave woke up, had his usual pre-party meal of a ham sandwich, Doritos, and a Coke. He took a shower, shaved, spent extra time grooming himself, and splashed on Chanel Per Homme cologne. He wore his black suit, a white dress shirt, a blue silk tie, and black cap-toed dress shoes. He packed his on-call bag with his shaving kit, clothes and shoes for tomorrow, then took a tab of Owsley acid, halved it with a razor blade, and halved the two halves again, and put the four quarters in an envelope in the bag. He drove to Sharon's to pick her up early so they would have time to check into the hotel, leave their stuff in the room, drop the acid, and get to the party by eight.

Sharon was waiting for him in the front room with her travel bag.

"Oh, Baby!" Dave exclaimed when he saw her. The dress was red satin and fitted down to her ankles with a slit on one side to her thigh, making her slender figure look even more elongated. Her slim waist was accentuated by a wide band of material that anchored a swath of material that covered her breast, leaving a deep V from her throat to her cleavage, and her back bare from the band of material up. Her long hair was curled into large deep ringlets that flowed over her shoulders and back. Her makeup was alluring with red lipstick that matched the color of the dress and dark eyeliner that made her eyes even more pronounced. The smell of her perfume was heady, and she had used a fragrant body lotion that left her skin soft, moist, and sparkling with glitter. In a word, she was exquisite.

Dave was sure there was nothing on under the dress except her thigh-high silk stockings. A little exploring with his hands as he greeted her proved he was right. She laughed and slapped his hands away. "Behave! Besides, I have a surprise for you when we get to that."

She covered her upper arms, shoulders, and back with a wide red satin wrap and went out the door with her flight bag before Dave could molest her further. She didn't wear a coat because she was out of the house into the car, then out of the car into the hotel quickly, and she didn't want to spoil the effect of her dress and wrap. Driving to the hotel, Dave couldn't keep his eyes off her; she had to tell him multiple times to watch out and pay attention to his driving.

When they arrived at the hotel, Dave had Sharon wait for him in the lobby with their bags while he parked the car. He returned to the lobby to find three men in suits standing with Sharon, talking to her. Dave ignored the men, walked between them, picked up the two bags, and Sharon took his arm as they walked away. "That should teach you not to leave me in a hotel lobby alone. I could have made a lot of money tonight. They were in a bidding war for me, and the offers were getting very tempting. The last bid was almost twice what I make in month, and the guy was kind of cute."

Dave stopped and looked at her "What!"

Sharon laughed. "They were trying to buy me for the night. How much can you offer me for a night of sexual pleasure tonight?"

Dave looked back at the three men who were still watching Sharon. "What?"

Sharon pulled his arm to her. "Calm down. You get so jealous. Let tonight be a lesson to you: don't leave me in a hotel lobby alone. I might change professions. I could have had a good time with him and made enough to buy a new car."

The three men saw Dave scowling at them and walked away quickly. "What? Didn't you tell them you weren't an escort, and you were waiting for me?"

Sharon pulled him around and started walking toward the front desk. "Yes, but they were a little drunk and very excited about me. They paid no attention to what I was saying. They were German, and their English wasn't that good." She laughed. "But now I know what sex with me is worth, and I don't think you can afford me."

Dave frowned at her. "I am not letting you out of my sight again tonight." Dave knew how desirable Sharon was, but it never occurred to him that another man would actually try to buy her. He knew there were wealthy men who buy high-end escorts, like a commodity, to be used for sex, the same way they would buy a set of golf clubs to be used to play golf. He never thought they would try to buy any woman they wanted, whether she was an escort or not. This encounter unnerved him considerably and reinforced his understanding that there were people who lived in a completely different world, with a whole different set of rules and codes of conduct than the one he lived in.

Dave kept Sharon at his side as he checked in and got the key. She flashed the desk clerk a big smile and he gave them a room upgrade, looking at her the whole time, never even glancing at Dave. They took their stuff to the room, dropped the quarter tabs of acid, and went back down.

There was a line of elegantly dressed people at a table outside the doors of the ballroom signing in, paying, getting their glasses of Champagne, and having their hands stamped. Dave and Sharon quickly found Connie, Audrey, Harven, and Jake. Like Sharon, Connie and Audrey were wearing new dresses that displayed their figures in an unabashed alluring way.

Once they were together, Jake looked wide-eyed at the three women. "Wow, there is no doubt we are with the three hottest ladies here tonight. What did Jackson say? 'A plethora of pulchritude.' Damn, we got a plethora of pulchritude right here. Ladies, please just allow me to take in the view."

They all laughed. "Where is Henry? He is the one who picked this party and made the reservations. Was he still at the house when you left, Harven?" Dave gave the envelope with the other two quarter tabs of acid to Harven so he and Connie could drop the acid before the party started.

Harven replied, "I haven't seen Henry since before Christmas. I think he met someone. He had a meeting with Sheffield to go over his plans to do his Medicine residency here, then apply for a fellowship in Infectious Disease at Hopkins, with the goal of doing pure research at the CDC. Sheffield told him he would need a background in Immunology to do that and recommended he meet with someone from the Immunology Department at the University. I haven't seen him since."

They were standing in the line talking when Henry and his date arrived. "Jesus, she is as tall as Henry! She must be over six feet tall without heels." Dave was looking back down the line as Henry and a very tall, blond woman walked toward them. Henry was dressed in a perfectly tailored tux and was grinning as he strode toward the group with the tall blond woman on his arm. She was dressed in a slinky long silver formal with a wrap, and as she got closer, Dave saw she was hauntingly beautiful and had little or no makeup on. Her hair was so blond, it was almost white; her eyes were pale blue, and she was not only tall, but her shoulders were broad, and the muscles of her arms were well defined and toned. She was beautiful and fit.

Henry and the woman walked up to the group. "Sigrid, these are the friends I told you about. Sharon, Connie, Audrey, Dave, Harven, and Jake, this is Sigrid. She finished her PhD in Immunology in Copenhagen last year and is at the university working on a joint research project between her university and ours. She hasn't been in the States long or met many people, so I asked her to join us tonight."

Sigrid released Henry's arm and stepped away from him to offer her hand to each of them. "I have heard a great deal about each of you, so I feel I know all of you already. I am so pleased to finally meet you." Her English was perfect with a Danish accent that made her sound decidedly sexy.

As Dave took her hand, he thought, *She is a lab rat just like Henry; she is a great, big, beautiful lab rat.* As he released her hand, Dave looked at Henry and realized in all the years he had known his friend, he had never seen him so happy.

The women Henry dated all fit the same mold: small, cute, rich, well bred, sophisticated, and deferential to Henry. Sherry had been the perfect example of Henry's type. Sigrid was the exact opposite of Sherry. Sigrid was tall, she was anything but cute with a deep universal beauty, she was the product of a European social democracy, and Dave could tell immediately she would not be deferential to anyone. As the evening went on, Dave would discover Sigrid was Henry's equal in every way, not only in size and athletic ability, but in intelligence, education, sophistication, experience, knowledge, and understanding of the world. Dave thought that at another time in history, Sigrid would have been a famous shield maiden. She was the embodiment of a Valkyrie.

Dave could not wait to talk to Henry alone as he mused over what Henry told him about Sharon. "You love her because you love yourself, and she is just like you." *Well, touché my friend*, Dave thought. But all that was for later. The acid was coming on, it was time to celebrate, and Henry's happiness only added to Dave's joy.

Henry took charge when they reached the reception table. They paid, had their hands stamped, received their glasses of Champagne, and found their table in the ballroom based on the number they were given. Henry stopped them from sitting down as he stood and with his glass raised, he said, "Here's to us, to friendship, and to our future. May we continue to share nights like this for a long time to come." They clinked glasses, took a sip of Champagne, and sat down at the large round table.

Sigrid looked around the table. "I want to thank all of you for allowing me to join you tonight." She raised her glass to them and took a sip of her Champagne. It was apparent she was warm, friendly, and personable.

Jake was sitting next to Sigrid. "I have to amend my previous statement; we are with the FOUR hottest ladies in the room. Our plethora of pulchritude has just been enhanced by one. Sigrid, collectively, we are known as the gang, and we are more than happy to welcome you. How did you and Henry meet, and please tell me you two are on a date, we are going to see more of you, and that Henry is not just being a good Samaritan to a beautiful lonely Danish girl who is new to our country."

"Be careful, Sigrid, he is a pilot and has an overinflated opinion of himself as a suave, charming jet jockey who has a way with women." Audrey added, "But yes, we are all dying to know where you met Henry and if you are dating. I am sorry, but we are sort of like a family, so naturally, we are going to grill you a little."

"Henry told me you are all very close, and there are actually more of you in this gang. He told me the three couples here tonight are all lovers who will soon be married." She looked at Sharon and Dave, and Dave could tell there was a fierce intelligence behind those pale blue eyes that were now sparkling with mirth. "And he told me you two made love at first sight."

Henry laughed. "No Sigrid, I said they fell in love at first sight."

Sharon was high and happy. "No, Sigrid is right; we did make love at first sight; everyone knows that. It took us a little longer to fall in love. We fell in lust at first sight." Everyone laughed. They were all happy because they were young, in love, their futures were unlimited, and it was New Year's Eve.

Sigrid looked mischievous. "And are you still in lust?"

Sharon gave Dave a sexy, come-hither look. "Little bit." They all laughed again.

Sigrid looked at Henry and touched his arm with her hand. "Is that the way it is with you Americans? You fall in lust first, and then you fall in love?"

The look Sigrid gave Henry and the way she touched his arm told Sharon everything she needed to know about their relationship, and the way Henry looked back at her generated enough heat that Sharon could feel it across the table. *Wow*, Sharon thought, *Henry is not just in lust, he is in love, and I think she is too.*

Still looking at Henry as he gazed back at her, Sigrid continued, "The leader of my research team told me I had to meet with an American doctor who wanted to know how Immunology research related to Infectious Disease research." Sigrid looked back at them. "I was very annoyed. I had a lot of work to do, and I did not have time to waste on some doctor who was too dumb to know how Immunology was related to Infectious Disease. I had to set aside an afternoon to meet with him on a day he chose because of his schedule, with no regard to my schedule. I had to meet with this moron the day after Christmas when I was already behind on my work because of the holiday. I decided to be unpleasant to him and end the meeting early so I could get back to my work." She looked back at Henry with a warm smile. "I was even more annoyed when this handsome, charming man showed up and distracted me to the point that I found myself not wanting to be unpleasant to him. We talked into the evening about how to deal with virus strains that attenuate so quickly they don't lend themselves to an immunological form of treatment or vaccine for prevention." She looked back at the group. "We argued because he is very arrogant and thought he knew all the answers, when in reality, he didn't know what he was talking about."

Harven interrupted. "I am shocked. Shocked to hear that Henry was arrogant."

"I am shocked. Shocked to hear Henry thought he knew everything," Dave added.

Sigrid laughed and continued, "It is obvious you both know him well. It got late, and we were still talking, so he asked me to go to dinner with him."

Harven interjected again. "Henry, you sly dog, you wooed her with immunologically resistant, attenuating virus strains."

Dave followed with, "How could she resist the temptation of a double-blind study on how a virus strain's rapidly changing protein coat effects its virulence?"

Henry responded, "Very funny. You two think you are so funny." But Henry was smiling and having a great time.

Sigrid turned to Dave. "What did you talk to Sharon about to get her to fall in lust with you at first sight?" Then she looked at Sharon. "No, you answer, Sharon."

"Literature, art, and travel," Sharon answered.

"Things you both like, correct? Was he arrogant and opinionated, and did you argue?" Sigrid added.

Sharon laughed. "Yes, yes, and yes. He tried to convince me his macho literary hero Hemingway was not a male chauvinist warmonger." Sharon looked at Dave. "But then, I found out his real hero and role model is Huxley, and that sealed the deal." She touched his arm the same way Sigrid had touched Henry's arm.

Sigrid smiled. "And you, Connie and Harven, and you, Audrey and Jake, did you not connect on the things you have in common and things you both like, then did you not discuss them to grow closer? Henry and I are researchers, that's what we have in common. So, we discussed infectious disease and immunology." She looked back at Henry.

"OK, that's enough grilling. I need a real drink, and I am trading this Champagne in for a Scotch. Anyone else want to hit the bar? Can I bring you something, Sigrid?" Henry stood up.

"No, I will go with you." Sigrid stood up as Henry rushed to pull her chair out for her, and they walked to the bar at the back of the room.

After they walked away, Dave laughed. "Henry is in love. I never thought I would see it in my lifetime. He is smitten. I just hope she is as smitten as he is."

"Oh, she is. She has him hooked, the hook is set, and she has reeled him in." Sharon eyes were dancing.

"For some reason, that sounds familiar. Is that what you did to me?" Dave took her hand.

"Pretty much. Only you scared me a little at first, and I wasn't sure I wanted to reel you in. Then you started that macho Hemingway BS, and I almost threw you back." Sharon pulled him over so she could kiss him.

"I like her. I like her a lot." Audrey watched them walking away.

"So do I," Connie added. "She is head and shoulders above Sherry, literally and figuratively." They all laughed.

"I can tell you one thing, she is smart. I think she may be smarter than Henry. And did you see her body? She is an athlete. I think she is Henry's match in everything. I like her too, and I can see why Henry fell so hard for her." Dave looked at Sharon.

"She completes us. Henry needed someone for us to be whole. Hot damn, we all have it going on. I am sorry, I don't want to get emotional, but I feel fortunate to be a part of this group. I yearned for things like this when I was in country." Jake raised his glass. "Man, I am glad to be alive, home, and with friends." He was a little choked up as they clinked glasses and drank.

Audrey took Jake's arm and put her head on his shoulder. "I love you."

"I love you, too." Jake put his arm around her and hugged her.

"You know, Jake is right. We are all very fortunate, and we should be grateful for the kind of lives we have, the love we have, and the friends we have. Happy New Year, everyone." Harven raised his glass and they toasted the New Year, then he leaned over to kiss Connie. That was the end of the Champagne, so the men joined Henry and Sigrid waiting in line at the bar.

Dave stood beside Sigrid. Even though her body was toned, and her shoulders were broad, she was not big; she was tall and slender. "Sigrid, I can't help but notice you must be an athlete, or you were an athlete at one time. Jake and I played American football, and of course Henry told you he was a world-class swimmer, so what did you play or do?"

Sigrid looked at Henry. "Henry, you are a swimmer?"

Dave looked at Henry. "You didn't tell her? Sigrid, I think he still holds some records. Henry, didn't you hold the world record in something at one time, and don't you still hold some American records? He also won a National Championship."

Henry looked annoyed. "I held the world record in the 200-meter fly very, very briefly, at one meet, and I may still hold the American record. I am not a swimmer anymore, and I don't follow swimming or keep up with it since I stopped competing." He put his arm around Sigrid. "I would rather do double-blind studies on viral receptor sites." He laughed as he hugged her.

Sigrid smiled. "I was involved in sports at university, but now I just work out regularly to keep in shape."

Henry added, "Me too, and if we ever get to this bar, I will show you what I do to keep my right arm in shape."

Sigrid untangled herself from Henry. "I think now that all the boys are here to keep you company, I will rejoin the girls. Get me a glass of a nice dry Riesling, please." She walked back to the table.

Henry watched her go. "Isn't she something?" When she sat down at the table Henry looked back at Dave. "OK. Give me all the shit you want. I am ready for it, but I am going to preempt you by saying you were right. You can go down the line of all the things I said to you, everything you said back to me, and right here and right now, I will say, you were right." Henry laughed. "Boy, were you right."

Dave replied, "Does she know how rich you and your family are?" Dave knew she had to know Henry had money from his car and clothes.

"She knows. I am playing this straight down the line by Dave Cameron rules. When I told her I had a trust fund and my family had a lot of money, she laughed at me and asked if money was all we Americans ever thought about. She accused me of being like all American men—obsessed with money and sex. I had to work to convince her I was concerned about doing research to promote the advancement of science for the common good. I couldn't believe a woman got mad at me for telling her I had money. She said my family and I were evil for hoarding money, not sharing it with those in need. It took me even longer to convince her I was a socialist, like her, and I intended to use my money to benefit others."

Dave laughed. "So, you convinced her you were not obsessed with money. Did you convince her you were not obsessed with sex?"

"No. I can't keep my hands off her. She said, 'You know, Henry, we can have sex anytime; we don't have to have sex all the time.' But I can't help myself. Go ahead and give me a hard time. I don't care. Tell me you were right, and I was wrong. I agree you were right all along, and I was wrong. But you should see the body she has, no you shouldn't, I mean, you know what I mean. Plus, she is brilliant. You joked about it, but it's true—I get turned on talking to her. When she talks about immunology, it's like she is talking dirty to me. I know you think I am crazy, but she is so damn smart, just listening to her makes me hot for her."

Dave cracked up. "Ohhhh, Cisco, you got it bad, man. You is smitten, man; you is way smitten with it. Cisco, you got the fever, man, you got the way high fever. You is burning up with it."

"Fuck you, Poncho. You is one big kettle calling this pot black. You got so much fever, I'm surprised you is not burned up from spontaneous combustion." Dave and Henry continued laughing and bantering about Henry's new-found love and Dave's love for Sharon while enjoying each other's happiness.

Audrey smiled at Sigrid when she sat down with them. "You two are an item; it is obvious from across the room. Henry is a great guy; they are all great guys, but Henry is special. I think you know that already."

Sigrid looked down and blushed a little. "What is it, an item? Does it mean if we are an item, we are lovers?"

Sharon answered, "Little bit." The acid was peaking, but it was a mild peak, and she was just very high and happy. She liked Henry a lot, so she was thrilled about Sigrid. "And if Henry is anything like his friend, Dave, it is probably more than just a little bit." The other two women laughed.

Sigrid's blush increased. "I think maybe he is a little like his friend. We have been together constantly since we met, unless of course he is at the hospital. I feel terribly guilty because I have neglected my work to be with him." She looked up. "He is very intense. Are all American men so intense?" All three of the other women laughed.

Connie got up. "Come on, girls." They all got up and moved around the table to sit on each side of Sigrid. "Sigrid, he is intense because of you; you make him intense. Normally, Henry is anything but intense. American men are like any other men—they get intense when they are an item."

Sigrid looked around at them. "Your men are also so intense?"

Connie laughed. "Sigrid, all men are intense when it comes to being an item."

Sigrid blushed more. "I have not had many lovers. I have always been focused on my academics, busy with sports, and now I am engrossed in my research. Then along comes this intense American man, and he changes everything."

Audrey was sitting on one side of Sigrid. "I think I can speak for all three of us when I say the same thing happened to us. We were all comfortably living our lives when along came a man who turned our lives upside down."

The men returned with the drinks and were met with a chorus of, "You guys sit over there; we are sitting over here with our new friend Sigrid." "No boys allowed." "She needs to be protected from intense American men." Sigrid laughed.

Jake shook his head. "Next, they will be hugging."

Dave added, "We are lucky they have those dresses and heels on, or they would be jumping up and down hugging."

Henry chimed in, "They group hug, they jump up and down, and they go to the bathroom together. I just don't understand women."

A love story and social commentary

Sharon led them, and despite their high heels and dresses, they stood up, formed a circle with their arms around each other, and jumped up and down together.

Henry sat down. "I fucking give up. It is international. She is from Denmark, and she does it too. At least they are not squealing."

Sigrid put her head back and the others joined her as she squealed.

Jake looked at Henry. "You had to say it, didn't you? You couldn't leave well enough alone."

The entire room turned to look when they heard the squeal. "Do you think you are a bunch of Dallas Cowboys cheerleaders?" Harven put down the two wines he was carrying. "Sit down and behave. You are making a pulchritudinous spectacle of yourselves."

The women sat back down laughing. Henry handed Sigrid her glass of white wine and she raised it. "To all my new friends, Skol."

Sharon raised her glass. "To Sigrid our new friend. Skol."

Connie giggled and raised her glass. "To love. Skol."

Jake raised his glass. "To love and friends. Skol."

Audrey raised her glass. "To love, friends, and the New Year. Skol."

Harven raised his glass. "To lust, love, friends, the New Year and let's put some emphasis on the lust. Skol."

Dave raised his glass. "To love, lust, friends, the New Year, Sigrid and Henry. Skol."

Henry looked at Sigrid and raised his glass. "To Sigrid. Welcome to America, welcome to our group of friends, but most of all, welcome into my life. Skol."

The orchestra filed on to the raised stage at the front of the room as they finished their toast. The tables were arranged in a horseshoe in front of the stage, leaving ample room for dancing between the tables and the stage. When the band was introduced and began to play "Moonlight Serenade," Dave led Sharon to the dance floor by the hand. Like all well-bred, Southern kids, they had taken ballroom dancing at age twelve when they were in the sixth grade, so they fell right in with the music. The acid carried them along as they glided around the dance floor in each other's arms with their bodies producing a palpable current where they touched.

Dave put his lips near Sharon's ear as they glided on the music. "I love the way you look tonight."

Sharon whispered back in Dave's ear, "I love you; I want to be with you forever like we are tonight." They stopped dancing for a moment and held each other with their lips touching each other's ear in a gentle kiss. The acid, the music, and the night put Sharon in a dream-like state as she swirled into the next dance only aware of Dave and the music.

They danced until the band took a break then walked back to the table arm and arm with their heads together, smiling at each other intimately. When they got back to the table, Dave noticed that Sigrid was watching them closely with her intelligent pale eyes that didn't miss anything. Despite the cold blueness of their color, her eyes conveyed warmth and understanding as she studied Dave and Sharon.

The night went by quickly as they danced, talked during the band breaks, and got to know Sigrid. Dave became more impressed with her the more he learned about her. She was brilliant and had progressed through school at an accelerated pace, earning her PhD in her early twenties. She was younger than the rest of them but seemed more mature than any of them. She competed in track and field at her university, making the national team, but not the Olympic team. She was a sprinter and long jumper, so she and Dave talked about that. She was a scientist, but she was also well rounded, well read, and had backpacked through Europe during the summers she was in college. She knew art, literature, and history, so she, Sharon, Dave, and Henry had a lively discussion during one of the breaks.

Jake said Sigrid completed them, and he was right. All eight of them were bright, well educated, well-read with a sense of purpose to their lives. They fit together as a group. Dave thought how privileged and fortunate they were compared to the patients he saw at University Hospital. That led him to understand Henry was right—because they were bright, educated, and principled, they were obligated to make a contribution. They were obligated to try to better the lives of others and not be centered only on themselves. Mama was right too; they were blessed, and they should never forget to share their blessings with others. The acid had made Dave wax philosophical, and now as he looked around the table, he experienced a warm, full, happy feeling of contentment. *Jake is right,* he thought. *We all got it going on now.*

Dave followed Henry to the bar during a break and pulled him aside. "Henry, you can't let that woman get away. You will never find anyone else like her. You are right, she is exceptional. Do whatever you have to do, but don't lose her."

Henry looked troubled. "I know, but she is only here for six months. She will finish her research project and go back to Denmark. She has a place on the university staff there and is planning to return to teach and continue her research. I don't know what to do. She has her career, I have mine, and the Atlantic Ocean is between us. I can't give up my dream, and I can't ask her to give up hers."

Dave looked Henry straight in the eyes. "Bullshit, Henry. You only get a chance for happiness like this once in a lifetime. Follow her to Denmark and do your training there. Use your family's influence to get her a position here. Find a way to make it work. I could never be happy without Sharon, and I will do anything to keep her in my life. Do whatever it takes to keep Sigrid in your life."

"Oh, Poncho, you do fuck with a man's head with all your romantic notions. It scares the hell out of me to think about changing my whole life for a woman. My logical mind rejects emotional decisions like that." Henry looked back at Dave intently.

"You are not changing your life for a woman or making an emotional decision. You are changing your life for love, and there is no decision to be made, emotional or otherwise. You have no choice. You choose love or live with regret for the rest of your life." Dave took Henry by the shoulders. "Choose love, Henry."

When they came back to the table, Sigrid looked at them with an amused expression on her face. "I saw you two talking. Should I be worried?"

Henry reached for her hand. "No. There is nothing to worry about. I can see that now."

Sigrid looked at him. "What?" Henry kissed her. "Henry!" He kissed her again, and this time, she kissed him back.

Harven said, "Now that's what I call some lust if I have ever seen it." They all laughed and raised their glasses to Henry and Sigrid as they kissed.

Sharon leaned over to Dave. "What was that all about?"

Dave responded, "Remember when you came out of the pool and stood on the ladder in the white bikini?"

Sharon smiled. "You mean he knows he loves her?"

Dave smiled back. "He would be fool not to, and if there is one thing Henry is not, it's a fool. Do you think she loves him?"

Sharon looked at them. "She loves him. She may not know it yet, but she loves him. They are made for each other."

Dave took Sharon's hand. "Like us?"

"Yes, like us."

After the discussion at the bar, the subject of free will came up at another break. Henry realized he was compelled to be with Sigrid. So, Henry brought it up. He pointed out that there was no free will. All decisions were predetermined by nature and nurture. Everyone was the product of their experiences and driven by their genetic memory, so their decisions were based on their paradigms, dynamics, and genetics. Dave countered that if there was no free will, there was no humanity, no human factor, and no soul. Dave believed all living things had a soul, an intangible something within them that defined life. Sharon added that humans did have free will because they could use deductive reasoning and didactic evaluations in their decision making. Sigrid sealed the argument against Henry by pointing out that humans could use intellectualization to decide. They did not have to be driven by their dynamics, paradigms, and genetic memory; they could override that with intellect. They could recognize their thoughts and behaviors were the results of those things and choose to think and act differently.

Audrey said she thought there might be some drives you could not override, no matter how much you intellectualized. Jake countered that the strongest drive in any living thing was the drive to survive, but he had seen guys override that drive and die to save someone else in Vietnam.

Harven ended the discussion by getting involved with Connie's assets and stating there was absolutely no way he could keep his drive for her intellectualized because there was no connection between his brain and the organ that controlled that drive. "Freud was right, everything is about sex, and Henry is right—there is no free will. There is only sex, and everything revolves around sex. We are sexual creatures, sex drives our will, nothing else, and our will is certainly not free."

Connie pushed him away and laughed. "I hate to admit it, but I believe in your case, that is true."

Midnight came, they kissed, toasted the New Year with the Champagne, sang Auld Lang Syne then danced until the party ended at one. Audrey, Connie, Jake, and Harven had taken a cab together to the hotel so they took a cab back to the park. Henry and Sigrid had driven to the hotel, but Henry vowed he was fine to drive. Dave and Sharon caught the elevator up to their room, and since they were the only ones on the elevator, Sharon's dress was on its way off before they got to the room.

The upgraded room was large with a king-size bed and a floor-to-ceiling double window looking over the city. Sharon took her bag, headed for the bathroom, and closed the door. She took her dress off and hung it on the door hook. As Dave had surmised, she had nothing on under the dress. She put on a long sheer red negligee that was tied with a silk ribbon under her breast.

Dave was undressed and in the bed when she opened the bathroom door and stood with the light behind her. She got exactly the response she expected as Dave exclaimed, "Oh, Baby!" He was out of bed in a single bound, but she ignored him and walked to the floor-to-ceiling window, pulled the curtain back and stood in the window with her arms out, her hands touching each side of the window opening. Their room was not that high, and if anyone on the street below had looked up, they would have seen the beautiful woman standing in the window gazing out at the city, but it was late, no one was on the street, so no one saw the apparition in the hotel window.

She was still tripping but it was mild, and she had reached the mellow thoughtful stage. Dave walked up behind her, put his arms around her, and put his face beside hers. Sharon put her head over so he could kiss and nuzzle her neck, but she did into move or turn from the window. They both looked out at the bright twinkling lights of the city. All the buildings had left their lights on for New Year's Eve, so the city was aglow with white and colored lights of all types. Through the lens of the acid, the city looked like a giant kaleidoscope of colors and shapes.

"This time will be over soon. Caroline will marry Ron and move to New York, because that is where Ron needs to be to advance his career. Audrey will marry Jake, he will get promoted, and they will move to a different base. Connie and Harven are going to California after they get married. Who knows what will become of Sigrid and

Henry? They are from two different countries, thousands of miles apart. We will all go our separate ways to fulfill our hopes and dreams. We will never be together again like we are now. Promise me we will stay in touch with our friends, no matter where we are. Oh, Dave, I love our life the way it is. I know it can't go on like this and has to change, but I am going to miss these times and nights like this." She turned in his arms and kissed him.

Dave was tripping too, and the feel of her body through the negligee was too much for him. He scooped her up and carried her to the bed. She started to take the negligee off, but he stopped her. "Please, leave it on." Dave stood beside the bed and looked at her lying there in the negligee. "Tonight is for you." He gave her a night of sensual pleasure and sexual ecstasy she would never forget.

Dave woke up from an incredibly erotic dream to find it was not a dream. Sharon was on top of him with her arms around his neck, nibbling at his ear with her hair down around his face, and he could smell the Chanel and her body lotion. "You were ready, so I started without you." She laughed. "Now it's my turn to take care of you." And she did. They made love with the morning light streaming through the big window bathing them in its warm glow.

They lay in bed cuddling and enjoying the feel of their bodies against each other until Sharon sat up. "Let's try out the tub." She left Dave in the bed and went to the bathroom to start filling the big tub. The negligee was long gone, and Dave watched her walk to and from the bathroom with an overwhelming realization that her body really was perfect, she really was beautiful, and they really would always be together like this. She came to the bed and pulled him up by the hand.

"Come on. God, you would think you had never seen me naked before. Come on, this tub is great. Stop ogling me, and let's go have some fun in the tub. You always wanted to go skinny dipping; well, let's go skinny dipping."

Dave grabbed her, pulled her down on the bed, and rolled on top of her burying his face in her breast. "Dave, the water might run over. Come on, you can play with the girls in the tub."

Dave stood up beside the bed. "I want to live here. We can live here and never get dressed or leave the room. We will make love all the time and order room service when we're hungry."

A love story and social commentary

Sharon took the opportunity to slip past him and run to the bathroom. The tub was full, so she got in. Dave was right behind her, slid in the tub beside her, and immediately returned his attention to Sharon's breasts as they frolicked in the big tub. They bathed each other and used the hand attachment to wash each other's hair. They got out, toweled off, dried their hair, and Sharon reached for the robes. "No. Bare skin or black negligee, no robes." Dave took the robe from her and put it back.

"Where is my negligee? I was not in complete control of my faculties when it came off, and I have no idea how it got off or where it is." Sharon walked back to the bedroom looking for her negligee.

Dave followed. "It evaporated. You are so hot, you vaporized it."

Sharon found the negligee buried in the sheets. "You know you spoiled me last night, so now I am going to expect that from you all the time." She came to him and kissed him. "Do you know when check-out is? We could order room service and have breakfast in bed, but you have to wear a robe. I have told you before, I am not eating with you with no clothes on."

Dave called the front desk and they told him check-out was normally noon, but they had extended it until one o'clock because all the guests were up late for New Year's Eve. The front desk transferred him to room service, and he ordered breakfast.

Sharon went to the bathroom and retrieved the robes. "I am going to put this on for breakfast and so are you. I am not greeting the room service guy in this negligee." She threw the robes on the bed and walked back to stand in the window looking out again. "What a wonderful way to start the new year. When last year started, I could never have imagined it would end the way it did last night, and in my wildest dreams, I could not have conceived of the next year starting the way it did this morning. I want to spend every New Year's Eve in a hotel. I wonder what cities I will look out over in the future?"

She came back and lay across the bed on her stomach with her chin in her hands. "I wonder where being with you will take me from here and how much more it will change my life." She rolled onto her back. "It has already been a wild ride far beyond my comfort zone. How much more is there to experience that I never even knew was out there? Sigrid was right about men like you. You are intense, the ride is scary and feels out of control sometimes, but it is wonderful and fulfilling, and I never want it to end. I wonder how dull and unfulfilled my life would have been if I had never met and fallen in love with you. I love your inquisitive mind, your need to know and your need to experience, to participate and be involved, your lust for life, and not just your lust for sex and for me, although that too, but your lust to live life to the fullest. Like I told you when I met you, it is what is above the shoulders, not what is below the waist. But you taught me about what is below the waist, Jesus, have you ever taught me about that, and last night was an incredible lesson. I love you for that too."

Dave lay down beside her and held her until room service came.

13
GYN ED

The OB/GYN ER was vastly different from the Medicine or Surgery ER. The OB/GYN ER was really the GYN ER with all pregnant women going to Labor and Delivery for their care. The shifts were staggered with one shift of twelve hours on and twelve hours off, alternating with a shift of twenty-four hours on with twenty-four hours off. Dave worked from seven AM to seven PM, returning the next day to work from seven AM until seven AM the following day, then back at seven AM after twenty-four hours off to work a twelve-hour shift again. There were no teams; Dave worked with whomever was on, and that varied from shift to shift with schedules of the residents, other interns, and students. One thing that really struck Dave on his OB/GYN rotation was that women's health was mostly in the hands of men. There was one woman on the OB/GYN teaching staff at University Hospital and only a few female OB/GYN residents.

The cases he saw were mostly boring and repetitious, consisting mainly of STDs, vaginitis, Bartholin's gland cysts or abscesses, pelvic inflammatory disease, excessive vaginal bleeding or dysfunctional bleeding, lower abdominal pain, painful intercourse, and UTIs.

Many of the patients he saw came from black or Latino neighborhoods where the people lived in dire poverty with no hope or opportunity. Others were homeless and lived in tents or cardboard boxes, suffering from drug addiction, alcoholism, or mental illness. In the rural areas outside the city where the black and Latino families tried to survive on the land, the living conditions were even more primitive with dirt roads, no sewer or water, and no electricity.

The results were the children went hungry and the old people were neglected. The worst case of neglect he saw was an elderly black woman whose family brought her into the ER because she said she had a problem with her breast but refused to let anyone look at it. It was another case where he smelled the patient before he saw her. The nurse came to get Dave after the old woman was in a hospital gown. "You have got to see this to believe it."

Dave put a mask on to cut the smell and followed the nurse to the exam area. When the old woman finally let him pull back the gown to see her breast, he gagged, not only on the smell, but at what he saw. Her right breast was completely replaced by a slow growing, fungating carcinoma with superficial infection and necrosis. The cancer had destroyed her breast. What was left was nothing more than a rotting mess. Dave put the gown back and paged the Surgery team on call, but there was nothing they could do for her except remove the breast and make her as comfortable as possible until she died.

These cases of neglect caused Dave to question how the richest country in the world could allow people to live in conditions that produced such things. It was as if the Great Depression Steinbeck described in *The Grapes of Wrath* still existed in the poor rural areas of the South and in the city slums. Both Dickens and Steinbeck emphasized the corrosiveness poverty had on a society, the damage it did, and how it infected the whole culture, yet Dickens child of Mankind, Want, was still alive and well in the richest country in the world. Dave confronted it every day at University Hospital.

He knew a lot of it was tied to racism, but since many of the impoverished were white, it couldn't all be based on race. Lack of education and opportunity were factors that crossed the color line and produced most of the misery. It was a type of social Darwinism or natural selection ingrained with the premise of survival of the fittest. It was the by-product of a capitalistic economy where individualism and the individual were overemphasized. The collective or common good was secondary to and subjugated by the myth that Americans were rugged individualists who could take care of themselves and didn't need any help. The myth that in America, individual freedom was more important than the collective good, was used by politicians to get people to vote against their own self-interests. Dave could not help but put what he saw in his country in juxtaposition with what he had seen in the social democracies of Europe.

But racism and bigotry were always present, adding to and fueling the issues produced by poverty and poor education. The worst case of racism Dave encountered in the GYN ED involved a poor white couple who lived in the same conditions as the blacks they hated.

There was a black RN on the three-to-eleven shift Dave liked to work with. She warmed up to Dave when she heard Dave on the phone with Sharon talking about jazz and the blues. She approached him after he said good night to Sharon.

"Dr. Cameron, I couldn't help hearing you on the phone with Baby. My dad had an incredible collection of blues and jazz records he left to me. That record collection and my love of music were about the only things he left me. Would you like to borrow some of my records?"

"You know you can call me Dave." Dave was sitting in the doctors' station after calling Sharon.

"No, I can't, and you know why. Would you like to borrow some records to play with Baby? Who do you like?" She was standing next to the ward clerk's desk, who was also black.

"I am old-school where jazz is concerned. I like Dizzy, Bird, and Trane but Be-Bop can get too far out for me. I prefer Coleman Hawkins, Sidney Bechet, Oscar Peterson, and of course Mister Louis Armstrong, not Hello Dolly Louis Armstrong, but Hot Five and Hot Seven Louis Armstrong, King Oliver Louis Armstrong, Do You Know What It Means to Miss New Orleans and Basin Street Blues Louis Armstrong. For the blues, you know Muddy Waters invented electricity, but John Lee Hooker is my favorite. I love St. James Infirmary. I am glade bands like the Stones, ZZ Top, and the Allman Brothers are covering some of their songs. Of course, the blues is the back bone of American music and will always be a part of any good rock and roll," Dave answered.

The black ward clerk turned to Dave. "You can hang with John Lee?" She and the RN looked at each other and laughed. The three of them got into a discussion about the blues, jazz, and their influence on rock and roll. They talked about jazz-rock fusion, like Steely Dan, blues-rock fusion, like the Rolling Stones, and the blues' influence on folk-rock. Their discussions about music continued when things were slow in the ER. The RN brought some great records for Dave to play with Sharon on their nights together at Dave's apartment.

They were in the middle of one of these discussions one night when the stud approached Dave. "There is a man who won't let me see his wife. He said he doesn't want a short-coat doctor; he wants a long-coat doctor."

Many of the patients who frequented University Hospital knew that students wore short coats and MDs wore long coats. "Let's go." Dave laughed and said to the black RN, "We will give them an RD, a real doctor, and an RN, a real nurse."

When Dave pulled the curtain back, the husband yelled at him. "Get that nigger out of here; she's not touching my wife, and neither are you. I told that short-coat doctor I want a real doctor. I am not going to let some nigger and a long-haired hippie take care of my wife."

Dave looked at the man and his wife. The man's breath smelled of stale beer. His fingernails were ragged and dirty, his skin was pallid, and his eyes had a watery bloodshot hue. His clothes were grimy and rumpled, as were his wife's. Dave said, "She is a registered nurse, and I am an MD, but if you don't want us, I will put your chart back, and you can wait until a white nurse and another doctor with short hair are available."

"We been waiting long enough; you get someone right now!" Dave realized the man was drunk, and one look at the wife told him she was abused. She sat shaking on the exam table.

Dave closed the curtain. "Get security."

When the black security guards showed up, the husband went off on them too; they zip-tied him and got him out of the ED in no time.

Dave sent the stud back with a white LVN to examine the wife.

"I am sorry. You didn't deserve that," Dave said to the black RN when they were back at the doctors' station.

She replied, "You didn't do anything, so you don't need to apologize. You think that is the first time something like that has happened to me? I deal with it all the time."

Dave felt ashamed. "You are an excellent nurse. Why don't you leave and go where things like that don't happen? I am applying to programs in California to get away from this kind of shit. Why don't you move out of the South?"

She looked at him and shook her head. "Do you think you can move away from racism and make a geographical solution to the problem? I am a single mom with two kids, and I take care of my mother, who worked two jobs to put me through nursing school. She cleaned white people's toilets as a maid for a white family in the day and worked for a janitorial service cleaning white people's toilet at night in a high-rise office building. My husband was killed in Vietnam. What am I supposed to do, move someplace without a job or any means of support with my mother and two kids? I am black. It was hard enough for me to get a job here. What makes you think it is any better somewhere else? The reality is it is hidden, not out in the open like it is here, but it's still there, Dave, and that is who I am talking to now, not Dr. Cameron. You said I am a good nurse, but would you hire me if you were in private practice and your patients were all white? No, I think not, because if you had a black nurse, you wouldn't have a practice of white people very long, no matter where you were. California, the promised land—do you really believe that fantasy? We are still a long way from Dr. King's promised land, and I doubt I will get there in my lifetime." She smiled at Dave. "But you are a good man and a good doctor. It is a pleasure working with someone like you—someone who can hang with John Lee." She laughed.

The GYN ED would have been easy for Dave without the rape cases. Every rape victim had to be examined for injury and a rape kit used to collect evidence. The victims of violent rapes often ended up in the Surgery ER or in the Trauma Unit, but a GYN exam still had to be performed and a rape kit collected.

It angered Dave to see what men did to the girls and women they raped. The violent gang rapes and the brutal rapes by psychopaths who tortured or mutilated their victims left many of the women critically injured as well as emotionally scarred for life. Then of course there where those the rapist actually murdered in the process of raping them.

His disgust increased significantly as he saw how the rape victims were treated by the police and justice system. The police told him most cases where the victim knew their assailant were never reported, and if they were reported, they were never prosecuted because it was a case of he said/she said. Even if there was evidence of trauma, the men simply said the girl or woman liked it rough. In cases where the victim did not know their assailant, unless there was a witness, the outcome was the same for the same reason. Even with the gang rapes, the men said the woman or girl wanted to pull a train. If she was injured, they said that she was into S and M, and again, it was her word against theirs.

A young college girl was brought in by her roommate after she was raped by another student she had seen multiple times on campus. He had been stalking her until he caught her in an isolated part of the campus at night. If she made a sound, he hit her. If she did not do what he told her to do, he hit her. If she was uncooperative, he hit her. Not only was she badly beaten about the face, but she also had vaginal trauma and tears indicating forceful penetration.

She told her story to the investigating officer, and Dave reported what he found on her exam, including the extent of her facial and vaginal trauma. She told the office that pictures of all the students were on file in the dean's office, and she was sure she could identify her assailant. The officer had only one question: were there any witnesses? When she said no, he told her that even if she identified his picture, there was no evidence against him, and it was his word against hers. He suggested that she dressed too provocatively and that may have provoked him into stalking and attacking her.

That was too much for Dave. He got in the officer's face, and went Texas Tom on him. "You are worthless as a police officer, and you are more worthless as a human being. Get the fuck out of my ER and send someone in to take over who is not a flaming asshole."

The second officer told Dave there were literally hundreds of rape kits sitting on a shelf in the evidence room unprocessed because the DA's office wouldn't prosecute a case they couldn't win, and it was very difficult to win a he said/she said case. The victim reports a rape, but the rapist states it was consensual sex, so with no witness, it is his word against hers. The police saw no reason to waste time investigating the rapes or processing the kits if the DA wasn't going to prosecute. Dave pointed out the facial and vaginal trauma, the history of stalking, and the girl's emotional state. The officer said it was still his word against hers, and he could get his friends to say he was with them at the time of the rape to give him an alibi. He added that if the rapist used a condom, there was no evidence in the rape kit to link him to the rape. Plus, he said it took a unanimous vote to convict someone, and the men on the jury tended to side with the male assailant.

The poor girl felt abandoned and undervalued. She cried uncontrollably. All Dave could do was call Psych to see her. Dave realized these poor women and girls were traumatized physically and psychologically by the rape, then they were further emotionally traumatized by their treatment after the rape. The rape kit exam was bad enough, but not to be treated as a victim but made to think it was their fault, then to get no help from the police or the justice system crushed them completely.

Dave was ashamed of his gender for the act of rape. He thought about the guy at the pool, the guys in the hotel, and all men who hit on Sharon almost every day of her life. His disdain for men who rape, men who thought they could buy any woman they wanted like a commodity, and men who hit on women pushing their unwanted advances on them escalated into concern for and worry about Sharon's safety. He thought about Bar hitting her and the poor college girl who was beaten by the rapist. The result was Dave decided the next man who crossed the line with Sharon in front of him would find Dave's fist planted squarely in the middle of his face, and God help Bar if he ever came near Sharon again.

The further outcome was Dave made Sharon start carrying a can of mace in her purse and have an airport security guard walk her to and from her car. She protested, but Dave told her it was not up for discussion. Dave was disturbed by the MVA cases he had seen in the Trauma unit, and he worried about Sharon driving on the expressway in her little Volkswagen, but the rape cases were worse and pushed his concern for her further.

Sharon tried to get Henry to do an intervention on Dave to calm him down, but that resulted in Henry buying Sigrid a handgun when he found out the rape was on the university campus where she was doing her research and that the rapist was still at large. He demanded she not work late, leave the campus before dark, and when she refused the gun, accusing him of being a crazy American cowboy, he got her a can of mace. It spilled over to Harven from Henry; Connie found herself with a can of mace and Harven walked her to her car after her shift if he was available or he made her use a security guard when he wasn't. The women got together and tried to confront their men, but they were argued down by the statistics Dave found on sexual assaults in a study done by a women's research group.

Dave pontificated, "I know the three of you think you are liberated, but I have news for you, you still have a long way to go. This study shows most women experience some type of sexual assault at some time in their life, and believe me, you are nowhere near equal in the eyes of the law on sexual assault. We love you too much to take any risk where you are concerned, and we are certainly not going to depend on the law or law enforcement to protect you. Hear me loud and clear, these precautions are necessary, reasonable, and prudent."

The study also showed students, nurses, and flight attendants were particularly vulnerable because of late-night shifts, late trips, or late-night study habits. So, the girls carried mace and never walked alone after dark, and the boys hovered over them, making sure they took every precaution.

Dave dealt with drug seekers on all his previous rotations, and he was accustomed to them, but he had never dealt with a situation like one he encountered in the GYN ER. The black RN smiled mischievously when she handed him the chart. "You are going to have fun with these two."

Dave looked at the chart, saw the chief complaint was vaginal discharge and assumed she meant he was in for an unpleasant task. He was surprised when he entered the exam area and saw a very pretty blond woman sitting on the exam table with another just as pretty dark-haired woman with her, but his surprise turned to apprehension when he realized the blond had the exam gown on backwards with the opening in the front, untied, and nothing else on except stiletto heels. He looked at the other woman who was wearing a tight skirt that was so short it barely covered her rear, a sweater that looked like it was painted on, and stiletto heels. "Hi, I am Dr. Cameron. I am sorry but you have your gown on backwards. The opening goes in the back and it needs to be tied. I will get the nurse to help you."

Before Dave could get out of the exam area, the blond jumped off the table, stripped off the gown, and held it out to him. "Can't you help me?" She had a voluptuous figure and a come-hither smile on her face.

Dave couldn't get out of the exam area fast enough. "She needs help with her gown."

The nurse laughed. "I told you it was going to be fun."

When Dave entered the second time, the dark-haired woman said, "He's cute, but he shy. We have to do something about that."

Dave tried to ignore her, but she walked over to him and pressed against his arm. He tried to stay professional with her right up against him and said to the blond, "You are here for a discharge? Is that correct?"

The blond got off the table to stand next to Dave, pressing against him too, so they had him boxed in. "Yes, I can't work like this. I use Massengill douche regularly, but now I have some kind of a problem."

Dave knew he was in trouble. Memories of his old sport fucking days came back to him as he pictured the two of them together. "That is probably what caused your problem, but let me get the nurse, and I will examine you."

A love story and social commentary

"Honey, you don't need the nurse." She pulled up the gown. "You know how many guys see this every night, but they pay to see it, and you're going to get to see it for free." She pushed her breast against Dave.

Dave understood, they were strippers. The blond was in her early twenties, the dark-haired one was a little older, both of them were hot and oozed sexiness. "Get back on the table, and I will get the nurse." When he left to find the nurse, Dave was sweating, and it wasn't because of the temperature in the exam area.

After Dave examined the blond, he kept the nurse with him as he explained, "The douche caused vaginitis. Never use a commercial douche, just use a little vinegar in water. Go home, take a bath and clean yourself inside, then start using a vinegar and water douche; the vaginitis will clear right up."

Dave started to leave with the nurse. "Hold on a minute, Doc." Dave stopped but the nurse left. "There is one more thing. I work nights and sleep during the day. It's hard to sleep during the day with all the noises. Can you give me something for sleep? I have taken Quaaludes before, and they work for me. Can you give me some Quaaludes?" The blond smiled sweetly at him.

When he hesitated, the dark-haired woman came up to him. "If you do that for us, we will do something for you. In fact, if there is someplace we can go, I will take care of you right now."

The blond jumped off the table again, joined the dark-haired woman, and they both pressed up against Dave. "If not, we will give you our number, and we will take care of you anytime you want if you take care of us."

"I know what you want the Quaaludes for, and it's not sleep. I am a doctor, not a drug dealer, plus I am engaged." They both had their breasts pressed against him. The blond reached down and took hold of him through his scrub suit. "You may be engaged, but it seems he isn't. It feels to me like he is interested in our offer."

The dark-haired woman added. "We won't tell her if you don't." Then she laughed.

Dave could feel that things were out of hand, so to speak. "Look you are both very hot, but I am a professional and I love my fiancée. So, let me go. I have to admit it has been entertaining, but it has gone too far and has to stop now."

Dave disengaged himself and got out of the room as fast as he could, but as he left, he heard them say, "I thought he would do it for sure." "Yeh, with that hair and the beads. He is cute too. It would have been perfect. I was ready to do him some place here tonight, or we could have done him together later." "Yeah, he could have kept us supplied, and we could have kept him supplied." They both laughed.

Dave went straight to the phone to call Sharon. "Hi, Baby."

"What's wrong?" Sharon responded. "It is too early for my call, and you sound weird."

God, are we so connected that she knows what happened? "Nothing is wrong. I just miss you, that's all."

"Don't lie to me, Dave. We promised we would never lie to each other. What is going on? You sound different. Did some little Florence Nightingale or some hot patient come after you?" Jesus, how could she know? "Do you feel guilty about something and needed to call me to cover your guilt?"

"Baby, the strippers came after me." Dave knew he could never lie to her.

"What? The strippers came after you? Dave, are you high at work?" She sounded annoyed.

"No, these two strippers wanted Quaaludes and offered to fuck me to get them."

"Two strippers wanted to fuck you for Quaaludes? What were you afraid of—them, yourself, or both?" She sounded more annoyed. Dave realized she was right; he was afraid of his old sport fucking self, and it was because of his old sport fucking self that he was afraid of them.

"I needed to talk to you, to hear your voice, to tell you I love you, and that I would never do anything like that," Dave answered. Dave thought about the guys offering Sharon thousands to fuck her on New Year's Eve, and he wondered how often she was approached at work with some kind of proposition like the one the strippers offered him.

"Dave, if I called you every time I got hit on or propositioned on the plane, I would be on the phone all the time. If you didn't do anything, there was no reason to call me. If you did, you better tell me now and not lie to me." She sounded mad.

"I didn't do anything, but one of them did. She grabbed me. I guess I do feel guilty. Another woman had a hold of me, and I feel guilty about it, but I didn't do anything."

Sharon continued, "Maybe you didn't do anything, but your evil little friend reacted, is that it?"

"I'm sorry, Baby. I love you, and I feel terrible about it. I had to call you. Please forgive me."

Sharon started laughing. "So, your evil little friend got you in trouble, and you had to call me to tell on him." Sharon was not the only one laughing; the RN and ward clerk were laughing too. They had heard everything. Dave laughed with them because he realized what a comical figure he was and how different he was since he met Sharon.

Dave finished his month in the GYN ED rested and in good shape physically but troubled by things he had to bury to survive emotionally. The graveyard was continuing to fill up. Dave said goodbye to the RN and ward clerk on his last shift. He told Sharon about her when he first brought her records to the apartment for them to listen to.

Sharon looked troubled. "She is a woman, and she is black. You and I can never know what she has to deal with every day, much less what her life has been like. God, she must have a lot of courage." Sharon made sure Dave thanked her for the hours of fantastic music she had provided them when he said goodbye. "Tell her thanks for the records from me. Let her know how much I enjoyed them, and how much I admire her courage."

When Dave relayed what Sharon had said to the black RN, she looked surprised then said, "Tell my white sister she is welcome."

His last day in the GYN ER was a day off after a twenty-four-hour shift. His last day on any ED shift had to be a day off, or he would be working straight through. Having the first day off on the next rotation had been just luck; his luck held and his first day in Labor and Delivery was an off day, so he had another two days off with a night between. Dave did not want waste the night off. Dave and Sharon combed through the entertainment section of the Sunday paper looking for something and found the New York City Metropolitan Ballet Company was on tour and one of their performances was in the city on his night off.

They planned an evening at the ballet with a late supper after the performance. The ballet finished at nine and there were restaurants around the theater. Dave drove home after his last shift in the ED and set the alarm to give him plenty of time to get ready.

Dave was dressed in his black suit when Sharon walked in a little after five. He was sitting in one of the beanbags waiting for her to walk through the door like someone waiting for some type of entertainment to begin. He loved to look at her when she was dressed to go out, and he knew she would make a special effort tonight because of the ballet. She had on a black low-cut cocktail dress with black heels, a short black satin jacket with no buttons, and black stockings. She looked like she was on her way to a Broadway show in New York. It was cold, and she had her top coat, but it was over her arm when she walked into the apartment because she wanted Dave to see her without it. He got up, walked to her, put his arms around her waist, and kissed her. "You look wonderful tonight."

"So do you. Dave, you have no idea how good you look with your hair pulled back, so it looks like it is short, and you are dressed up." Sharon touched the side of his face. Dave had heard this from her before, and he knew she was giving him subtle hints that she wanted him to cut his hair, but he wasn't ready for that yet.

Dave walked her to one of the beanbags, and she sat down with some difficulty because the dress was short and tight. She had to extend her long legs with Dave standing over her to help her down and as Dave gazed down at her legs, the usual yearnings began to grow. There was no doubt in his mind as he looked at her that sex and drugs were keeping him in his scrubs.

Dave put Prokofiev's Romeo and Juliet on since that was the ballet being performed. They took a few tokes of the potent Jamaican weed while they listened to Prokofiev's masterpiece. Dave looked longingly at her as she sat in the beanbag in her sophisticated stylish dress and jacket. He loved every part of her, but it was her beauty and her perfect body that drove his desire, and it was that desire that blotted out everything else, no matter how horrible it was, from his consciousness. He loved her deeply and she was the great love he had yearned for, but she was more than that—she was a part of him now, a part of his very existence, and he could not function without her.

After they finished the weed, they had a glass of wine while listening to the rest of the music from the ballet. Dave helped Sharon up and held her top coat for her, kissing and nuzzling her neck from behind as she put it on. She turned and kissed him as they held each other for a moment before leaving to drive to the city.

A love story and social commentary

They had another glass of wine standing in the lobby of the theater watching all the people arrive. A ballet always brings out the most attractive people in a city dressed to be seen and admired. Sharon's eyes were sparkling as she sipped her wine and watched the couples file in.

"Oh, Dave, I had forgotten how glamorous the ballet was. I loved the ballet, then I walked away from it and buried myself in my studies at college. I want to be a part of it again. Not to dance of course, but to be a part of it, like tonight. I am so glad we came."

Dave had his arm around her waist, and he brushed her ear with his lips before whispering, "I would take you to the moon if it made you as happy as you are tonight."

The ballet was excellent. Dave marveled at what good athletes the dancers were, and Sharon was amazed by the grace and beauty of movement they exhibited. Of course, it was all very sensual and stimulating in a subtle romantic way, emphasizing the human form in a fantasy of unrealistic stylized movements.

Dave and Sharon walked with one arm around each other's waist to a romantic little café near the theater for another glass of wine and a light supper. The café was full of couples from the ballet holding hands across the table or sipping their wine gazing at each other as they waited for their food. It was a popular rendezvous spot for the lovers, sharing one last moment with the world before retiring to consummate their love. Dave and Sharon ate in an atmosphere of beauty, love, and romance. Sharon hummed the music from the performance as they drove to Dave's apartment.

Their lovemaking that night was like the ballet—romantic and filled with subtle overwhelming passion. When their passion was spent, Dave lay holding Sharon in his arms wondering, as Sharon had in the hotel, what would have happened if they had not met and fallen in love. She drove him crazy with desire, and their lovemaking took him to heights he never dreamed were possible until he met her. He snuggled her closer. *Invictus*, he thought again. *"I thank whatever gods may be," and boy do I ever thank them for Sharon.* He fell asleep holding her tight.

Sharon woke up before Dave, got out of bed and put on a negligee, one of several she kept at Dave's apartment now that she called "her little numbers." She padded to the kitchen and started breakfast even though it was close to noon. She was aware Dave was watching her. "Go put your robe on. Why can't you get it straight about eating with no clothes on?"

"It is straight, alright, believe me. It's as straight as it can get." Dave laughed.

Sharon turned to look at him and exclaimed, "Oh my!" Sharon took Dave by his handle and led him back to the bedroom. "I guess we had better do something about it right away." She laughed as she pulled him on to the bed.

"You know the eggs are burned by now. The bacon is OK, but the eggs are tiny little crisps in the pan. You sexually harassed and molested the cook before she was finished." Sharon was snuggled under his arm with her head on his chest and her leg over his. "Can I finish making breakfast now, or is your evil little friend going to cause more trouble?" Sharon got up and put the negligee back on. "What do you want to do today, and he doesn't get a vote?" Sharon pointed at Dave.

Dave got up and put his robe on. "I was going to call Henry to see if he is off and maybe they can come over to hang out, listen to some music, and order a couple of pizzas for dinner."

"Great." Sharon bounded off to the kitchen to make more eggs to go with the bacon. By the time they finished breakfast and cleaned up the kitchen, it was past noon, so Dave called Henry.

"Hey, Cisco, you up? If you are, I can call back later." Dave laughed.

"Very funny. I was up early, if you must know. Ouch! Damn, she hurts when she hits. What's up with you, Poncho?" Henry replied.

"Since it sounds like you are off today, do you and Sigrid want to come over, listen to some music, and order a couple of pizzas for dinner?" Dave asked.

"Wait, let me ask Sigrid. She is mad at me because I kept her from going to the lab this morning. That thing you were taking about, you know, being up. Ouch, stop hitting me!" Henry asked Sigrid if she wanted to take the rest of the day off since it was more than half over already and go hang out with Sharon and Dave. "She said she will go hang out with you guys but not with me because I am a bad man who prevents the advancement of science in order to gratify my sexual desires. I swear to God that is what she said. Give us some time to clean up and for me to get treatment for my bruises. She hits like Ali. Sigrid, stop hitting me. She said I deserve it for corrupting her and making her neglect her research. Who knew Danes were so abusive? See you later, Poncho."

Dave could hear Sigrid in the background telling Henry she was a wholesome pure girl until she met him, then both of them laughing as Henry hung up the phone.

Sharon and Dave took a shower together and washed each other's hair. Sharon pulled Dave's hair back in a ponytail and tied it with the thong with the trader bead. They both dressed in jeans and pull-over sweaters. Dave had plenty of beer, a bottle of red wine and a bottle of white wine, plus some chips and dip. He rolled a J and left it in the ashtray on the small table between the beanbags, then he put the chips and dip on the bar. He put The Band on the turntable, queued up ready to go.

Sigrid and Henry arrived around two in the afternoon with two more bottles of wine. Henry was dressed like Henry always dressed, only he had on a down jacket. Sigrid had on a beautiful white ski sweater with dark and light blue patterns woven into it that accentuated her eyes, a blue wool scarf, and skinny jeans. But it was her boots that caught Sharon's attention. They were calf-high, fur-lined, lace-up boots with wide heels and a band of fur at the top and under the laces.

"Oh, I love your boots! Where did you get them?"

"They are Danish. I got them in Copenhagen. Everything I have on is Danish. I am dressed exactly the way a Danish girl would dress on a day like today in Denmark." Sigrid smiled. Her hair was down, and she had on no makeup except a light-colored lipstick. Her eyelashes and eyebrows, like her hair, were so blond they were almost white, adding to her haunting natural beauty.

Dave ushered them in and took the bottles of wine. "Jesus, Henry, we are ordering pizza. Are you sure you want to drink these with chips, onion dip, and pizza?" Henry had brought a bottle of Grand Cru Bordeaux and a bottle of Pouilly Fuisse.

"Open the Pouilly Fuisse first. We will drink the Bordeaux later." Henry took his coat off.

Dave indicated a beanbag for them to sit in and went to the kitchen to open the wine. The beanbags were oversized so Sharon and Dave fit easily in one, and even though Henry and Sigrid were bigger, they would have fit too, but Sigrid made Henry to sit on the floor in front of her. She sat down in the beanbag and took her scarf off. "I needed to go to the lab this morning, but he wanted to play, so he overrode my wishes and we played, but his play time with me is over; I am here to visit with you. He can sit alone and play with himself now."

Dave came out of the kitchen with two glasses of wine. "He can't play with himself in front of me." He handed one glass to Sigrid and the other to Sharon who sat down in the other beanbag.

"What kind of a guy takes advantage of a poor foreign girl's lack of understanding of the language to make a joke about his friend?" Dave came back with two more glasses of wine and handed one to Henry. "Sigrid's English is better than mine; I think she is the one who made the joke. I just delivered the punch line."

Dave raised his glass. "Skol." They all repeated "Skol" and took a sip of wine. Dave started the stereo on a volume that would allow them to talk and went to sit with Sharon.

"If Henry has to sit on the floor alone, so do you." Sharon was in the middle of the beanbag.

"What did I do?" Dave sat down on the floor.

"You harassed me while I was making breakfast, like Henry kept Sigrid from going to the lab, so you two harassers can sit together on the floor and play with each other." Sharon turned the joke on Dave and laughed.

"Do you partake of the Devil's weed, Sigrid?" Dave asked.

"Devil's weed? Oh, you mean do I smoke pot. Yes, a little like Henry, but not like his roommates. They smoke like Dutchmen. When I am at Henry's, I feel like I am in Amsterdam."

"There is a number in the ashtray on the table beside you, if you want to light it." Dave indicated the table. Sigrid lit the joint and passed it to Sharon.

They passed the joint around while they listened to The Band. When The Band finished, they were pretty high, so Dave put the Rolling Stones on. Henry greeted the music with his usual "Stones, Mother!" Followed by "I refused to be exiled any longer" as Exile on Main Street began. He slid in beside Sigrid and she snuggled into his arms, so Dave joined Sharon in the other beanbag. They were high and happy, the music was good, and the wine was excellent. The hospital and all it represented was on another planet a million light years away, as the two couples cuddled, talked, listened to music, and drank French wine.

Sigrid sat up. "It is so good to relax with some wine, music, and friends. It reminds me of home. In Denmark, the days are so short in winter, and it is so cold, we spend a lot of time indoors passing the time in good company visiting and talking. Henry has to do something all the time. We go out to dinner, we go shopping, we go here, we go there, we go somewhere and do something all the time, and if we aren't going and doing, we are an item." Sigrid lay back and snuggled close to Henry. "That part is OK, but I wonder why we can't have more time like this too."

Dave knew why. Because just like Dave, Henry had to find ways to blot out what he saw and dealt with every day.

Sharon said, "It is because he needs to be distracted. Dave is the same way. Intense. That's what you said. They are intense. I know how you feel. I feel the same way. I even thought there might be something wrong with us because I thought we did it too much." Sharon laughed.

"Yes!" Sigrid said.

"Then I realized the beauty of our lovemaking replaced the ugliness he is exposed to, so I embraced it, and boy does he need a lot of embracing, but like you said, that part is OK." Sharon smiled, nuzzled and hugged Dave.

Sigrid sat up and looked at Henry. "Is that why you are so intense? You need distracting."

In the almost nine years Dave had known Henry, he had never seen Henry vulnerable, speechless, or emotional, but Henry's face softened considerable as he put his arms around Sigrid and hugged her.

Sigrid cuddled Henry as he held her. "OK, I keep you distracted, don't worry, but can we do this too? I like your friends, and I would like an afternoon like this from time to time."

Henry got up to open the second bottle of wine. "You are right, Sigrid. I forgot how good it is to simply hang out with friends, talk, listen to music, and share a bottle of good wine." He came back and filled their glasses, looked at Dave, and lifted his glass. "Skol, brother, we definitely have to do this more often."

Dave responded. "Skol, brother."

Dave and Henry had forgotten how much they depended on each other. They both realized they needed to get together more often and spend more time together in order support each other. Sharon took a sip of her wine. "This wine is over the top. Henry, we can do this as much as you want if you bring the wine." They all laughed.

Henry said he was moving out of the Park house. Now that he and Sigrid were together, he wanted his own place, and he had located a flat in a high-rise apartment building in the city.

Sigrid added. "I am glad he is moving, because Mike keeps walking in on me when I am in the shower. I think he listens for the shower then comes in. In Europe, there are topless and nude beaches, so I am used to being seen without clothes, but this is different."

Sharon agreed. "I am used to being looked at too, but you are right, with him, it's different. He doesn't make me feel admired."

"Yes, I want to cover up when he looks at me, not like on the beach when you feel proud if you are looked at," Sigrid added.

They spent the evening drinking wine, eating pizza, and listening to music wrapped in a warm blanket of friendship that warded off the cold dark horrors of the hospital Dave and Henry dealt with there.

14
Labor and Delivery

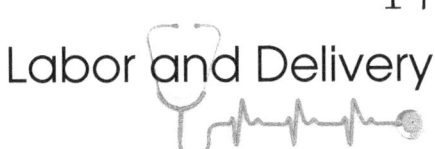

Labor and Delivery was a straight twenty-four hours on, twenty-four hours off. The interns started the shift doing circumcisions and postpartum bilateral Tubal Ligations and spent the rest of the twenty-four hours doing deliveries. Again, there were no teams, and he worked with various residents, interns, and students depending on their schedules. Unlike the GYN ED, the attending staff were always around directing and managing the residents.

Dave enjoyed delivering babies. It was a huge relief dealing with newborn babies, rather than sick, dying, broken, damaged adults and all their psychological problems. Despite the screaming, yelling, and mess, there was joy and happiness in the delivery room. New life brought new hope, and Dave found bringing life into the world brought him happiness.

He would always remember Big John. His mother ended up naming him John because the nurses had been calling him Big John since Dave delivered him, or really fumbled him, into the world. His mother was a small black woman who looked like her abdomen was about to explode when she presented to L and D. At first, Dave was sure she had full-term twins, but her exam showed only one fetus and one heartbeat. It was her first baby, so she labored long and hard. She was nearly exhausted when Dave finally took her to the delivery room.

Newborn babies are slippery. Dave was always very careful not to drop the baby every time he did a delivery. But Big John was something else. When he crowned, Dave did a large episiotomy, but when his head came out, it was so big it tore everything all to hell and gone anyway. Then he just kept coming, shoulders, body, and all. Dave tried to get a grip on him, but he was just too big, too heavy, too slippery, and coming too fast. He slipped from Dave's hands, so Dave kept grabbing at him trying to get control of him as he slid toward the kick bucket at the foot of the delivery table. Dave never dropped him but fumbled him into the kick bucket as if he were trying to help him into it in the first place. The second John hit the kick bucket, he let out a scream.

He was huge and the contents of the kick bucket made him more slippery, so Dave had trouble getting him out of the kick bucket as he kept screaming at the top of his lungs.

"Where is my baby?" the mother asked.

"He is right here, and we will have him with you in a minute." But Dave could not get him out of the kick bucket. The nurse came to Dave's aid and finally they were able to get him over to the warmer to clean him up. He never stopped screaming the whole time.

"Where is my baby? Is he all right?" the mother asked again.

"He is fine. He is a fine, big healthy boy. We just have to clean him up, weigh him, and get his vitals," Dave replied.

"What Apgar?" the nurse asked.

"Twelve!" Dave replied and they both laughed. John weighed in at sixteen pounds even. He immediately became the nurses' favorite, and they called him Big John, so the mother had no choice but to name him John.

The interns and the students did all the deliveries with the residents, only intervening when the mother needed a C-section or when there was a problem like a breach presentation. At first, Dave assisted the resident when a baby got in trouble with declining heart rate and needed an emergency C-section. After doing a few, the resident assisted Dave, and finally, Dave did the C-sections alone with a student assisting him. Dave liked doing C-sections. He became very good at getting the baby out in about two minutes and within five minutes of making the decision to take the mother to the OR. It was exciting and aroused his sense of competitiveness. He was in a race against time to get the baby out before it suffered any permanent damage, and he got a lot of secondary gain from winning the race.

But there were problems in L and D: still births, babies with birth defects or deformities, babies with CP, and mothers with Preëclampsia or even worse, eclampsia (toxemia). Dave had to deal with diabetic mothers, mothers with drug or alcohol addiction, and babies who suffered from the effects of their mother's issues. Most of the mothers were black or Latino, so of course the specter of poverty and all it brought with it loomed over the delivery room. There was no place Dave saw Dickens' children of humanity, Ignorance and Want, more clearly then in L and D. For the most part, Dave felt he was making a positive impact, so he was encouraged, and of course, there were the cute babies and their proud, happy, loving mothers. He slogged through the poverty, lack of education, heart ache, tragedy, and the disasters he encountered doing what he could to help.

There were emergencies and emergency surgeries in L and D, like placental abruptions, placenta previas, and ectopic pregnancies, but the residents handled those cases. Dave's only involvement was in assisting at the surgeries.

Dave had a hard time with the birth of a deformed child. He had lived that tragedy; it was one reason he became a doctor, and each time it happened, he experienced it over again just as he had with his own sister. It is difficult to comprehend the angst caused when what was supposed to be the happy, joyous occasion of the birth of a child turned into a tragedy of major magnitude that impacted a whole family permanently.

Even in L and D, there were cases that left a lasting impression on Dave. Death always left an impression on him, but death in L and D, where it was supposed to be about new life, whether it was the death of the mother or the child, was particularly unsettling.

One night, he received a call from Trauma 1. They had a mother near term who had suffered a lethal head injury in an MVA. When Dave and the resident got to Trauma 1, they found the mother on life support with a flat EEG, but the baby had a good strong heartbeat, so they did a C-section and delivered a healthy baby boy. The resident went back to L and D and left Dave to deal with the father, who was in the ED waiting room.

Dave and the trauma resident took the husband, and now new father, to the side room in the ED waiting area to have him sign papers to remove his wife from life support and to tell him he could see his newborn son in the nursery. Dave wondered how someone would deal with the dichotomy of losing their wife and gaining a son at the same time. One was the most wonderful thing that can happen to a man and the other was the worst thing that could happen to a husband. Dave would never forget the expression on the man's face or the play of mixed emotion he exhibited at hearing both things simultaneously. The whole incident left Dave with the impression that life was far too complex and complicated for him to figure out. It made him stop asking why. He came to this conclusion: it is what it is, so acknowledge it and move on. He acquired one more tool to help him deal with the tragedies he was exposed to—another type of shovel to use to bury them in his graveyard of the unthinkable and unacceptable.

Valentine's Day for Sharon and Dave came and went with Dave working a shift in L and D and Sharon flying. Dave sent her flowers and a card she got that night when she got back from her trip, and she took Dave a box of candy with a card the next day when she went to his apartment. That night, they had a candlelight dinner of pizza and wine then Sharon put on a new little number and they made love in candlelight listening to the music from the ballet.

After Valentine's Day, Dave was involved in a case that brought him the satisfaction of being a doctor and the joy of making a difference. She was seventeen years old. The young man who came with her and checked her in was about the same age. Neither spoke any English. The interpreter told Dave she got pregnant in Mexico. She and her husband had walked from Monterey, Mexico, across the border into Texas and then found their way here. They left Mexico because they weren't married when she got pregnant, and they wanted a better life for their child. She had not had any prenatal care.

Married or not, it was obvious to Dave they were very much in love as they said goodbye to each other in L and D. The interpreter had to pull them apart in order to move her into a room. Her labor was going fine until Dave was doing a routine check and heard the heart rate of the baby drop drastically. He didn't hesitate. He yelled for the nurse and started wheeling the bed to the OR, yelling orders as he went.

She was moved to the OR table screaming in fear because she could not understand what was being said or what was happening. Anesthesia arrived and crashed her as a quick prep was done on her abdomen. Dave had the baby out in no time. The infant girl was blue because the cord was wrapped around her neck twice, and it was obstructed. As the baby moved down the birth canal during labor, the cord had tightened and occluded. If Dave had not been listening when it happened, she would have been still born. If Dave had not gotten the baby out so quickly, she would have had brain damage. But because he had been examining her at the time the cord occluded and had acted quickly doing the C-section, he was able to present the young man with a fine healthy baby girl. Dave went home the next morning with a full heart and a sense of pride because he had made a difference.

Dave was able to eat, rest, and sleep on his shifts, so he gained weight. Even though babies seemed to prefer to be born at night and even though Dave did a lot of deliveries on each shift, plus the C-sections, circumcisions, and BLTs, there was down time. He was able to go to the call room and sleep in a bed at night between deliveries and rest in the doctors' lounge during the day.

Henry had moved to the high-rise building downtown and invited everyone over for a wine and cheese get-together as a sort of house warming on the day after Dave's last shift in L and D. Dave had gotten some sleep his last night at the hospital, so he was up, showered, shaved, and dressed when Sharon got to his apartment a little after noon.

It was the end of February and cold. Sharon had on jeans, boots with high heels, and a ski sweater with a puffy down jacket over the sweater. When he saw her, Dave thought, *I want to take her skiing.* They drove to Henry's apartment all bundled up against the cold.

The whole gang was there when they arrived. Henry's flat was spectacular, and Dave almost burst out laughing when he walked in and saw the interior. He pulled Henry aside. "She is not a bird or a fish."

Henry smiled. "Biology is biology, Poncho. I have got to keep her here until I finish my training." In certain species of birds and fish, the male builds a nest to attract a female. The better the male is at building the nest and the better the nest is, the better his chances are of attracting the female of his choice. Ever the biologist, Henry had built a nest to attract the female of his choice and to keep her from returning to Denmark.

It was a big flat, and Henry had spared no expense in decorating it in a purely Scandinavian style. It had three bedrooms, one of which Henry had turned into a study with a desk and book shelves lining the walls; another he had laid out like a lab with book shelves, a large table and chair ready for a microscope and instruments, and bright lighting. The master bedroom had a king-size bed with matching dresser and chest along with two walk-in closets with shelves. There was a living room, a formal dining room, and spacious kitchen with a breakfast nook. It was all furnished in simple Scandinavian furniture of light wood and glass. The lamps, fixtures, and decorations were tasteful and original prints by Chagall, Miro, Picasso, and Matisse adorned the walls.

Dave looked at the prints. "Who are her favorite artists? Let me guess, could they be Miro and Chagall or is it Picasso and Matisse?"

Henry looked at his flat. "I love her, Dave. You are the one who told me not to lose her and to do everything possible to hold on to her."

Now Dave did laugh. "You have recreated Copenhagen for her."

Henry laughed with Dave. "I want to spend the rest of my life with her, but the devil is in the details. She doesn't like the United States. She loves and misses her family, likes Denmark, and wants to go back. I have to get her to stay here long enough for me to finish my residency and do my fellowship, then I will go to Europe with her. I can work for the International CDC; that's where the real challenges will come in the future. We could even become a research team. I don't want to take her away from her family or her country, but I want to finish my training."

Dave looked his friend in the eyes. "Marry her, Henry. Get her to move in here with you first. Your family donates a lot of money to research, and they can get her an extension on her grant to carry on her research wherever you are in training. You can afford for her to fly home first class, spend some time and see her family as often she wants until you can permanently move to Europe. Tell her that. Tell her you want to spend the rest of your life with her, that you want the two of you to become a research team to fight the coming epidemics together. Woo her, Henry. Woo her with double-blind studies like we joked about. You built her a nest, now woo her."

While Dave and Henry were talking, Sigrid sought out Sharon and found her talking to Connie in the living room. "Sigrid, I love your style. Are all your clothes from Europe, or did you buy some here?" Sigrid was dressed in an ice blue cocktail dress that matched her eyes with a darker blue silk scarf around her neck, and dark blue heels that matched the scarf. "You look like a Nordic ice princess and I mean that in a good way."

"Thank you, Sharon. I brought everything with me from Denmark. Henry keeps trying to buy me clothes here, but having him buy things for me makes me uncomfortable. That's what I want to talk to you about—Henry and this flat." Sigrid moved closer to Sharon.

"Should I leave?" Connie asked.

"No, you can help too." Sigrid looked around. "Look at this flat."

Sharon looked around. "It is obvious it is a shrine to you. So, what is the problem?"

A love story and social commentary

"I don't want to stay in America. I want to finish my project and go home. I miss my mother and father, my brother, and all my friends in Denmark. I don't like it here, but I love Henry, and I know he wants me to stay here. I know he decorated this flat to entice me to live with him, but I want to go home. I don't know what to do. I can't do both." Sigrid looked stricken.

"If you love Henry, you need to be with him. Love is hard to find, and if you find it, you shouldn't give up on it, but you have to be happy too. Love should fulfill your happiness, not take it away from you." Sharon wondered how hard it would be to maintain a long-distance relationship across the Atlantic Ocean.

Sigrid looked at Connie, but Connie said, "Don't look at me. I can't add anything to what Sharon said. But I agree with her, don't give up on love and don't lose hope. You will find a way. You are two of the smartest people I know. If anyone can figure it out, it's you two."

Sigrid smiled at them. "What should I do about moving in with Henry? My research grant pays for room and board at the university, a car, and expenses until May when the project is finished. It would be a waste for me to move here, so again, I don't know what to do."

"Keep your place at the university and stay there when Henry is at the hospital. Move some stuff here and stay here when you can be with Henry. That is what we do. Sharon stays at Dave's when they can be together, then she stays at her house when Dave is at the hospital. I do the same thing; except we stay at my place when Harven and I can be together because it is nicer, and I live alone. That's a simple solution and it works; we can both vouch for that." Connie looked satisfied with herself.

Dave and Henry walked up to the group of women. "Let's get some wine, Baby, then I want to take a complete tour of Henry's new nest."

Dave and Sharon went to get wine, and Connie went off to look for Harven, leaving Henry and Sigrid alone to talk.

They sipped wine and mingled. The major topics of conservation, besides how fabulous Henry's apartment was, had to do with the three upcoming weddings—one in April, one in May, and one in June.

When Sharon and Dave were asked about their plans, they responded that they were simply trying to get through the rest of Dave's internship, then get into a residency program and grad school in California. If they were pressed, they changed the subject to the amazing wines Henry was serving or the original prints that adorned the flat.

Everyone said goodbye and left around six. Dave and Sharon stopped for Chinese take-out on their way to the apartment. They ate, smoked part of a joint, listened to some of their favorite albums, and went to bed.

Sharon's applications were in, and Dave had listed his match preferences. Match Day was April 30. He had listed the four California programs first then University Hospital last. They planned their vacation time for May so they could spend a week finding a place to live and getting everything set to move, hopefully to the Bay Area or LA, but they needed to be ready for Dave to start his residency in July, no matter where they were.

Sharon had increased her savings by modeling for Neiman Marcus catalogues. She also did some work for Bob and Phil. By the end of April, they would know where they would be for the next two years, and by the end of May, they would have a home.

15
The Wards

The OB/GYN wards for Dave were the GYN wards. All pregnant women admitted for control of their diabetes during pregnancy, bed rest for twins, toxemia, or any other OB complication were admitted by the residents, and Dave had little or no contact with them. He admitted minor GYN cases only. Again, there were no teams, and Dave worked with different students, interns, and residents based on their schedules with the attendings, always overseeing everything closely.

The schedule was like the Surgery wards with every third day on call, the day after call off once rounds were finished and all the patients were stable, elective surgeries in the morning with rounds between the surgeries, then clinic in the afternoon on the day before call with rounds, admissions, and emergency surgeries on the days on call.

The cases Dave admitted from clinic or on call were limited with the residents doing all the significant surgeries and admitting all major GYN issues. In clinic, Dave did cervical cone biopsies and cervical cryosurgeries; he saw the same things he had seen in the GYN ER. On his Surgery days, Dave did bilateral tubal ligations, D and Cs for dysfunctional uterine bleeding, and assisted the residents on hysterectomies, salpingo oophrectomies, and cancer surgeries. On call, he did D and Cs for bleeding, assisted the residents on emergency surgeries, and admitted patients with sepsis due to a gynecological source of the infection or PID. The OB/GYN Department of University Hospital did therapeutic abortions for medical reasons only.

Dave saw a lot of STDs in the GYN clinic, more than he saw in the GYN ER. He treated everything from pubic lice, commonly known as crabs, to gonorrhea, and even one case of syphilis. He was surprised that he saw women from higher socioeconomic levels. These women came to the University Hospital GYN Clinic because they thought or knew they had something, and they were too embarrassed to go to their private doctors, plus they did not want to have an STD noted in their regular medical records.

He treated a woman for gonorrhea who went to a club alone. She blacked out and woke up the next morning in a motel. She had vague memories of either one man having sex with her a lot of times or a lot of men having sex with her one at a time. She was not sure if the memories were real or not. She had no idea who the man or men were or how many there were if there was more than one, so there was no way to trace her contacts.

He took care of a married woman with chlamydia who was an account manager for a large firm who was having sex with her boss in order to keep her high-paying position. She didn't know if her boss or her husband gave her the chlamydia, and she refused to give Dave the boss's name or any way to contact her husband, even though she knew they both had it now. She said she would work it out on her own.

A college student came in with trichomonas she contracted from a musician she had a one-night stand with because she didn't want to go to the university clinic with an STD. There were multiple cases of herpes in young women who contracted it from casual sex with men they didn't know, and he saw women with condyloma or venereal warts who didn't know they were contagious. Many of the women he saw didn't know who gave they them the STD because they were having sex with several different men. Dave thought about his own past and was extremely grateful he had not contracted anything.

He treated working girls, mainly lower-class street prostitutes, with every type of STD known. There were also high-end escorts who came in to be tested. One was very pretty, well dressed, and well educated. She told him she was checked on a regular bases because she could not afford to pass anything on to her high-profile clients, and she didn't want anything in her private medical record about frequent STD testing. Dave wondered why someone like her did what she did, so he asked her. She said she liked sex, enjoyed what she did, and made a lot of money for doing what she would normally be doing anyway. She was fascinated by men and liked how they were all different sizes and shapes.

Dave got to sleep at night and rest when he was on call and was off for at least half the day after call. His clinic day was a long hard twelve-hour day but then he went home and slept with Sharon in his own bed. He had the afternoons and nights after call available to do things, so he and Sharon met with their friends, and those get-togethers helped him deal with his issues. Of course, he worked for thirty-one days straight and had to be at the hospital at seven AM every one of those thirty-one days, but it wasn't bad compared to some of the other rotations.

Even though he did not have a lot of contact with them, other than assisting at their surgery, the GYN cancer cases caused him the most emotional duress, especially the ovarian cancer cases. A lot of the ovarian cancer patients were fairly young, had young families, and the disease was universally fatal.

The thing that bothered him about the GYN cancers was that cervical cancer and uterine cancer were completely curable if they were diagnosed and treated early. Universal cervical and uterine cancer screening with a PAP smear and pelvic exam yearly could save lives on a huge scale. Yet the uninsured and poor had no access to these simple screening tests. Some patients at University Hospital received free screening, but they were a fraction of the vast majority of the poor and underserved women in the community.

Dave couldn't understand why there was no funding for universal women's cancer screening. He felt that not providing free screening for curable cancers that could be detected by simple tests and exams was not only negligent, but it was also criminal. To him, withholding lifesaving women's health screening to fund other government programs was murder on a grand sociologic scale by the politicians.

Dave hated politicians who wrapped themselves in the flag, presented themselves as devout Christians, and voted down any measure having to do with health care. They voted huge sums for the military to fund an unwinnable endless war, but they refused to vote for a health care bill. They voted to kill on a mass scale yet refused to vote to save lives on any scale. They were inherently evil and voted for death over life yet presented themselves as God's servants, doing God's work, for purely patriotic reasons, protecting and promoting the American way of life. The word *hypocrite* was too mild to describe them.

The other thing that bothered Dave was the sterilization procedures. Women were asked right after delivery if they wanted to have something done to prevent them from having more babies. The GYN clinic also pushed BTL as an alternative birth control method if the woman had two or more children. At first, Dave thought it was racial because most of the women in L and D were black or Latino, but white women were also asked if they wanted to stop having babies and were told about BTL.

Dave began to think it was socioeconomic. It seemed a concerted effort was being made to stop women who lived in poverty from having babies. Dave could see why and how this could be true, but he thought maybe he was just overreacting. Yet if there was funding for BTLs for the poor, why wasn't there funding for universal cancer screening for the poor?

There was an undercurrent in the male dominated OB/GYN Department that made Dave uneasy. It wasn't only the impression he got that the department thought it had the moral authority to control the birth rate in the poor; it was a subtle attitude that permeated the interactions with all the patients. He had not encountered anything like it in Surgery or Medicine, and it wasn't confined only to the attendings; he saw it in the residents and straight OB/GYN interns as well. There were some women on the OB/GYN house staff, but Dave didn't have an opportunity to work with any of them, so he didn't know if they were tainted by it too, but he doubted it. He thought it was a gender-related, unstated belief that women were inferior and could be dealt with in the offhanded dominant way by the male staff and attendings.

Dave developed a deeper understanding of the courage and strength of women while on the OB/GYN service. He had gained some insight into what women had to deal with through his relationship with Sharon. His OB/GYN rotation had expanded his insight considerably. He had seen the strength it took to be a mother from the terminal cancer patient on the Medicine wards protecting her children from foster care. He got a better grasp of the kind of courage women had from Carol, the decorated night nurse on Medicine 3. But it was the whole process of bringing a child into the world that crystalized how strong and courageous women were for him. A woman's strength and courage reminded him of Melville's description of Starbuck's courage in *Moby Dick*. It was a commodity, a staple, a solid dependable resource always there when needed, never to be flaunted, squandered, or wasted but to be used judiciously when it was necessary.

A man might display courage in a given situation, but a woman had to constantly possess courage in order to just be a woman. Dave had worked with male nurses who had been medics in Vietnam. The majority of them were excellent nurses, and Dave knew about their courage from the media coverage of the war. They went into combat unarmed to take care of the members of their unit, but they were taking care of men they knew, their buddies, and their brothers. Carol went under fire to take care of patients she didn't know and had never met. The courage she displayed was motivated by an entirely different instinct—a woman's need to care for and nurture. A woman carried another human being in her body, went through the risk and pain of expelling that human being, to then nurture and care for it until it matured. The strength and courage it took to be a woman was only exceeded by the strength and courage it took to be a mother.

It pained Dave to think about what Sharon went through every day at work and the strength she had to have to ward off the unwanted attention and advances, to deal with the sexual harassment, and to keep things from getting out of control. She had to walk a fine line and not create a problem through her actions, do a good job, and still protect herself. It was hard to be a woman because you were undervalued and over judged. It was harder to be an attractive woman because you were also hit on, and you had to deal with the situation in a way that prevented the rejection from escalating into something ugly. Then there was the black RN in the OB/GYN ER who had to have even more strength and courage to deal with not only being a woman but also with being a black woman and a single mother.

Dave had mixed feelings about his OB/GYN rotation and the discipline in general, but he had acquired a deeper understanding of some fundamental truths about the complexity of human existence. He was in a great mood on his last day on call, because April brought the change to Pedi, Match Day on April 30, and his last three-month rotation.

Part 5: Pediatrics

16
The Match Game and the Wards

The Pedi ward schedule was exactly like the Medicine ward schedule. He was on call every third day with clinic and afternoon rounds on the day after and the day before call with all the patients stabilized before he could sign out. If he was not on call on the weekend, he only went in at eight or nine to make rounds. There was a Pedi attending who met with the interns and students after morning rounds every day and a supervising resident over the interns. Grand Rounds were on Saturday at noon, but there were no rounds with the chief the day after call.

Dave did not receive an invitation for an interview with UCSF or Stanford. He did receive an invitation for an interview from UCLA Medical Center and LA County Hospital, the USC program. Sheffield didn't do a formal interview with Dave for University Hospital but spoke to him and let him know he was on their match list. Because of the distance problem, he did a phone interview with UCLA and USC. Dave thought the interviews went very well, especially the interview with USC. After the phone interviews, Dave was sure he would be at USC unless UCLA came through. Sharon was hoping for UCLA because the UCLA Medical Center was on the UCLA campus. The one drawback to UCLA was Dave would have to drive to Torrance for some of his rotations.

Sheffield told Henry and Mike they could continue at University Hospital for their residencies. Harven received invitations for interviews for a straight Medicine internship at Stanford and UCLA but not UCSF. George had applied to programs in the Southeast and received several interview invitations. The month of April was a waiting game for all three of them.

From the first day, Dave had trouble with the Pedi wards. The good news was his service was small; the bad news was the children were very sick with a variety of ailments. Dealing with sick, suffering children was hard for Dave, but at least he did not have to take care of children with cancer because they were on the Pedi Oncology service.

He only saw them in their rooms as he made his rounds. Children dying with cancer tore at Dave's heart. The old questions with the elusive answers he thought he had gotten past these last few months came back to haunt him again. What the hell? What was the purpose of suffering and death in a child? Where was a benevolent, caring God in all this? What kind of a God gave a child cancer? Why did loving parents have to be tormented by seeing their child suffer and die?

The Pedi ward rotation allowed for down time, time to sleep, and time to eat, but Dave found it very difficult emotionally and psychologically. The one positive thing was the staff, from the attendings down to the nurse's aides. They were all kind, gentle, caring people. Also, he found more women in Medicine. His supervising residency was a smart, knowledgeable, slightly overweight woman with a cheerful disposition and a warm, open personality. She was patient, helpful, and thoroughly engaged in helping Dave supervise his studs and manage his service.

But it was the oncology staff that really impressed Dave. He respected all oncologists, but pediatric oncologists were a breed apart. To Dave, being an oncologist was the toughest job in medicine, but being a pediatric oncologist required dedication, commitment, and a special kind of empathy beyond the capacity of most physicians. To face each day knowing most of your patients were going to die, while continuing to strive to fight for their life and remain positive, was a significant challenge, but to do it with children was beyond anything Dave could imagine.

If Dave was awed by the Pediatric oncologists, he saw the Pedi Oncology nurses as saints. Oncology nurses in general are special people, but the Pedi Oncology nurses were the most dedicated, caring, resilient women he met during his internship. Every day they dealt with suffering and dying children, knowing all they could do was make the day as pleasant as possible for them. The Pedi oncologists bought the children time, and the Pedi Oncology nurses tried to make that time meaningful. Both knew they would lose in the end and fail, but they never stopped trying, no matter how tough it got.

A lot of the Pedi Oncology nurses were young. He talked to the Pedi Oncology charge nurse about them. She told him a lot of them burned out after about five years and had to move on to another service, but some like her just couldn't walk away knowing how needy the children and their families were. She said it took hold of her, wouldn't let her go, and she had to keep working with children with cancer no matter how hard it was on her. Dave could not imagine the courage it took to walk in to those rooms smiling, happy, and cheerful every day doing everything in your power to make one more day fun and pleasant for a child you knew was dying. Dave was affected by the pathos of Pediatric Oncology, but he was lifted up by the knowledge there were people in the world like the Pedi Oncologists and the Pediatric Oncology nurses who demonstrated to him what caring, love, and empathy could do in the face of the worst of circumstances.

During his summer jobs in medical school, Dave had learned that the real work of health care was done by nurses. As he progressed through his internship, his respect and admiration for nurses continued to grow. Doctors gave orders, but it was the nurses who carried those orders out and many times good nurses helped stop bad orders and saw that good orders were instituted when necessary. Dave had learned there was no substitute for a good nurse, and patient outcomes often depended on the quality of nursing care rather than the physician's skills or knowledge. The work of the Pedi Oncology nurses further bolstered his opinion that nursing was a calling that required as much dedication as a physician and a depth of empathy that exceeded that of most physicians.

Dave was struggling when something happened that finally broke him. Everything inside him collapsed, leaving a vacuum that nothing rushed in to fill as if he had been hollowed out. He was a little sick from the Pedi Clinic because he had been seeing children with cold and flu symptoms. His resident told him he was lucky it was April, or it would be worse. She said during the winter, at the peak of the cold and flu season, the Pedi staff were sick all the time. So maybe the fact he was sick had something to do with why it hit him so hard, but in reality, he knew it hit all the doctors and nurses on the ward just as hard.

She was simply a beautiful little girl with bouncing curls, an infectious smile, a joyful laugh, an inquisitive mind, and an engaging personality. She was involved in everything, observant and bright, so she had to know everything, constantly asking "What dat? What dat noise? What dat for?." She refused to stay in her bed, dragging her parents all over the ward, clutching her beloved teddy bear in her left arm. The nurses fell in love with her immediately and indulged her every whim. They let her stay in the nurses' station sitting in their laps while they did their charting or follow them as they made their medication rounds, always clutching her teddy bear in her left arm. She was outgoing, talking to everyone and brightening their day with her special glow.

She also had a lump in her left lower leg that was malignant, and she had been referred to University Hospital Pediatric Oncology Service by her pediatrician for amputation of the leg and a work-up for metastasis. It would turn out to be an osteosarcoma, a common type of cancer that occurs in the bones of children. There was a good survival rate if it had not metastasized but only a one in three chance of survival if it had. She had been admitted the day before her surgery for a metastatic work-up and pre-op evaluation before the surgery early the next morning. She went through the work-up without complaint, never letting go of her teddy bear the whole time.

She didn't just charm the nurses; she charmed everyone on the floor, including Dave and all the doctors. He never knew her name because everyone, including her parents, called her Little One, Sweetheart, or some other term of endearment. She must have been about five. She did not know she had cancer or that tomorrow they were going to cut her leg off; she just thought the whole thing was a great adventure. But her parents knew. They were heartbroken, but they kept up a brave face, smiled and played with her as if nothing was wrong. Dave was on call the day she was admitted and was making rounds the next morning when she went to surgery.

When she left for surgery, everyone was there to see her off. She was clutching her teddy bear and smiling, although Dave could tell she was a little confused by all the attention. It was when she came back from recovery that she tore Dave's heart in two, along with everyone else's on the floor. She was sedated but still holding onto her teddy bear. When Dave looked at her lying on the gurney, he saw the outline of one leg under the sheet but on the other side, nothing. They all knew that if the work-up showed it had metastasized, she only had a one in three chance of living. And even if she had no mets, she faced a long rehab with PT, pain, and an ever-changing prostheses as she grew. She would never be able to run and play as she had on the ward before the surgery, and she would face a lifetime of wearing and managing a prostheses. That was a lot to ask of a child, if she survived at all; of course, dying was a lot more to ask of a child.

There was not a dry eye in the hall as they watched her being wheeled into her room. Veteran Oncology nurses who had seen it all and had been hardened by years of exposure to children with cancer were crying, as were the poor child's parents as they followed the gurney. Seeing her tiny body on the gurney still clutching her teddy bear with no leg under the sheet hit Dave like a hard punch to the stomach.

As he drove home that day, the same questions kept repeating in his head. How do you tell a child when she wakes up with no leg that the doctors had to cut her leg off? How do you tell a child she has cancer, and cancer is why they had to cut her leg off when she has no idea what cancer is? How does a child process that? How do you explain the pain she has now, and the ghost pain she will have later? She thought she was on a wonderful adventure, but now her leg was gone, and she was in horrible pain. How do you explain that to her? How do you tell her she is dying or may die? How do you explain death to her or why she might die?

A sickening sadness engulfed him, producing an aura of dark gloom around him that was almost palpable.

Dave drove to his apartment and lay on his bed gazing up at the ceiling. What kind of a malevolent force does this to a child? What underlying evil caused his sister and this exceptional child to suffer, and for what reason? Does being a doctor make any difference when you are not able to stop or do anything about these types of things? Dave was emotionally exhausted and psychologically drained. It had been a long, hard ten months, and he was at the end of himself, driven over the edge by the heart ache he felt for the little girl.

He realized he was depressed. He had dealt with depression on his Medicine rotation, along with other psychosocial issues. Mental illness along with patients with personality and character disorders made up the majority of patients he saw in both the Minor Medicine ER and the Medicine Clinic. Dave had been somewhat skeptical about the symptoms of depression and frankly angered by his encounters with patients with personality and character disorders. Now he understood the symptoms of depression were real and produced suffering. He reflected on the frightening fact that the statistics proved half the population suffered from some form of mental illness, and even more had personality and character disorders. Yet the health care system was geared to handle mainly organic problems with little or no effort made to treat psychosocial issues. That's why the patients with psychosocial problems clogged up medical treatment facilities. Dave was empty and flat as he looked up at the ceiling, feeling as if he were sinking into the mattress with the weight of the depression pressing down on him.

That is the way Sharon found him when she got to his apartment. She knew something was wrong when she came in and found Dave lying on his bed fully dressed with his shoes on. She walked into the bedroom and sat on the bed. Dave didn't acknowledge her but just kept staring at the ceiling. "Are you alright?"

"It was a rough day, and the kids keep giving me bugs, so I am a little sick." Dave sat up, put his arms around his knees, and looked at Sharon. "I guess I am a little sick from the whole last ten months. It hasn't been just a rough day; it has been a rough ten months. Something happened that broke my heart today. I can't tell you about it, I can't talk about it, I don't even want to think about it, but I don't think I will ever be able to forget it. I have about a half-dozen things like that inside me now. Things I can't talk about or think about, but things I can never forget. Things that hurt my heart and left a permanent indelible mark on my soul. I don't know how many more things like that I can take. You just get numb. Maybe that is what has to happen; you have to get numb so you don't feel the pain anymore, and you can deal with anything without it hurting you." Dave looked at Sharon. "I am sorry, Baby." Dave got up.

Sharon was worried. "I don't want you numb. I don't want your heart hurt, or your soul marked. I want your soul just the way it is and your heart unharmed. I want this internship over. I don't want you permanently damaged." Sharon was aware he was on a raw edge. "Dave, you need to get some rest and you need to get away from this for a while. In a week, you have some time off. You are burned out physically, emotionally, and psychologically; you need some down time to recover. You desperately need some R and R."

Dave looked at Sharon sitting on the edge of the bed with a worried look on her face. "It's pretty warm out even though it is late, and I think you are right. I need some R and R. I haven't been in the water

A love story and social commentary

for months. Let's go to the pool." He took her hands and pulled her up. "Look at you. Why am I whining and feeling sorry for myself when I have you? Put your bikini on, and let's go wash these blues away." There was more sadness in his eyes than she had ever seen before and a feeling of despair that surrounded him she had never felt before.

Sharon fell into his arms. "Do you think I am your toy to play with?" It was bad, really bad, and she knew it. She had never seen him like this. *I will pull him out of it,* she thought. *I have done it before, and I can do it again.* She knew just what he needed; he needed her.

Dave smiled. "You bet." Seeing how beautiful she was, how perfect her body was, and feeling her against him lifted some of the black fog from his psyche, but something intangible pulled at him that he could not shake. It was a feeling of emptiness, an emotional flatness, a black shroud over his whole being. He needed some way to rejoin the human race, but he didn't know how to go about it. "Can you wear the white bikini? I don't think anyone will be at the pool. I know you said you would never wear it again, but I realize I loved you in that bikini."

Sharon leaned back from him. "I think there is more lust than love associated with that white bikini, but OK, if that will cheer you up." She had never seen him so down, seen his face so sad, or felt the aura of gloom around him she felt now, and she knew whatever had happened, it was worse than she thought.

Dave led her to one of the beanbags, and they cuddled in it while they smoked a number. By the time they finished half the joint and had snuggled for a while, Dave was starting to feel more normal, if being stoned and turned on by Sharon's body could be considered his normal state. They put their swim suits on, Dave grabbed a couple of beers, some waters, the towels, and they headed for the pool.

When they got to the pool, Dave threw the stuff he was carrying on a table, kicked his flops off, ran and dove in the pool, and then he began to swim laps vigorously. Sharon stood by watching him for a while, then pulled two lounge chairs together, put the towels down on them, took her cover-up off and lay down on one. She had seen this kind of behavior from Dave before when he was really stressed, but she had never seen him depressed or sad like this. Even when he was stressed, he was still usually happy, upbeat, and positive. She opened herself a beer and waited for him to finish his baptismal and purification ritual.

It was a glorious spring evening with a clear blue sky. All the flowers in landscaping around the apartments were in bloom, and the air was warm, pleasant, and fragrant. The water in the pool was sparkling and transparent. Sharon watched Dave swim back and forth while she sipped her beer. She looked around and saw a few people at the pool and recognized several regulars from last summer. From their smiles, it was apparent some of them recognized her as well.

Finally, Dave got out of the pool, walked over to Sharon, picked up his towel from the lounge chair, and dried off. "I needed that swim desperately. I didn't know how much I needed it. What I really need is to be sailing on a day like this, but I don't have a boat or an ocean, or to be spring skiing, but I don't have a mountain."

Sharon stood up in front of him. "You don't have a boat to sail; you don't have a mountain to ski; you don't have any toys to play with, except me." She smiled and put her arms around his neck.

Dave threw the towel on the lounge chair and scooped her up and fell on the lounge chair with her, burying his face in her breast.

"Dave you can't molest me in public. Jesus, you are causing multiple wardrobe malfunctions."

Dave had his hands all over her. "You said you were my toy and I intend to play with my toy." Dave stood up, picked her up, and walked to the side of the pool, as she tried to adjust her top to cover her breasts and get her bottom back in place.

"Don't you dare. This suit will come completely off if you throw me in the pool." Sharon tried to get out of his arms.

"Good. I want to be there when that happens." He jumped in the pool with her in his arms as she protested.

They came up and Sharon put her arms around his neck hugging him to cover her exposed breasts, and she wrapped her legs around him to keep her bottom from sliding down further. "You can be such an asshole sometimes. Now I am stuck to you like a barnacle, because that is the only way I can stay covered. This water is crystal clear."

Dave smiled at her, holding her rear with both hands. "I like having a barnacle stuck to me." She smiled back at him. Sharon felt some sense of relief because she could see the man she loved was starting to return. She knew he was trying to bury whatever it was that was troubling him with the help of the weed, the swimming, and her body.

"Can you get your hands out of my bikini bottom and put my top back where it is supposed to be?" Sharon pulled back a little from him.

"Dave, really. Stop groping me in public and put my top back." Dave took his hands out of her bikini bottom and pulled her top back over her breasts so she could stand up to pull her bikini bottom up. "If you don't treat your toys better, they will be taken away from you." She put her arms around his neck again. They frolicked around in the pool for a while before getting out. Seeing Sharon get out of the pool in the thin, tiny white bikini reminded Dave of the day he first realized he loved her—a day that seemed so long ago it was like it was in another lifetime. They lay back on the lounge chairs and sipped their beers in the warm glow of the perfect spring evening.

Dave looked around at the glistening clear water of the pool, the half-dozen or so attractive people sitting at the pool, the cloudless blue sky, and all the vividly colored blossoms in the landscaping around the pool. It occurred to him it was Thursday—a sweet Thursday, just like Steinbeck described in the book. Dave thought, *This can't be the same world I was in just a few hours ago.* He looked over at Sharon lying next to him with one knee cocked up and one arm over her head in the skimpy white bikini that barely covered her.

He was with a beautiful woman who looked like a model right out of the pages of a magazine, the epitome of sensuality, while a wonderful little girl was lying in a hospital bed with only one leg in terrific pain. How could those two things exist in the same space and time? Did all that really happen this morning? Was it real or only a bad dream? Was this sweet Thursday just a fantasy? How could they both be real.

Dave's depression was situational, and it began to lift as he started to see things differently. He thought about the veteran Oncology nurses crying over the little girl, and he realized they were reacting appropriately. They knew how to deal with tragedy; they dealt with it all the time. They were dealing with it by getting in touch with their emotions and appropriately expressing them by crying. It was a terribly sad thing, they grieved for her, so they cried. By getting in touch with their emotions and expressing them, they were able to cope with it in a healthy, healing way. Dave didn't cry. He choked up, but he didn't cry. He didn't grieve; he held his grief inside, unexpressed. He was unable to get in touch with his emotions because that was too painful, so he stuffed them and tried to bury the event with denial, like he had all the others. They were all inside him buried in a toxic dump site that corroded his psyche from within and consumed him psychologically as he tried to keep the toxicity at bay. He could not continue to deal with tragedy that way. He had to talk to someone and deal with his feelings in a healthy, healing way. He had to accept that it was fine to cry if he were sad. He had to learn to grieve, and let the grief cleanse him so he could heal. He had to have the courage to deal with the pain and accept the reality, rather than denying it because it hurt too much.

Bad things happened to good people. He knew that intellectually, but not emotionally. That is why he had become a doctor, to help good people when bad things happened to them. That is why the Oncology nurses and doctors do what they do. They helped good people when bad things happened to them. Understanding this emotionally was like lifting a dark cloud from his soul. He finally realized he could not fix everything or overcome every tragedy. He realized he had forgotten his primary directive, try to help, but if you can't help, at least do no harm. Do no harm and do all you can to help—that was what he was supposed to do.

Dave realized neither world was a fantasy; they were both one real world, his world, the world he had chosen. The world he had to become comfortable in if he was going to be a doctor. His naiveté and idealism had prevented him from seeing things clearly in a mature and realistic way. It had taken a little girl losing her leg and some Oncology nurses to teach him how to cope; not by stuffing and denying his emotions in order to avoid the pain, but by having the courage to face the pain by embracing his emotions and allowing them to be expressed in a healthy, healing way.

Sharon had finished her beer and was lying back with her eyes closed dreamily, enjoying the warm fragrant air and soft caress of the fading spring sun. Dave rolled over on to her lounge chair and put his arms around her. "I want to talk."

Sharon opened her eyes. "Does what you want to talk about have anything to do with the way you are holding me? If it does, we need to take this conversation inside."

"No, I want to talk, and I want to hold you while we talk. I want to talk to you about what I do and how I deal with it."

Sharon looked into his eyes. She saw a spark that was not there before. "I am listening. I am here, and I am listening. I want to help. I have wanted to help for a long time, but you have shut me out."

Dave continued, "Like I said, it has been a rough ten months, but I understand a lot now that I didn't until today. Actually, until just now. I was afraid this year was going to change me, and it has. It changed me in a bad way, just as I was afraid it would, and it has been getting worse. But today, I understood I was changing myself for the worse by the way I was dealing with the tragedies I encounter. Today, I dealt with something I could not stuff or deny, it was too sad and overwhelming. I realized I needed to deal with my emotions, not stuff them, and that I need to talk to someone and get some help with expressing my feeling, healing my wounds, and dealing with the pain. I think every training program should make therapy available to their house officers; in fact, I think house officers should be required to meet with a therapist on a regular basis to keep them from being permanently damaged by the stress and emotional duress they deal with on a daily basis. If I can't get a therapist to see, I will find one to talk to who wants to do a paper on how fucked-up interns are."

Sharon reinforced his thoughts. "I agree. Remember, I asked you if you had someone you could talk to about what you dealt with when we first met."

Dave went on, "I have difficulty with death, trying to understand it and feeling guilty when I can't do anything about it. I also struggle with trying to understand why terrible things happen and feeling helpless because I can't stop them from happening. Well, to put it in the vernacular, shit happens, and it is my job to help, no matter what happens or why it happens. As a doctor, I need to try to help if I can. To try to help and to do no harm, that means to do no harm to myself as well. Do all you can to help, then acknowledge and move on to the next one, because there is no end to the suffering of humanity. There are plenty more that need my help, so I can't harm yourself to the point I can't help any of them."

Sharon felt a sense of relief. This was the old Dave, the Dave she loved, the Dave she wanted to spend her life with, the man she admired and respected. "Oh, Dave, I am so glad to hear you talking like yourself again."

Dave smiled. "Don't think I am the same person I was, because I am not. Before this internship, I was a doctor in name only. I had the degree, but I wasn't a doctor; now I am a physician. It was one hell of a rough road to get here, but it is also absolutely necessary anyone who wants to be a doctor must travel that road."

Sharon was feeling good again, when only an hour ago she was so worried. "You are almost at the end of the road."

Dave held her closer. "When I first became serious about being a doctor, I read a book about the road to becoming a physician. But somehow, I lost my way on the road and forgot what that book had taught me about the road. Today, I remembered and found my way again. The road came close to consuming me until I remembered why I was on the road in the first place and that it was a long, tough, hard road that had to be traveled."

Dave sat up. "I have some thoughts about the road. You have to see the cases, you have to have the experiences, you have to do the procedures—in short, you need to travel the road in order to become a competent well-trained doctor. But the road could be made easier and less damaging. Certainly, having therapy on a regular basis would make the road easier, but I think if you weren't sleep deprived and exhausted, some of the things might not affect you so drastically. But you have to do the on-the-job training, you have to put in the hours, see the number of cases, handle the problems, and do everything over and over again until it becomes second nature to you. You have to develop the clinical skills and become proficient in the art of medicine as well as science. That takes a lot of time, a lot of cases, a lot of practice and repetition. I know how to take care of sick adults and sick children now; I know my way around the ED, the OR, and the wards; I can deliver babies, and I can do a number of surgeries; I know my way around the human body; I know how to approach and work a problem to properly diagnose and treat the patient."

Sharon sat up beside him smiling. "You certainly know your way around my body."

Dave looked at her. "I made an A in anatomy in medical school and received some special training outside the classroom."

Sharon frowned. "You know I don't want to hear about your extracurricular training."

Dave looked pensive. "I still have two more months of internship, then two years of residency. It takes three years of training for Medicine and a lot longer for some specialties. If you eliminated the sleep deprivation and exhaustion by cutting the hours, that would decrease the training by forty hours a week for fifty-two weeks, or a full year, so you would have to increase the training period by a year to maintain the current quality of training. The introduction of straight internships is a move in the right direction, but it is not enough. The training periods are long as it is, so no one will want to make them longer. How do you eliminate the sleep deprivation and exhaustion but still maintain the necessary number of hours for an adequate level of training?"

Sharon made some suggestions. "You could go down to add extra training time by making more years of med school clinical and move the classroom work of the first two years of medical school to college; or you could narrow the scope of the specialties and make more of them, so it took less time to become proficient in a narrower field. But I don't know enough about it to know if either suggestion would work."

Dave looked at her. "Jesus, Sharon, great ideas, but I am afraid what is going to happen is those in charge will take the path of least resistance and just cap the number of hours a house officer can work. That will result in a decrease in the quality of physician training, the quality of doctors the training produces, and a major deterioration in the overall quality of health care those doctors deliver. I can't believe how smart you are. How can you be so beautiful and so smart? I am not sure what turns me on more—how smart you are, how beautiful you are, or your perfect body." He nuzzled her neck and cupped her breast in one hand. "OK, it is the perfect body, but the beauty and brains are a close second and third."

Sharon pushed his hand away. "Stop groping me in public. You are getting too feisty with all your new-found epiphanies. We went over your inability to deal with an attractive woman who was smart the night we met."

"The bottom line is something needs to be done before the politicians fuck it up. They don't care about anything but their phony baloney jobs and will do anything to keep them. They will turn things over to the pharmaceutical companies, the for-profit medical companies, and the insurance companies. The politicians in this country don't care about the quality of health care or if people even have health care at all. Frankly, I think they are too incompetent to do anything else, so they run for office, and they will do anything and everything they can to stay in office. It's disgusting, and the uninformed, uneducated, unengaged masses keep re-electing them.

God help us if medicine and health care ever fall into the hands of the politicians and the corporations. The politicians don't govern in the best interest of the people, but for their own self-interest. They are puppets for the wealthy and for the corporate interests that keep them in office" Dave stood up. "At least I know how to do this now. Like you said, it is only two more months, then two years of residency." He held out his hand to her. "Come on, I want to get back in the water."

"OK, but no groping. Everyone out here can see what you are doing because the water is so clear." Sharon got up and took his hand.

Dave led her to the pool. "I will settle for watching you get out of the pool in that suit again."

Sharon laughed. "Right, you and the other guys out here. I can barely keep it on and even when it is on, it barely covers me; when it gets wet, I might as well be naked."

"So?" Dave jumped in the pool and pulled her with him. They swam and played in the pool for a while, then Dave got out, and stood in front of the ladder to watch Sharon get out again.

She stopped and stood on the ladder looking at him. "You know you are a pervert, don't you? What is it with you and water? In the shower, in the bathtub, in the pool—you get in water, and you turn into a pervert."

Dave got a towel, put the towel around her shoulders as she got out, and hugged her. "Water is my natural habitat, and I thrive in it or on it, liquid or frozen. Let's dry off and go in. I want to listen to some music and finish that number. We can order a pizza for dinner and let nature take its course."

Dave had Sharon's bikini off as soon as they were in the door of his apartment. He stripped his own suit off and threw both of them in the kitchen sink. He put the Moody Blues on the stereo, led Sharon to one of the beanbags, pulled her down with him, and lit the remainder of the joint. When the joint was finished, Dave started on Sharon. He felt relieved, so he was insatiable. Sharon was just as turned on because he was almost back to normal, so they spent what was left of the evening in a torrid lovemaking session that was only interrupted from time to time to change the music or their location from the beanbag to the floor, to the bed, and back again. They devoured each other in an unbridled sexual pas de deux choreographed to their music.

It was dark, they were lying on the floor of the front room, and the music had stopped. They cuddled in the dark and silence, letting the night wash over them through the window. Neither of them said anything for some time. There was nothing to say, nothing needed to be said; they had said it all with their lovemaking, and they had woven a spell they didn't want to break. From the very first time they had sex on the night they met, their lovemaking had been overpowering and all consuming; now almost a year later, it had only grown in intensity.

At last, Sharon sat up. "We need to shower and order the pizza. You have to work tomorrow, and I am leaving for Caroline's wedding. I wish you were going with me. Not having a plus-one is an invitation for a lot of unwanted attention. I have been to enough weddings to know how these things go. I want to enjoy Caroline's wedding, I want to dance, and have a good time, but I know there will be a lot of single guys there looking to make it with someone."

Dave sat up beside her. "You can have a good time. Stick close to Jake, and don't let anyone corner you or get you alone. Have a good time but don't drink too much Champagne or you will look like an easy target."

Caroline was getting married in her hometown and Jake was driving Audrey, who was Caroline's maid of honor, Helen and Sharon, who were both bridesmaids, to the wedding for the rehearsal and rehearsal dinner Friday, then the wedding followed by the reception on Saturday. They would drive back Sunday morning so Sharon could be back in time to meet Dave on Sunday when he got off. Sunday was April 30, match day, so by Sunday, they would know where they were going to be next year.

Dave had a clinic day on Friday then was on call Saturday. He started the Nursery on Monday, but his luck was holding so his first day in the Nursery was a day off. When Sharon got back from Caroline's wedding, they would have a free night with the next day off to celebrate their future.

The next week, Dave had Sunday off after a twenty-four-hour shift in the Nursery with his vacation starting on Monday and running seven days and nights until the following Monday morning, but that was an off day too, so he had nine days and nights off. Sharon had taken ten days as vacation time. She made reservations for standby employee tickets for her and a companion for Sunday to LAX.

They showered, Dave put on his robe, Sharon put on a negligee, and Dave ordered a pizza. They ate their pizza with another beer, listened to Steely Dan, and went to bed.

Dave's last few days on the Pedi wards were uneventful. He did not see the little girl again because the amputation confined her to her room post-op. On Sunday morning, he went down to the administrative offices to check the main bulletin board for the match list. He matched with UCLA, Harven matched with Stanford, and George matched with the program at Duke. He contacted Harven and George. "Let's have a match party tonight at the Park house. Nothing big, just get together for some beer, wine, and the party tape. We have a lot of beer and wine left over from Halloween. I will talk to Sharon; she can contact Helen and Audrey. Caroline and Ron are on their honeymoon, Henry can call Bob and Phil, they can call Sam and Rachael."

Harven and George headed home to get the house ready for the party.

Dave would not be going to LA for a residency at UCLA if he had finished his internship a year or two earlier; he would be on his way to Vietnam as a GMO for a two-year tour of duty. Unless a doctor was in the Berry Program or Early Commission Program, he was drafted and sent to the war as soon as he finished his internship. If he joined one of the programs, he was allowed to do his residency first, then enter the military in the specialty he trained in, but either way, until the war started winding down in the early '70s, a doctor was bound for Vietnam. Once the troop reductions started and the draft lottery was instituted, the need for doctors decreased to the point the two programs were closed to new enrollees, and interns were free to continue their training uninterrupted.

Dave went home, showered, shaved, and changed to wait for Sharon. When she came in, Dave told her he matched with UCLA and about the match party. She immediately called the airline to confirm the flight to LA. They decided to stay at Sharon's after the party then come back to Dave's to spend the next day at the pool.

Sharon was so excited about UCLA; she could not sit down. She began to dance and twirl around the room. Dave stood up and corralled her. "Westwood, Baby, Hollywood straight away. It is time to make that California trip. The coast is the most. Then we are going to find the perfect town in Northern California to make our final stand.

We can keep a boat on the Bay, ski in the mountains, take advantage of everything San Francisco has to offer, I can be the town physician, and take care of our friends and neighbors while you become a respected and successful businesswoman. We will go to Europe every year for vacation. Oh, Baby, we have the whole dream, we are just like Bogie and Bacall, we've got it all. Ain't nothing to it but to do it." He spun around holding her up with her legs out then fell back into the beanbag with her in his arms.

She could not stay in the beanbag but got up to continue to dance and swirl around. "Next week, I can't believe it. Next week we are going to find our first home together, and in two months, we are going to be living in California. Wow, it is really happening. I can't believe it." She stopped. "Oh my God, I have to tell my mother. I have to call her. I haven't told her anything except I was dating a doctor. Oh, Dave, calling her and telling her I am moving to California to live with someone I am not married to is going to be tough. Me moving to California is going to be hard enough on her, but me living with someone I am not married to is going to be too much for her. When I told her I was dating a doctor, she wanted to know why I hadn't just stayed with BAR since he was from a rich and influential family."

Sharon started to twirl around again. "I don't want to call her now and spoil how I feel. I will call her later. Tonight, I want to celebrate." She came to Dave and lay down beside him in the beanbag. "If you ever doubted that I loved you, understand this: I am going against my own mother to be with you."

Dave reassured her, "Don't worry. I will charm her."

Sharon snuggled against him. "You don't know my mother."

Dave got up and put the Doors' "LA Woman" on since they were on their way to LA. "How was the wedding?" He lay back down with her.

Sharon's mood changed a bit. "It was fine. Jake is a really good guy. Their wedding is next, but I am not going alone. I will ride up with Helen for the rehearsal and rehearsal dinner the night before, you can drive up the next morning after you get off and sleep in my room until the wedding, then we can drive back that night after the reception."

Dave hugged her. "Did you have trouble because you were alone?"

She smiled. "Ron's friends and family are like him—cultured, well mannered, and polite. His parents are really nice. Caroline's parents, family, and friends are down to earth, outgoing, and friendly, just like she is." She sat up and looked at him. "But that's another reason you should have no doubt that I love you. I danced with a lot of guys who were quite taken with me. I could have had my pick. The groomsman I was paired with was handsome, charming, witty, and he tried to give me his room key at the reception. But I don't want to go through that again. I want you with me at Audrey's wedding, so the other men know I am not available. I want to dance with you, not a bunch of guys on the make."

Dave sat up with her. "If you dance with me, you will definitely be dancing with a guy on the make. But I hate jerks like that. It is OK to pursue a woman if she is free, but anyone who goes after another man's girl is a jerk. I am sure he was a narcissistic player with a very high opinion of himself. You told him you were with someone, and he still tried to fuck you?"

Sharon laughed. "I told him I was engaged, and Ron told him I was engaged, so yes, he knew I was with someone. He was really cute and outgoing, so I was having a good time with him, until he tried to give me his room key. I thought he understood I wanted to enjoy my friend's wedding and he was just showing me a good time; especially since he knew about you. But he came on strong from the beginning, telling me how beautiful I was and keeping my Champagne glass full. It was a planned seduction all along. He gave me the same line the strippers gave you. He said he didn't know you and would never meet you so he couldn't tell you, so if I didn't tell, you and no one else would ever know we fucked. He had a good line about me being engaged and didn't I want to get it on with someone different one last time before I got married, especially since no one but he and I would know. That's why he wanted to give me his room key, so I could come to his room after everyone had gone to bed. He said what you didn't know wouldn't hurt you, plus it was obvious the two of us were into each other, so why not enjoy ourselves and take advantage of a chance to have a good time together with no strings attached. No one would ever know but the two of us, and it would give me something to remember after I got married. He got very intimate and said he was sure he could give me an exceptionally memorable night. He turned out to be a real player. He reminded me a lot of the guys I dated before I met Bar. They were good looking and witty too; some were professional athletes, others were wealthy or well-known, still others were from prominent families like Bar, but they didn't care about me; all they wanted was to fuck me. They never tried to get to know me; they only wanted my body. Just like this guy, they were narcissistic and superficial. They tried to charm or impress me into fucking them, never engaging with me or trying to connect with who I am."

"You know that's all a standard line. He has used it many times before probably with good success. How do I know he wasn't successful with you? How do I know you didn't fuck him?" Dave couldn't control his jealousy.

"Dave, you have to stop being jealous. If I had fucked him, would I have told you about him? I told you when we first got together, if I ever want to fuck someone else or if I ever fuck someone else, I will tell you. I meant it then and I mean it even more now. I love you. I love the way you fuck me. I haven't and I don't want to fuck anyone else. Jesus, look at you. You are positively green, and I haven't done anything." She put her arms around his neck.

"You experienced the same thing I did with the strippers." He put his arms around her and pulled her down with him.

"Yes, and like you, I didn't do anything about it." She snuggled against him.

Dave thought, *But I considered it and you probably did too.* "I guess we have both been tempted and we both resisted the temptation."

"You may have been tempted, but I wasn't. I never even thought about having sex with him. I left him standing there with his key in his hand, a stupid grin on his face, and walked away without saying a word. Having sex with some else could never come close to what we have, so why would I want to fuck anyone else? Plus, I love you. Why can't you get that through your head and stop being jealous? I love you, and I don't want to make love to anyone else." She pulled back and looked at him.

Dave knew she was right.

They talked and listened to some more music, Sharon called her roommates about the party and left to get ready. Dave ate a ham sandwich, rolled a large spilf from a big Jamaican bud, then took a short nap. Dave was happy he had matched with UCLA. By doing a rotating internship at University Hospital first to prove himself in a good program, he had gotten into an excellent residency program. But one thing nagged at him, especially after Sharon told him about the guy at the wedding—he wished she would marry him. He would never pressure her, but if she married him, everything would be perfect for their move to California.

Sharon let him in when he got to her house, laughed, then ran upstairs. "Great idea. It will only take me a minute to change. Helen and Linda are in the kitchen." Dave was dressed the way he was the night they met, in jeans, his Gandalf T-shirt and tire tread sandals, with his hair down to his shoulders.

Dave went to the kitchen to find Helen and a dark-haired woman in her early thirties sitting at the table. Even though her attire was feminine, the woman had short hair, short nails with no polish, and no makeup. She made Dave think of Sam.

"Linda, this is Dave, Sharon's fiancé. Dave this is Linda." The woman nodded to Dave as he sat down with them. "Linda moved into Caroline's room while we were at the wedding this weekend. She is a flight attendant I have been working with since Sharon started bidding around your call schedule. We are going to get an apartment together when Sharon moves out. Are you and Sharon going to get married here or in LA?"

Dave looked a little uneasy. "That is entirely up to Sharon."

Helen looked serious. "You know Sharon has a phobia about getting married?"

Dave nodded. "I know. That's why it is up to her."

Sharon came into the kitchen. "What is up to me?"

She had changed into the same outfit she wore the night they met—the short black skirt, the white top unbuttoned and tied at the bottom, and black heels. She took Dave's breath away, just as she had the night they met, and all he could say was, "Wow."

"You are X-rated children." She turned to Linda. "They are wearing the same things they wore the night they met. That is why she changed, to match him. This is a party to celebrate the guys matching with their training programs. Dave matched with UCLA, and they are moving to California. They are wearing what they wore the night they met, like they were in high school."

Linda looked admiringly at Sharon. "I can see why he was all over you; you are stunning, and not just the shoes, but your whole outfit says, come fuck me. I guess he got the message."

Helen continued, "Believe me, he got the message, but she was all over him too, I mean literally all over him. Needless to say, they left the party early, and I am willing to bet they leave this party early too."

Linda responded, "The way she looks, I'm surprised they are even going to the party."

Sharon held her hand out to Dave. "Let's go. I want a glass of wine, I want to get stoned, I want to dance, and I want to celebrate." She looked at Linda and Helen. "Then I want to do what we did the night we met." She pulled Dave up, flipped her hair at Helen and Linda, and started for the door.

Dave jumped up. "I am on it. I got it. Wine, weed, dance, celebrate, fornicate, in that order. Come on, ladies."

Helen got up laughing. "Like I told you, Linda, they are X-rated children."

As they walked to the house next door, Dave and Sharon held hands, and Sharon skipped along beside Dave like a little girl, swinging their hands back and forth.

Helen and Linda fell in a little behind them. "Look at them. They are so cute, it's disgusting. I am going to miss her terribly. I am going to miss all three of them, but I am going to miss her most of all. I want to dislike Dave for taking her away from me, but look how happy she is. When she came back from finding out where he matched, she danced up the stairs singing 'California Dreaming.' There used to be a sadness about her, but since she met him, it is like the dark cloud that was surrounding her lifted, and her inner light began to shine through."

Linda looked at Helen and nodded at Dave and Sharon. "I guess that's true love."

Helen looked back at her. "I wouldn't know. I have never been in love. Have you?"

Linda responded, "No, not true love. Not like that." She nodded at Sharon and Dave again.

They continued looking at each other, walked on, and caught up with Sharon and Dave on the front porch of the other house. Helen looked at them as she and Linda walked up. "I wonder what it is like to feel like that about someone?"

Linda answered, "I don't know, but I would like to find out." She looked at Helen as Dave turned to them. "Stop lagging, it's party time. We need to get on with the wine, weed, dance, and celebration parts."

Helen laughed. "I know, so you can get to the last part."

Dave smiled at Sharon. "You bet. Look at her. Do you blame me?"

Linda looked at Sharon. "No, like I said, I am surprised you didn't skip all the other parts and go straight to the last part to begin with. I know I would have." The last thing she said was lost on Sharon and Dave, but not on Helen, who turned to look at Linda.

The first thing Dave heard as they walked through the door was, "Hey, Poncho, I'm gonna miss your ass. You taking that little girl with you? Damn, Sharon, you almost got dressed. I get it, I have seen you two before." Henry grabbed Dave in a bear hug.

Dave hugged his friend back. "Hey, Cisco, I hate to leave your ass behind, man, but I got to make that California trip. This little girl is gonna make it with me." Dave looked over his shoulder at Sharon. "You think I would leave that behind?"

Sharon interjected. "I am not a *that*. I think the real Poncho and Cisco were much more respectful of women. I think if someone wants to make it to the last part tonight, like we talked about, they had better not call me a *that*."

Helen introduced Linda to Henry and Sigrid. Sigrid had on a cream-colored pants suit that consisted of a vest cut like a man's suit vest with nothing on under it and wide leg slacks, long enough to cover her high heels and reach the floor. The pants made her legs look even longer, and the heels made her as tall as Henry. "Why do you call each other Poncho and Cisco? I know they are American TV characters you grew up watching. But why are you Cisco and Poncho?"

Henry looked at Dave. "Should I tell her?" Dave nodded. "They were our Hell-Week names. The actives gave us names for Hell Week. I was The Cisco Kid and Dave was Poncho the Sidekick."

Harven and Connie heard the Poncho, Cisco exchange at the front door and joined them. "If you ever plan to motor west," Harven sang, "Travel my way, take the highway, that's the best." Connie joined in. "Get your kicks on Route Sixty-Six."

Dave sang poorly, "It winds from Chicago to LA. More than two thousand miles all the way."

Sharon followed in perfect pitch and a nice voice. Then all four of them harmonized, "Get your kicks on Route Sixty-Six." Sharon took off. "Now you go through Saint Louie, Joplin Missouri. And Oklahoma City looks mighty pretty. You'll see Amarillo, Gallop New

A love story and social commentary

Mexico, Flagstaff Arizona. Don't forget Winona, Kingman, Barstow, San Bernadino." Sharon finished up in a high ringing voice. "Won't you get hip to this timely tip. When you make that California trip." Then all of them together again. "Get your kicks on Route Sixty-Six." The four of them laughed and high-fived each other.

George and the grad student walked up. George was animated and excited. "Not everyone is going to California. Some of us aren't getting above our raising and are staying right here in the sunny Southland."

Mike and Janice joined them all at the front door. "And some of us are staying put with a good thing."

Henry responded. "Right on."

Sigrid pulled on Henry's arm. "What did he say about raisins?"

"Not raisins, Sigrid, raising," Henry answered.

"What is his raising? What does he mean?" Sigrid looked puzzled.

"He is speaking Appalachian. There is no English translation." Henry laughed.

Dave pulled the joint out. "I have here a magical Jamaican Match Day joint."

Bob, Phil, Rachael, and Sam, had not arrived yet. Dave called to everyone, "Arm yourselves with the adult beverage of your choice and let us retire to the zoom room to partake of this fine Bob Marley weed. For the uninitiated, this is one toke, and the world turns round weed; take two tokes and you will be severely fucked-up; take three tokes, and you will be in La La Land."

Six of the people who filed down the hall to the zoom room were impacted and their lives forever changed by a piece of paper hanging from the hospital administration's bulletin board. That piece of paper had determined their future, and tonight they were going to celebrate embracing that future the piece of paper had dictated. Two couples were going west, and one couple was going east. That piece of paper was the hinge on the door of their futures.

Harven had the party tape queued up, but he didn't start it. Instead they all stood in a circle and passed the joint around until it was finished. Then Harven triggered the tape, and Brown Sugar filled the room followed by Henry's yell of "Stones Mother." Gradually, the couples left the zoom room to get more to drink, to talk, or to dance in the front room with the others, but Helen and Linda remained behind.

Phil, Bob, Rachael, and Sam must have heard the music, because they showed up shortly after it started, and of course they were already stoned. Phil asked Henry for an update on things. Henry told him, "Mike and I are staying here, George is going to the program at Duke, Harven is going to Stanford, and Dave is going to UCLA."

"It is going to be a lot different with all of them gone. Oh well, I suppose a new group of grad students, medical students, or whatever will move into the two houses, but this group was special." Phil danced with Rachael while Sam and Bob sat on one of the couches, sipped wine, and watched. Linda and Helen emerged from the zoom room to dance together.

After dancing for a while, Henry and Dave went to the dining room to get refills. Henry told Dave Sigrid was moving in with him at the end of the month. She had received a special grant to continue her research at the university, arranged by Henry's family, and Henry had promised her she could go home anytime she wanted to stay as long as she pleased to be with her family and friends. Henry planned to ask her to marry him and to promise her they would live in Europe after he finished his training. The two friends were high and happy celebrating how well things turned out for them both. Harven joined them, and they all three pledged to stay in touch over the next few years as they completed their training. Harven suggested they take their vacations at the same time each year in January and meet somewhere to ski. Henry volunteered his family's lodge in Colorado where he and Dave skied when they were in college.

Dave and Henry returned to the front room to find Mike and Janice sitting with Sharon and Sigrid. Only a few couples were still dancing, and the others were sitting or standing around talking. The celebration was winding down. They wanted to enjoy each other's company and talk, rather than dance.

Dave had heard Mike was trash-talking him to the other house officers at the hospital, and he thought it was because of Sharon. His reputation was being tarnished by the rumors Mike was spreading, and he considered confronting Mike about it, but he decided he was leaving soon, so it didn't matter, yet it bothered Dave to think his peers thought ill of him because of what Mike was saying. They listened to Mike because they knew Dave and Mike were friends, so they thought the things Mike was saying had to be true.

Dave handed Sharon her wine then put his hand out to her. She took his hand and stood up. Henry took the hint and did the same thing with Sigrid; the four of them walked off to find Connie and Harven. Dave had not spoken to Mike or acknowledged him in any way since he heard about the rumors Mike was spreading.

They found Connie and Harven in the hall on their way to the to the zoom room. "I want to go to the zoom room and turn the music down since hardly anyone is dancing. Besides, if we go to the zoom room, maybe Sharon will take her clothes off again since she has on the same thing she had on that night and she has been smoking Jamaican weed."

Connie smacked him. "Behave."

They closed the door and lounged on the cushions in a small circle. Harven explained his idea of meeting every January for the next few years to ski, and Henry added that they could use his family's ski lodge in Colorado. Sharon wanted to know if there was enough room to include Audrey, Jake, Caroline, and Ron. Henry responded that there were six bedrooms, so there was plenty of room.

"Six bedrooms!" Sigrid was shocked. "That is not a ski lodge, that's a chateau. How many other places like that does your family own?"

Henry looked embarrassed. "Granny owns a twenty-thousand-acre ranch with a ranch house in Texas, a beach house with private docks in the Keys, the ski lodge in Colorado, and of course, my grandmother, my parents, and my aunt and uncle own their own homes as well."

"Twenty thousand acres! The beach house and the ranch house—they are as big as the ski lodge?" Sigrid asked.

Henry responded. "No, they are bigger."

Sigrid looked at Henry. "It does not bother you that so many are homeless, yet your family has so many big houses and so much land?"

Henry took her hand. "I intend to use my share of the family money for good. Don't get me wrong, I want to live well, but I will do as much as I can to help others."

Dave spoke up for his friend. "Henry's grandmother, known affectionately as Granny, controls the family fortune and distributes all the proceeds, plus she controls the properties. Henry started receiving a distribution from his trust fund when he was eighteen. He has control of that, but nothing else. The family donates to various charities, and

Henry has championed some causes on his own, but Granny calls the shots."

Henry added, "And no one tells my grandmother what to do, period, not with her money, or anything else."

"Wow, I knew you were rich, Henry, but I did not know how rich." Sigrid was surprised.

Henry looked at her. "Does it make a difference?"

She paused for a moment, then answered, "I guess not, if you truly intend to use all that money for good." Henry pulled her to him and put his arm around her. "I do." Henry looked into her eyes. "You might as well know all of it. There is an apartment in Paris my sister lives in and one in New York City my cousin lives in. There is also a yacht with a captain, cook, and crew that is available to members of the family, but it isn't used much, so Granny is thinking about selling it. Sigrid, my family once owned a great deal of land, and that land has oil on it. The family sold most of the land but kept the mineral rights so there is a considerable annual income from those oil leases. That income and the income from the family's other investments are distributed by Granny to all the family members yearly, plus we all have trust funds that give us significant incomes. I have reinvested a lot of the money I have received so I have a lot of my own money. You are right, my family is very rich, indeed."

Dave had been to all the properties Henry's family owned, plus Henry's parent's house and Granny's house. They were not houses in the true sense of the word. The beach house was really a compound on acreage with a private beach, a large pool, and a dock for a sailboat and a sports fishing boat. Dave and Henry spent Spring Breaks there with Henry's cousins during college. The ranch house looked like Tara from the movie *Gone with the Wind* and had an air strip with a hangar. In college, Henry flew Dave there for weekends when they wanted to get away. The ski lodge was like a condominium complex with a steam room, sauna, large hot tub, and an indoor heated pool. Henry's parents lived in the Garden District of New Orleans in an antebellum home that looked like it belonged on a large plantation. Henry's grandfather was dead, and Granny lived in Dallas on Turtle Creek in what could only be described as a mansion. Henry's family was one of the old Texas big oil families, and they were very rich.

Harven tried to change the subject. "So, we are committed? We will meet at Henry's to ski in January."

"You bet," Dave answered and they all nodded in agreement with him.

Turning the music down led to the end of the party, and everyone began to leave. Connie stood up. "Some of us have to work tomorrow, and Sharon has kept her clothes on, so let's go upstairs, Harven." She held her hand out to Harven, who took it and stood up.

"Next year in Colorado," Harven said as they left.

Henry stood up with Sigrid. "I guess it is time to take my shield maiden home. We will see you guys when you get back from California."

"I am not a shield maiden. You are an earl with all your houses and money. An earl would not have a mere shield maiden. But you had better be a good earl and take care of people." She said, "Goodbye," to Sharon and Dave, and they left.

Dave tried to get up, but Sharon pulled him back down. "I want to finish what I started the night we met."

Dave looked at her, and her top was untied. "There are still people here. Someone might walk in on us."

She stood up and walked to the door to close it. "I don't care. I intend to finish what I started that night." She walked back to Dave, pushed him down on his back, straddled him and began to undo his belt.

Dave helped her get his pants off. "Did you plan this?"

She slipped out of her thong and sat down on him with her skirt up around her waist. "Little bit, but not until I saw you in that stupid Gandalf shirt with those tight jeans, and I remembered how hot I was for you that night." She leaned down and put her breast in front of his face took the back of his head in one hand and pulled him to her, burying his face in her softness. "Dave, I am very happy tonight, and I want you to make me go woo, woo, woo big time right here where it all started."

Dave locked his arms around her, rolled over on top of her and did just that until she cried out as she grabbed the cushions with both hands, digging her fingers into them, and then beating them with her fist. Dave was in her before the sound had time to die away, driving her into the cushions as she grabbed them again to hold on.

Dave held her wrapped around him. "Was it us or was it the weed?" He laughed.

"Perfect," was all she said.

They cuddled with Sharon snuggled under Dave's arm with her head on his chest and her leg over his. They were intoxicated on sexual fulfillment in a dream-like state for some time. They were beginning to stir when the door opened.

"Is there anyone in here?" It was Mike's voice.

Dave answered. "Yes." Sharon pulled her skirt down and retied her top while Dave looked for his jeans, sandals, and Sharon's thong. All he had on was his T-shirt.

Mike and Janice walked in and left the door open. "I thought you might be smoking some more weed."

Dave stood up in front of them with his jeans and sandals in one hand, and Sharon's thong in the other. Sharon took the thong and walked past Mike with the thong dangling from her finger. "No. We were fucking." Dave pulled his pants on, followed Sharon out and put his sandals on in the hall, then Sharon and Dave walked down the hall and out the door, with Sharon still dangling the thong from her finger.

Outside, Sharon leaned into Dave, and he put his arm around her. "I know that was tacky, but he deserved it. He was just dying to get a look."

Dave hugged her, and she put her arms around him. "Janice certainly got a good look."

Mike and Janice watched Dave and Sharon walk down the hall to leave, and Mike said, "She is such a slut. I can't believe Dave is going to marry her, but he is just as bad. They deserve each other." Mike was humiliated.

Dave and Sharon walked back to her house arm and arm. "Poor Henry. He has always been so careful to date only women who were rich so he could be sure they weren't with him for his money. Now he is in love with someone who has a problem with him being wealthy. Wait until Sigrid meets Granny and sees the place in Dallas, or the ranch, not to mention the beach compound with the boats, grounds, pool, private beach, and a yacht anchored in the cove. The ski lodge is the smallest and least impressive of them all. You enter the ranch house through a large room with a cathedral ceiling and a huge fireplace. Above the fireplace is an oil painting of Granny straddling a calf with a branding iron in her hands about to brand a calf. The calf's legs are tied, and it has a rope around its neck, leading to her horse in the background. She is dressed in chaps, a leather vest, and boots with a cowboy hat. Henry grew up going to that ranch on weekends. Sigrid didn't know it, but she was right when she called him a cowboy. Not only does he sail, water and snow ski, but he can also ride, and he flies his own plane."

"She loves him in spite of his wealth, not because of it. I like her a lot. She has such a fresh straightforward view of things, and she definitely has her priorities straight. I am so glad we are all making an effort to stay in touch no matter where we are." Sharon laughed. "I understand Henry. He was afraid he would be loved for his wealth, not for who he is. I know how that feels. I was afraid I would be loved for my looks, and not for who I am."

"Yes, but your looks are an asset, not a deterrent. Sigrid sees Henry's wealth as a deterrent. That's different," Dave pointed out.

Sharon laughed again. "Henry's wealth is an asset. The kind of wealth Henry has can open doors for her she never dreamed of, to do things that she would never be able to do without his financial backing. She will see his wealth as an assent soon enough. She is still trying to get her head around it; she still doesn't understand how wealthy Henry really is, or how that wealth can help her do what she wants to do and more than she ever conceived of doing with her career and her research."

They walked on to the house, went upstairs, and got straight in bed. Dave still had a day to rest and relax before he started his next rotation in the Nursery, and Sharon was looking forward to the trip to California. Once they had a place in California, they still had two weddings to attend, then the move to accomplish, all while Dave finished his internship and Sharon continued to fly. Sharon knew the next two months were going to be very busy. They slept late, showered, got dressed, had breakfast, then drove to Dave's to spend the day relaxing by the pool, before having dinner, listening to their favorite albums, and going to bed early.

17
The Nursery and the California Trip

The Nursery was a straight twenty-four on and twenty-four off. He had a supervising resident and only one stud to manage. Most newborn babies are welcomed, and their arrival is a happy occasion for the parents. There are unwed and teenage mothers, many of whom give their babies up for adoption, but even that brings joy to a couple who couldn't have a child on their own.

The problems in the Nursery arose with the babies of alcoholic mothers or mothers with drug addiction. Fetal alcohol syndrome was terrible, and the drug addicted babies went through withdrawal, had seizures, and suffered permanent brain damage. These unfortunate babies would never have a chance at a normal life because of the actions of their mothers. Then there were the poor babies with Down syndrome, CP, and other birth defects who would suffer their whole life through no fault of their own.

But Dave didn't try to deny the pathos of those situations or bury the pain anymore. Instead, he let it wash over him in a tidal wave of emotion. There were times when he was working with these unfortunate babies and he had tears in his eyes. The heartache he felt for them and their parents was unmeasurable, but he had learned a lot from the oncology nurses, and he was applying what he had learned. He let himself suffer and heal, instead of carrying a festering wound buried deep inside him that would never heal. He had learned that denial as a defense mechanism doesn't work in the practice of medicine.

When it all got too much for him, he would go to the doctors' lounge and apply cognitive thinking, replacing the horror he was experiencing with positive thoughts of the wonderful life he had. When he was off, he applied cognitive behavior, swimming laps until he purged the negative toxic thoughts from his mind and flushed the stress-related physical effects out of his body. He had found a psychiatry resident to have lunch with on a regular basis who listened to him as he talked out his most troubling issues. He still relied on getting high on weed as a form of self-medication, and on having sex with Sharon to take him away from the surrealistic world of the hospital, but the sex and weed now only brought him pleasure; he no longer depended on them to cope.

The Nursery rotation turned out to be the best thing that happened to him during his internship. It was a catharsis that cleansed him of all the things that had accumulated in him over the previous ten months. He literally cried out his emotional pain, and the tears healed his wounds, not only from his experiences as an intern but from his experience with his sister.

The most stressful cases Dave had to manage in the Nursery were the preemies. Dave had no experience with the tiny babies since the OB/GYN residents did all the premature deliveries in L and D. They were so small and fragile, Dave was afraid to touch them. But his supervising resident was kind, gentle, and caring; taking time to reassure Dave and to help him calculate the micro doses of meds, oxygen, and fluids necessary to maintain the small infants. Many did not make it, succumbing to hyaline membrane disease or other problems, but Dave was able to deal with their deaths better because they barely had the organ base necessary to survive. Each one he saved seemed like a miracle, and that overshadowed the ones he lost. Many of the problems, like the babies with jaundice, were solvable, and the major cases were transferred to specialty services, so the pressures and demands on him were self-limited.

Sharon notified UCLA's graduate school that she was accepting the place they had offered her. Dave and Sharon spent the days after his shifts getting ready to leave, packing, making reservations, contacting UCLA, lining up a rental car, and planning things to do after they found a place to live.

After one of his 24-hour shifts in the Nursery, Dave called Sharon and told her to come over a little later than usual. Dave cut his hair that day. He went straight to a barber shop from the hospital. He didn't have it cut short, it was still long, but it was groomed and styled to look well-kept and neat. He did it for Sharon, he did it for their future, and he did it so he could get along in the world a little easier. Sharon and their life together were more important to him now than any political, antiwar, or civil rights statement. He did it because it was time to grow up, assume the responsibilities of a physician, and join the ranks of his profession. But mainly he did it for Sharon, to take care of her, to assure her of the future she dreamed of and wanted.

When Sharon saw him, she clapped, jumped up and down, twirled in a circle, then ran to him and jumped into his arms. He said, "Does this mean there is going to be some good wu chang lang tonight?"

She kissed him then leaned back to look at him. "You are really a nice-looking man. I never knew you were so hot. You are better looking than any of the guys who are always hitting on me. And yes, I will wu your chang with more than a little lang tonight."

It was obvious to Sharon that Dave was coping better, was more mature, more realistic, and less naive, but he had not changed fundamentally. His body and muscles were coming back from swimming, so a lot of Sharon's fears dissipated. She was excited about finding a place to live in LA. Her natural domestic instincts were bubbling over as she reviewed her plans for their apartment and fine-tuned just how she wanted each room to look. They had the money they needed to move and get resettled and to cover her grad school expenses, while giving them enough left over to do the things they wanted to do, like go on a ski vacation with their friends and maintain a reasonable lifestyle in a very exciting place.

Dave's shifts in the Nursery were busy, but there was down time and time to sleep intermittently. He made rounds with his stud and resident in the mornings, admitted normal newborn babies to the Nursery when they came from L and D, answered calls from the Nursery to handle problems, was present to take the baby at C-sections, and answered calls from L and D to admit and handle problem babies and preemies. He managed to sleep at the hospital, although it was up and down, then he slept until noon when he got back to his apartment.

During a down time in the doctors' lounge, Dave calculated the number of hours he worked during his year of internship. He had averaged a hundred hours a week in the hospital on his every third-day on call rotations and eighty-five hours a week on his twenty-four hours on, twenty-four hours off rotations. With his time off, the shorter days and shifts, plus the extended hours he worked, he worked about five thousand hours under very stressful and emotionally taxing circumstances, or an average of over ninety hours a week.

Dave slept on and off for about four hours on his shift the day before they left, but he could not get any more sleep because they went straight to the airport to stand by for a flight. They got on a morning flight that put them into LAX in the early afternoon. Sharon knew the flight crew, and there were seats in first-class, so after takeoff, the flight attendants moved them up front. They were completely unaware of the other passengers around them, lost in their own world, and the first-class flight attendant kept refilling their Champagne glasses.

A passenger asked if they were on their honeymoon. Dave told them they were engaged and going to LA to find a place to live. Some toasts were offered, a lot of advice was given, and a small party for Sharon and Dave ensued. The Champagne flowed; a passenger told Sharon how beautiful she was, another told Dave how lucky he was, and several related their own love stories. All of them wanted to know how Sharon and Dave met, what they did, and why they were moving to LA. They became a happy, noisy group. Some other passengers complained to the flight attendant, and she asked the partying passengers to respect those who wanted a calm, quiet trip, and things got back to normal, but by then, Dave and Sharon were buzzed on Champagne and overwhelmed by the outpouring of goodwill. It was a great way to start their trip to LA and their future life together in California.

They arrived at LAX on time, retrieved their bags, picked up the rental car, and drove to the UCLA campus. It was a Sunday, but school was in session, and there were a few people in the Administration Building, so when Sharon and Dave found the grad school offices, a young man was there to greet them. He told them a lot of the staff were working weekends to get ready for graduation and offered to talk to Sharon about her place in the MBA program. He reviewed Sharon's file quickly, welcomed her to UCLA and the MBA program, then gave her the forms and paperwork she needed to complete. He told her classes started on September first with orientation beginning the week before. He asked if she had any questions. Sharon asked about a place to live, and he replied many students lived on campus because housing in the area was so expensive. Sharon thanked him, and they left him standing at the conference room door, smiling as he watched Sharon walk away.

They drove to the hospital, went to the administrative offices, asked about the location of the Medicine wards, and picked up the paperwork and forms Dave needed. Dave and Sharon went up to wards and one of the nurses directed them to the doctors' lounge where he found a few guys sitting around on couches. They seemed annoyed when Dave first introduced himself, until they saw Sharon, then they were up smiling, introducing themselves, offering places to sit, and asking how they could help. One of them, a student, fell all over himself trying to show Sharon a place to sit, getting her a Coke, and sitting beside her while Dave talked with the other house staff.

Dave asked where they should look for a place to live. A resident told him somewhere around the San Diego freeways because it would take him to Torrance for his rotations there. The resident advised him to get a rental agent first thing tomorrow morning or he would waste a lot of time.

By the time Dave and Sharon left to locate their hotel, Dave was dead tired, but Sharon was energized by being in such a famous and glamorous place. They were surrounded by Bel Air, Brentwood, Beverly Hills, and Hollywood, with streets named Sunset Boulevard, Santa Monica Boulevard, Wilshire Boulevard, Hollywood, Vine, and Mulholland Drive. Sharon and Dave had grown up in towns with populations of a little over a hundred thousand, and even though they had lived in large cities in the South, big cities in the South didn't have place and street names they had heard all their lives connected with fame. Even though Sharon had spent a lot of time in New York and LA on layovers, she was star struck. Dave would have been too, if he wasn't so tired. When they got to the car, Sharon was flush with the reality that this was her future. "Dave, I can't believe I am here, and I am going to live here."

Dave drove to the hotel. "I will call a rental agent in the morning. I hope we can find something fairly quickly. I want to take you to Disneyland, and I would like to spend a day or two relaxing at the beach. When we get back, we have to pack everything, have our stuff moved, and drive out here. At least you will have two months to get things ready before you start classes. It's going to be busy, and oh yeah, you have to keep flying, and I have to finish my Pedi rotation. No problem."

Dave had booked a hotel in Santa Monica that was within walking distance of the beach and pier. When they got to the room, Dave took his clothes off and climbed onto the bed. "I have to take a little nap." He had slept on and off for four of the last thirty-six hours, and he'd drunk a lot of Champagne.

Sharon reminded him that they needed to eat. "We will eat when I wake up. I'm only going to take a short nap." He slept straight through until the next morning.

When Sharon realized he was not going to wake up, she called the front desk, and the desk clerk told her they did not have room service or a restaurant on site, but there was a deli in the lobby where she could get something to eat. She went down and ordered a sandwich, chips, and a drink at the counter and sat down at one of the small tables to eat and pout a little. It was their first night in California, and she was eating alone at a deli while Dave was asleep in the room. Not a very exciting way to start their life in California, but then she remembered the flight, how nice the other passengers had been, their visit to the UCLA campus, and how helpful and friendly the administrator and the house officers had been, so she stopped pouting.

A nice-looking young man came in, ordered, took his food, and walked to her table. "Can I join you?"

Sharon looked up at him, smiled, and said, "No. I am with someone."

"I don't see anyone. Where is he? I doubt a guy would let a beautiful woman like you eat alone in a hotel deli. I think you are alone." He sat down. "My name is Erich. What's yours?"

"Excuse me." Sharon picked up her food and moved to another table. "Bitch," she heard the man say under his breath as she walked away. She finished eating as quickly as she could and went back to the room hoping the man wouldn't follow her. She had flown all over the country and never had a problem, but she always had gone out with other members of her crew, never alone. This encounter made her realize how vulnerable a lone woman was in a large city. Then she laughed as she remembered the can of mace in her purse.

Dave woke up early. "God, I am starving."

Sharon reminded him, "You forgot to eat last night."

"I haven't felt this rested and relaxed for a long time. How long did I sleep?" Dave got out of bed.

"About fourteen hours. Stop that, we have to find a place to live." Sharon was trying to dress, and everything she put on, Dave tried to take off. "Being rested and relaxed makes you too frisky. Let me get dressed so we can have breakfast and call a rental agent to find a place to live." She put her arms around his neck. "We have work to do."

Dave let her dress, showered, shaved, and put his own clothes on. They walked to a diner near the hotel and had breakfast before Dave began calling rental agents from the Yellow Pages of the phonebook in the room. On the fourth call, he found someone he liked that sounded intelligent and reasonable, so he put Sharon on the phone to talk to the agent. She told Sharon to enjoy their morning, she would pick them up at their hotel at one o'clock, and she would be available to show them apartments this afternoon and tomorrow.

Sharon hung up, looked at Dave and said, "Rodeo Drive." They drove to one of the most famous shopping streets in the world, Dave parked the car, and they walked along Rodeo Drive, window shopping. Sharon found a stylish dress shop and pulled Dave in with her. The clerk looked at them without a smile as Sharon browsed the dresses on the racks. Dave and Sharon were dressed in jeans, T-shirts, and sandals, unlike the other shoppers on Rodeo Drive who were dressed in expensive couture. Sharon found several dresses she liked and had the clerk pull them for her. The clerk took Dave to an expensive comfortable chair in the back of the store in front of a raised dais with fitting rooms behind it and went into one of the fitting rooms with Sharon and the dresses.

Sharon emerged in a beautiful dress that accentuated her figure and walked with her model's walk to the dais and did her thing for Dave. She tried two more dresses with the clerk commenting to her and Dave about how beautiful she looked in each one and how they brought out her best features.

"Which one do you like best?" Sharon asked Dave as she stood on the dais in the last dress.

"That one. That is the most beautiful dress I have ever seen, but where are you going to wear it?" Dave looked at the clerk. "How much is it?"

"It was five hundred dollars, but there is a seasonal markdown to three hundred." The clerk smiled at Dave.

"I have something in mind. I'll take it. It is going to need a few alterations; can you have it ready in a week?"

"Of course," the clerk replied.

Sharon waited on the dais for the tailor to mark the dress for alterations. Dave could tell she was having a wonderful time as she followed the clerk to the counter, paid for the dress, and took the pickup slip.

A love story and social commentary

The clerk said, "You seem so rural, but you act like a model."

"You know, you are right, we are rural, but I model for Nieman Marcus."

"I thought so, I could tell immediately you were a model by the way you walked and carried yourself, and of course you are quite beautiful. Your dress will be ready Saturday. Have a nice day."

They left the shop with Sharon holding Dave's hand and skipping along beside him the way she did when she was very happy. "Now it's your turn. How old are your suits? Let me guess, you bought them when you were in college, so they are at least five years old. You need a new suit, and this is the place to get it."

They found an exclusive men's shop, and Sharon led Dave in, smiling at the older gentleman who welcomed them. "He is looking for a suit."

The man smiled back at Sharon and explained they did custom-tailoring, but they did have a few off-the-rack suits from top designers in the back. He took them to a rack of fine suits on the back wall, then pulled a few in Dave's coat size. "The problem will be the pants. His shoulders are big, but his waist and hips are much smaller, so the pants that come with the coat will not come close to fitting him."

"I know. I like him that way. Can you alter the pants to fit?" She flashed her most alluring smile at the gentleman.

"I am a tailor, and I can tell you, if I alter the pants that come with the jacket to fit him, they will not look right. I could swap the pants with a suit with a smaller coat size and hope someone who is heavier buys it," the man said to Sharon.

"Oh, could you? That would be great. I like the dark blue one with the very fine pin stripe. It brings out his eyes," Sharon gushed.

"You have excellent taste. That is a very fine suit indeed. I will be happy to do it for such a lovely young woman. Is he your husband?" The man took the coat from one suit and the pants from another identical suit in a smaller size and ushered Dave to a fitting room.

"No, he is my lover," Sharon answered, smiling mischievously.

"I normally would not do this, but I can't deny such a beautiful young woman. I am Italian, and we Italians understand amoré. Consider this suit my gift to you." He opened the door to a dressing room for Dave and sat Sharon down in a chair nearby. "You can wait here while I mark the suit."

"Ciao, Bella," the man said to Sharon as they left.

When they were outside the shop, Dave took Sharon's hand again. "I think he liked you. Now we can dress like movie stars. Is that what you wanted?"

"Little bit." Sharon hugged his arm as they walked along. "I don't think we are going to find a place to eat lunch here the way we are dressed. I want to see the Sunset Strip, Hollywood and Vine, then go somewhere to eat."

Dave drove to Hollywood and Vine, down the Sunset Strip, then back down Santa Monica Boulevard to the hotel. They walked down to the Santa Monica pier and got hot dogs for lunch on the pier before going back to the hotel to wait for the rental agent.

They were waiting in the lobby when a white Mercedes convertible pulled up in front of the hotel and an attractive bottle blond in her forties dressed in a tight dress and stiletto heels got out. She clicked into the lobby, walked straight up to Sharon, and put her hand out. "You must be Sharon. My, but you are a beauty, aren't you, but I am not crazy about you're ensemble. One piece of advice for you, dear; dress to display your best assets, and your looks will carry you a long way in this town." After shaking Sharon's hand, she turned to Dave. "And you must be David. I am Gloria. I have three apartments to show you this afternoon, and I have more to show you tomorrow. Don't worry, I have found apartments for a lot of graduate students and doctors at UCLA Medical Center. I am sure I can find just what you are looking for in your price range." Despite her brash, brassy approach, she had an infectious smile and warm intelligent eyes.

She led them to the convertible, opened the passenger's door, pulled the seat back forward, and motioned for Dave to get in the back seat. "You sit up front with me, Sharon."

Sharon turned and smiled at Dave in the back seat. "I like her already."

Gloria looked at them, shook her head, and started the car. "You really are two babes in the woods, aren't you? Well, don't worry, Gloria will take care of you."

She put on an expensive pair of sunglasses, and as she put her hands on the wheel, Dave notice a diamond watch, bracelets, and rings, but no wedding ring. She was quintessential LA, but she was also a consummate professional. "You were lucky I had a couple of days open when you called. I am an independent realtor as well as a rental agent, so I stay busy. I have a lot of repeat clients because I am honest, good at my job, and I take care of my clients. The properties I am going to show you are five hundred a month. They are in safe neighborhoods, have easy access to the San Diego and Santa Monica freeways, and are as near the campus as possible. They are all modern and well maintained with nice pools. All the units I am going to show you have two bedrooms with two closets in the master; a kitchen with dishwasher, disposal, and meal area; a large front room with a patio or balcony; separate tub and shower with two sinks in the bathroom; and plenty of storage. There is a laundry in the building or nearby with washers and dryers."

Sharon looked back at Dave again. "They sound perfect." She turned in her seat. "Oh Dave, our first home."

Gloria looked at Sharon over her sunglasses and smiled warmly. "All you two kids have to do is pick one, put down a deposit, and sign the lease."

That's exactly what Dave and Sharon did. There wasn't much difference between the apartments themselves, but the buildings, tenants, and locations varied. They picked one that was a little older, had mature landscaping, a warmer feeling, and more long-term tenants. It was also the best location. The units were one-story cottages that resembled old Hollywood bungalows, and each one had an enclosed patio. Sharon's enthusiasm was bubbling over because it was exactly what she had pictured.

Gloria dropped them at their hotel Tuesday afternoon after they had signed the lease, paid the deposit, and paid Gloria their half of her commission. Gloria took her sunglasses off and looked at Sharon as she got out of the car. Her eyes were slightly sad. "I have one more piece of advice for you, Sharon. Don't succumb to the siren call of Babylon. This is a decadent town with a lot of temptations. With your looks, you are going to have guys all over you, offering you everything you could possibly imagine in your wildest dreams, but what they really want to give you is what I am sure Dave gives you quite frequently. All they really want to do is use and exploit your beautiful body, and they will promise you anything in order to do that. Don't be seduced by the fame and fortune of Hollywood." She put her sunglasses back on and drove off.

Dave and Sharon watched her drive away with one arm around each other's waist. "I think she is speaking from experience."

"I know she is, but I have been down that road. I have been dealing with that sort of stuff for years in first-class from professional athletes, entertainers, celebrities, and wealthy businessmen. No one is going to use or exploit my body, not the men I meet on the plane, not the men I dated before you, and not even you. I am in control of my own body, and I choose what I do with it." Sharon put her head on Dave's shoulder. "I already have everything I could possibly imagine in my wildest dreams." She smiled seductively. "I chose the guy who gives it to me, and I choose when he gives it to me." As they turned to walk into the hotel, Sharon added, "In fact, I think I would like for him to take me out to dinner tonight to celebrate, then like Gloria said, give it to me, and I do mean everything I could possibly imagine in my wildest dreams." They laughed together and hugged as they walked into the hotel.

Dave called the Disneyland Hotel and booked a room for Wednesday through Friday nights, then he called a place he had picked out in Newport near the beach to book a room for Saturday night, and lastly he booked a room in Marina Del Ray for Sunday night so they could get to LAX early Monday morning. They would drive to the Disneyland Hotel, spend the afternoon at the pool, spend two days in Disneyland, then drive to Newport Saturday morning for two days on the beach, and back to Marina Del Ray on Sunday for their last night, before flying home early Monday morning.

Sharon made the dinner reservation, spent extra time getting ready, and told Dave he had to wear a coat and tie. She made Dave shower alone and get dressed first, and then she took a long bubble bath and would not let Dave in the bathroom while she was getting ready. Dave was sitting on the bed waiting patiently when she emerged.

"You look fabulous," Dave said as he stood up. "No, you look magnificent."

He started toward her, but she skittered away from him. "I want to continue to look fabulous and magnificent." She had on the quintessential black cocktail dress with black stiletto heels; her hair and makeup were perfect.

"You are dressed like Gloria." Dave tried to get his hands on her again.

"I like fabulous and magnificent better. But yes, she said to dress to display my best assets in LA, so that's what I tried to do, and voila!" She posed with her hands on her waist. The dress and shoes displayed her long slender legs perfectly, and the dress was just tight enough to accentuate her rear. It was sleeveless and displayed a tantalizing view of the swell of her breasts and cleavage.

Dave moved toward her again, but she wagged her finger at him. "You can look but don't touch. The restaurant has valet parking, but I want to park and walk to the restaurant." She took his arm. "Let's go. This is our town now; let's go enjoy it."

Sharon was vibrant and luminous as she strode down the street on Dave's arm, with her head up, looking straight ahead, smiling. Beautiful women were common in the area, but she still turned heads, drew attention, and even slowed traffic. When they got to the restaurant, the maître d' was overly attentive. "Welcome, Dr. Cameron. I have a nice table for you and the lady." He took two menus and led them to a table, pulled out Sharon's chair and fawned over her as he placed her napkin in her lap and gave her the menu. He stood behind her as the busboy brought waters and the waiter arrived to introduce himself.

Sharon flashed a smile at the waiter. "Two Champagne cocktails, then give us a little time to enjoy them before you take our order." Sharon gave Dave the same smile. "We have something to discuss before dinner." Sharon had picked the restaurant and made the arrangements.

Sharon motioned for the server to put the Champagne cocktails on the side when he brought them and reached across the table to take both of Dave's hands. "Well, are you going to ask me to marry you?"

"What!" Dave exclaimed.

"I said, are you going to ask me to marry you? Do you think I would quit my job and move thousands of miles with someone if we weren't married?"

"What!" Dave was overcome.

"Do I have to ask you to marry me, rather than you asking me to marry you?" Sharon looked into his eyes.

"Do you mean it?" Dave responded.

"Do you want to marry me or not?" Sharon asked.

"Of course, I do," Dave answered.

"Then ask me." Sharon laughed.

"Oh God, yes." Dave pulled both of her hands to him and kissed them.

"I am the one who is supposed to say, yes. You are the one who is supposed to ask." She squeezed his hands.

Dave choked out, "Will you marry me?"

"Yes, Dave. I will marry you." Sharon's eyes were deep glistening pools as she looked across the table at Dave. Dave couldn't stand it any longer, he had been dying to hold her since he first saw her in the little black dress in their room. He stood up, walked around the table, pulled her up, and kissed her holding her so tightly she couldn't breathe. They were surprised and embarrassed by the smattering of applause. *What the hell—it's Hollywood*, Dave thought, so he reached back for the two Champagne flutes, they clinked glasses, and took a sip.

They sat back down and were holding hands across the table with one hand, sipping their Champagne with the other, when the waiter appeared with a bottle of Dom Perignon. "Compliments of a couple who want to wish you all the best." Sharon and Dave finished their Champagne cocktails, asked the waiter to thank their benefactors, and started on the bottle of Dom Perignon.

When they finished the meal, the waiter brought the dessert menu. "For dessert, I recommend baked Alaska flambé. It will go perfectly with the Champagne." He smiled.

Dave was glad they were walking back to the car, because they were both more than a little buzzed on Champagne. They strolled along slowly, arm and arm in the clear Southern California spring night, smelling the salty sea air off the Pacific Ocean, as happy and content as two people could possibly be. The blood, gore, stress, fatigue, and heartache of University Hospital were far away and forgotten. It was as if they had landed in some magical land where nothing like that existed.

Sharon squeezed Dave arm. "I have to say this: Toto, I don't think we are in Kansas anymore."

Dave kissed her. "We never were in Kansas, but I can tell you, for two kids who grew up in small Southern towns, we are a long way from home. Can you believe it, Sharon? This is going to be our life. I am so thankful we are going to spend our lives out here and not back there. God, we are lucky to have been born with intelligence and to have had the advantage of a good education. I am a little drunk on Champagne, so forgive me if I pontificate a bit, but intelligence and education are everything. Never stop learning, never stop questioning, never stop improving your mind, and always stay informed with valid information—that's what I believe leads to a full, well-spent life."

Sharon kissed him back. "Enough about what is above your shoulders. I am ready for what is below your waist. You turn me on when you talk like that, especially after all that Champagne, or maybe it's all that Champagne that turned me on. Either way, I am ready for you to give it to me."

Dave picked up the pace. "You bet!"

Dave woke up with a headache and a dry mouth. *All that Champagne*, he thought. The bed was a wreck, and their clothes were scattered near the door. He looked over at Sharon who was still sleeping tangled in the sheet. The other bed covers were on the floor. Dave chuckled to himself as he remembered last night. *Wow*, he thought, *every time we make a commitment, get sort of engaged, or get really engaged, it gets better. I can't wait for our wedding night.*

He tried to get up, but that made his head hurt worse, and the morning sun was pouring in through the window, setting his eyes on fire. *Coffee, I have to have coffee*, he thought. *Water first, then coffee, lots of water, then lots of coffee.*

He tried again and managed to struggle up to the bathroom to drink several glasses of water. Then he called housekeeping and asked for more packets of coffee for the coffee maker in the room. None of this disturbed Sharon's sleep, and even when the maid came with the extra coffee, she slept on partially covered in the tangled twisted sheet.

Dave drank more water and started the coffee, then went through all his stuff looking for aspirin. The way he felt reminded him of the mornings after a fraternity party in college, and he remembered why he had stopped drinking like that. The smell of the coffee finally caused Sharon to stir, and she rolled over, leaving herself mostly uncovered and exposed. "You got me drunk on Champagne and took advantage of me. Jesus, did you ever take advantage of me. You are a bad man."

Dave got her a glass of water, which she drank, then handed him the glass for more. Dave asked, "Do you have any aspirin or Tylenol?" Dave brought her more water, and she sat up in bed to drink it, looking around the room and at the bed.

"No, but is the coffee ready? I am depending on the coffee to bring me back to life." She stood up and walked to the bathroom for more water. "God, what a wonderful night."

Dave poured two cups of coffee. "You planned it all, didn't you? The dress and the suit—that's your wedding dress and my wedding suit. You picked the restaurant and made the reservation because you knew famous celebrities went there. You wore that dress because you knew I would tear it off and go crazy once I had you alone. You even talked dirty to me to encourage and tease me." When she came out of the bathroom, Dave handed her a cup of coffee.

She took the coffee and smiled at him over the cup of coffee. "Little bit."

Dave smiled back. "Don't call me a bad man. You are a devious, cunning woman." He put his free arm around her and hugged her. "So, you are the future Mrs. Cameron, wife of the esteemed Dr. Cameron. What changed your mind? I am curious."

Sharon looked serious and sat down on the side of the bed with her coffee. "A lot of things, but mainly getting married is for you, or actually for us. I think what really changed my mind was you cutting your hair. You cut your hair for us, for me, for our future, and I know that. You realized as a doctor, you would not be successful with shoulder-length, straggly, Woodstock hair. You knew our future depended on you being successful, so you cut your hair to ensure it. I realized the same thing. We cannot continue in a bohemian lifestyle. We have to become Dr. and Mrs. Cameron in order to have a bright future. There are a lot of other factors, but that is the main one." Sharon put the coffee cup down on the bedside table, stood up, and walked into Dave's arms.

"I love you. I want to grow old with you, I want to have that full, well-spent life you talked about, and I need to be your wife to do that. I know you are nothing like my father, and you would never treat me the way my father treated my mother. I have to admit all my friends getting married had something to do with it, too. I asked myself what was wrong with me that I couldn't be happy and marry the man I loved, like they did. So, I planned the perfect seduction and asked you to marry me. Do you mind terribly that I did it that way?"

Dave put his coffee cup down. "I love that you did it that way. I will never forget last night." He walked her to the bed, and they both sat down on the side of the bed. "But Sharon, with the expense of the move, the apartment, and everything else, I don't know how I can buy you a ring. There will be no honeymoon, and how can we find time to have a wedding?"

She put her arms around him and nuzzled his neck. "I don't want a ring. All I want is two simple, matching gold bands, signifying we are together. We will have an early honeymoon here and now, at Disneyland and the beach." She pulled back. "And no big wedding. I have my dress and you have your suit. We will get married at the house with our friends, my mother, your mother and father, and your brother. Oh Dave, I could never have imagined how much my life would change when you walked into the party that night."

"Nor could I, but I couldn't be any happier." They sat on the side of the bed holding each other for some time. Then they showered, dressed in shorts, T-shirts and sandals, checked out, and drove to Anaheim.

On the drive, Sharon brought up something she wanted to discuss. "My application and acceptance to UCLA is for Sharon Kelly. My contract with Niemen's is with Sharon Kelly. If you don't mind, I am going to keep my name for modeling and school, so I don't have to redo everything or make any changes to my identity. Is that alright with you? Where we are concerned, I will be Mrs. Cameron, but where I am the only one concerned, I will be Sharon Kelly, married but using my name."

Dave answered, "I know how you feel about giving up your name and freedom. As far as I am concerned, you can keep your name. I don't care. We will be married, and that is all that matters, so become married Sharon Kelly, that's fine with me. I don't need for you to take my name, and I will never take your freedom away. I won't own you when we are married. I will simply be your husband. Stay Sharon Kelly and stay free. I love you, Sharon Kelly. You are who I fell in love with, and you are who I am going to spend my life with, not your name." Dave thought about what happened on New Year's Eve with the men trying to buy her and how it made him feel.

Sharon smiled and leaned over to nibble his ear. "I knew you would understand. That's why we belong together, and why I am marrying you; we understand each other. You know me for who I am and understand me. No one else in my life ever has."

Dave drove up to the Disneyland Hotel around noon. Sharon had never been to Disneyland, and she was as excited as a child as she bounded into the lobby to be greeted by Goofy. She squealed with delight, ran to him, and hugged him. Goofy seemed just as glad to see Sharon. He hugged her back and kept his arm around her as he led her to the reception desk. Sharon was a quick study, and she knew the drill now; she flashed a smile at the desk clerk to make sure he was looking at her not at Dave as they checked in. The result was a very nice room with a view of the park.

Sharon could hardly wait to get to the pool. "I'm at Disneyland. I can't believe it. Stop lagging, and let's go!" She was out the door, and Dave had to chase after her. On their way to the pool, they encountered Donald Duck, who like Goofy, was exceedingly glad to see Sharon in her bikini and cover-up. He gave her a big hug, and led her to the pool with his arm around her. Dave followed behind as Sharon skipped along beside Donald. The pools were crowded with children and their parents, so it took a while for Sharon and Dave to find a place with an umbrella. Once they were settled, Dave went to the food window and got two beers, two sandwiches, and chips for lunch. Kids were everywhere, playing, yelling, and having a good time in and out of the pools.

Sharon watched the chaos as she ate and drank her beer. "What a great place for a family vacation, and what a wonderful place for children. I wish I could have come here as a kid. We never took family vacations. In the winter, we went skiing because my father liked to ski. In the summer, my father took golf vacations, to famous golf places, so he could say he had played golf there and brag about his score. If I ever have children, I can assure you they will come to Disneyland."

Dave choked on his beer. Sharon had never mentioned the possibility of having children before. In fact, she had sworn she would never bring a child into this world, but she had also sworn she would never get married, too. Dave swallowed his beer and looked at her as she sat watching the children play. Children, a real family—Dave was afraid to even think about it, but he had thought they would never get married and now they would be married in a few weeks. A tiny spark of hope ignited in his chest, but he was afraid to let it grow, because he was afraid of having a child with problems.

Sharon finished her sandwich and beer, lay back on her lounge chair, and closed her eyes. She felt a presence near her and opened her eyes to see a cute chubby little girl of about four, standing there patiently waiting to be acknowledged. "Are you somebody? My sister said anybody as bootiful as you are has to be somebody."

Sharon sat up and looked at her over her sunglasses. "We are all somebody, sweetheart."

The little girl continued, "But my sister said you must be somebody. Who are you?"

Sharon smiled. "I'm sorry, sweetheart. I am not a celebrity."

Dave interjected, "But she is a model. Do you know what a model is?" The little girl shook her head, no. "She poses in clothes in catalogues so people can see if they want to buy them. Do you know what a catalogue is?" Again, a negative head shake. "A catalogue is like a magazine; do you know what a magazine is?" A positive head shake. "She poses in something like a magazine in different clothes for people to see."

"Dave," Sharon protested.

Sharon lay back down as the little girl skittered away to run back to her sister and announce proudly to her and everyone around, "She's not somebody but she wears clothes in magazines."

"I would like to see her in one of those magazines where she doesn't wear any clothes," a man sitting behind the little girl's parents said and was promptly reprimanded by his wife.

"What's wrong with you? There are children here. What are you thinking? Don't answer, I know. I just hope the guy with her didn't hear you."

Sharon was dozing, when she felt the presence again. She opened her eyes to see the little girl was back. "Will you go swimming with me?"

"Can you swim?" Sharon asked.

"I have my wads," the little girl answered and pointed to the water wings on her chubby little arms.

"I am sorry," the little girl's mother said to Sharon, then called to the little girl. "Come back here, and leave her alone."

"It's OK. She is precious," Sharon answered. "I will go swimming with you." Sharon got up to walk to the pool, and the little girl reached up to take Sharon's finger in her hand. Sharon stopped and looked down at the little girl holding her finger, then bent down to take the little girl in her arms. "You are too cute for words. Do you know that?" The little girl nodded, yes. Sharon laughed, stood up, and walked to the pool holding the little girl in her arms.

She jumped into Sharon's arms from the side of the pool, pretending to swim while Sharon supported her. She laughed and giggled the whole time, occasionally stopping to just hold Sharon around the neck. Then she stood on Sharon's shoulders to jump in the water while Sharon held her hands. Sharon was laughing and having a great time along with the little girl.

Finally, the little girl got out of the pool and ran to her mother to get dried. Sharon got out and walked to Dave, who was holding a towel for her. Dave wrapped the towel around her and pulled her to him while he dried her off. They had avoided any PDA, including the traditional application of sunscreen, because it would have been inappropriate in front of all the children, but now Dave kissed her as he held her in the towel. She took her towel, put her sunglasses on, and lay back down on her lounge chair with her long hair draped over the back of the chair to dry.

Sharon was lost in her own thoughts when she felt the little girl climb onto the chair. She situated herself in her lap, and lay back on her. "Well hello there. Are you comfortable?" The little girl nodded, yes and smiled at Sharon.

It was the father who retrieved her. "I am sorry, but she seems to have adopted you. Thank you for taking care of her, but we have to go now. Come on, little one. Say goodbye and let's go. We have to get ready for dinner."

The little girl put her arms around Sharon's neck and hugged her then got up and took her father's finger as they walked away, but she stopped after a few steps and turned to wave at Sharon smiling. Sharon waved back.

"She is the cutest, sweetest thing I have ever seen." Dave had never seen her with a child or around children, and he was surprised by her behavior. Sharon didn't say anything else, and they relaxed in silence after the little girl and her family left.

Sharon rolled onto her side and reached over to take Dave's hand as she looked at him lying beside her. *What had this man done to her,* she thought. She had never intended to get married, promising herself over and over she would never marry, and now she was going to marry him. The last thing she would ever consider doing was have a child, but that little girl had touched something in her heart that caused a longing in her. She had felt a similar nagging about marriage before she gave in to it and decided to marry Dave. God help her, was she thinking about having a child? No way, it was just her biological clock ticking, and she was feeling an instinctual longing based on her age. But she had told herself similar things about marriage. She had resolved that conflict and was exceedingly happy with her decision, but this was different. There was no conflict and no decision to make. She was downright terrified even of the idea of having a child and it was never, ever going to happen, so she relaxed.

Dave looked over at her. "Are you alright?"

She smiled at him. "I have never been more alright in my life. Will you go swimming with me?"

"You bet. I thought you would never ask." Dave got up still holding her hand and pulled her up.

They spent the rest of the afternoon swimming, playing in the shallow end, and Sharon did some diving, much to the delight of several adolescent boys who watched her intently. In the late afternoon, they went in to clean up for dinner, much to the disappointment of those same young boys, then went to the hotel restaurant to dine with the Disney characters. Snow White, Alice, and Cinderella were wandering around the tables to the shrieks of the little girls who raced up to them to get their autographs in their books. Later, Mickey and Minnie came in to greet everyone and to welcome them to the happiest place on earth, then along came Wendy and Peter Pan with Captain Hook.

Sharon was having a great time clapping for the other characters and booing Captain Hook right along with the kids, until Captain Hook came after her shaking his hook at her. She scooted her chair around next to Dave, and he put his arm around her to protect her, so Captain Hook moved on to terrorize some little girls at another table, but Peter came to their rescue. Everyone shouted encouragement as Peter drove Captain Hook off in a sword fight.

Sharon did not scoot her chair back, but put her arms around Dave's neck, bit his ear, and then whispered, "I don't want to live in Santa Monica. I want to live at Disneyland in the Disneyland Hotel."

After dinner, they went back to their room, watched the fireworks from their window, made love, and went to sleep. Dave woke up to Sharon jumping up and down on the bed. "I want to go to the park. I want to go to the park now."

She was bouncing so hard, Dave had to get out of the bed. Of course, Sharon had nothing on, which led to Dave jumping on the bed in time with her until he could grab her and fall back on the bed with her.

"We don't have time for that. I want to go to the park. I want to ride the rides in the park, not you." She giggled and squirmed in his arms. Dave tried to pin her arms and legs, but saw it was no use, so he let her up to start bouncing on the bed again. "Let's go to the park. Let's go to the park." She fell back on the bed laughing and Dave pulled her into his arms at last.

They got up, showered, and dressed, laughing and playing with each other the entire time. They were some of the first people in line at the Monorail that morning, and they rode one of the last trains back that night. The second day was a repeat of the first, except they slowed down to take in all the shows, ride their favorite rides again and go to Tom Sawyer's Island. They ate in the park, watched the parade and fireworks, then danced to the band in Tomorrowland both nights.

They were sitting at the top of Tom Sawyer's Island in the afternoon of the second day. "This is the happiest place on earth. It has been the perfect place for a honeymoon. I couldn't have asked for anything more."

Dave thought about Caroline and Ron going to an exclusive resort on Saint Lucia, Audrey and Jake planning to spend a week at Los Breezes in Mexico, Connie and Harven having two weeks in France, and all he and Sharon had was two days in Disneyland. Two more years of residency, a year to establish his practice, and then they would be able to go anywhere they wanted. He had friends with MBAs or engineering degrees who were married, had children, owned their own homes and a resort property, and he was basically still in school for two more years.

They walked along the trails of the island holding hands. "My parents brought me to Disneyland the year it opened when I was nine years old. We spent several days here, and I will never forget it. I played on this island until dark every day; my father would have to

A love story and social commentary

come find me. We took two-week car trips for vacations when I was a kid. That year, we drove to Las Vegas for a few days then here, to the national parks in Southern California, then back home. We came back here when I was a teenager, and then went to San Francisco and the parks in Northern California. I was here a third time as a Lieutenant Governor in Key Club for the national convention in Long Beach, so this is my fourth time, but it is still magical for me."

They sat down in the fort on Tom Sawyer's Island and planned their wedding.

"I want to wait until Connie and Harven get back from Europe. I think Caroline and Ron will fly in from New York. Audrey and Jake will be there, Bob and Phil, Sam and Rachael, my mother, your mother, your father, and your brother. Helen can stand up for me and Henry for you, with of course Sigrid, and Helen's plus-one—that's twenty with us."

Dave added, "Mike and Janice may just show up. We will have a Justice of the Peace do a civil ceremony. I think you are right; we should plan on twenty. We will have a buffet dinner catered in the dining room and have the ceremony in the front room. For a reception, we can go to the black dance club. You can call them and reserve a couple of tables. We can have everything moved from my apartment and your room, keep what we need for a week, and stay at your house after the wedding. I want to spend our wedding night at the hotel where we went to the New Year's Eve party, maybe in the same room."

They kissed. "That's it then. We get married, then it's Hollywood straight away." There weren't many kids and no adults in the fort, so Dave cupped Sharon's breast and whispered in her ear, "Do you want to do it on Tom Sawyer's Island to celebrate?"

Sharon pushed his hand away. "You are such a pervert. Of course not. I am not fucking you on Tom Sawyer's Island. Sometimes I wonder if you are alright mentally."

Dave persisted. "There are some secret places I know about. You did it in the zoom room with a house full of people and in the yard beside your house."

Sharon laughed. "That was different, I was very stoned one time and tripping the other time. Do you want some little kid to see us and be psychologically scarred for life? Do you want to see the headlines; Dr. and future Mrs. Cameron arrested at Disneyland for fucking on Tom

Sawyer's Island? We will celebrate that way tonight in the privacy of our own room." Sharon stood up and put out her hand. "Come on. This is our last day, and I don't want to waste it fucking around, literally or figuratively. I want to ride every ride again; I will ride you and fuck around with you later tonight."

They headed for the rafts to leave the island. "Oh Dave, I love this place. Promise me we will come back often. We will be living just up the road."

Dave kissed her. "You bet."

They were up early, had breakfast, and got on the road for Newport. Dave had on his bathing suit, a T-shirt, and flip flops, and Sharon had her bikini on under her shorts and T-shirt along with her flip flops so they could go straight to the beach. They checked in, left their bags in the room, grabbed some towels, the sunblock, and walked to the beach. It was mid-May and a little early for good beach weather, but it was the weekend, so the beach was still crowded. They found a good spot and settled in for the day.

They ate hot dogs and drank beer from the beach stand, tossed around a Frisbee they found, and joined in a beach volleyball game. The ocean was too cold, so they went back to the hotel to swim. They ate seafood that night at a restaurant near the hotel, then went back to the beach to cuddle on a blanket to watch the moon on the water.

Dave wanted to make love on the beach, but Sharon told him doing it on the beach fell into the same category as skinny dipping in the apartment pool or fucking on Tom Sawyer's Island—it wasn't going to happen. They lay on the beach watching the elongated pearl-colored reflection of the moon on the water and the white foamy cascade of the breaking waves as they crashed on the beach surrounded by the natural beauty of the Pacific Ocean. Dave thought about all the nights he had spent on the beach at his grandfather's beach house, but that was the Gulf; this was the Pacific. He was in California, not a small Southern beach town. He realized Sharon was right, this was a whole different world from the one he grew up in and was used to. He reflected on how lucky he was and what a wonderful life awaited him with Sharon.

That night, after they made love in the room, Sharon complained of a burning sensation when she went to the bathroom.

"You have cystitis. Drink a lot of water and some cranberry juice. We have to go to a clinic and get you an antibiotic tomorrow."

Sharon refused. "No way. I am not spending our last day sitting in a doctor's office. You can write me a script when we get back. You broke me, so you can fix me. We are going to spend the day at the beach like we planned, drive to Marina Del Ray for the night, and fly back the next day."

Dave warned her, "You need an antibiotic. That's the only thing that will work."

Sharon replied, "I'll get some cranberry juice tomorrow and drink a lot of water. We will get me an antibiotic when we get home."

18
Sharon's Fight for Life

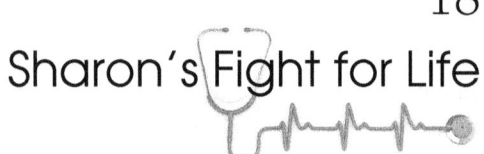

They spent the next day at the beach, and then drove to Marina Del Ray for a romantic dinner and made it to LAX the next morning in time to catch an early flight out. They had just reached cruising altitude when Sharon developed back pain and a fever.

"Dave, I feel terrible." Dave thumped her on the back over her kidney and she jumped, then he felt how warm she was. "You have a kidney infection."

"I will be alright once we get home." But Dave knew this was a gram-negative infection. Gram-negative sepsis was serious; it could lead to gram-negative shock, and septic shock was life-threatening. He would take her straight to the hospital for an antibiotic once they landed, but it was a three-hour flight.

When they would normally be preparing for descent, the unthinkable happened. The captain announced there were thunderstorms with high-wind shear, and they would have to wait until the weather cleared to land. Dave called the flight attendant and informed her he was a doctor, his fiancée had a serious infection, and they needed to get on the ground as soon as possible. They were held for two more hours.

"Dave, I feel awful. I have never felt this bad in my life."

Dave felt her and she was on fire, so he called the flight attendant again and asked if they had a thermometer and some aspirin. Then he asked to talk to someone from the flight deck. He talked to the first officer, asked for an ambulance to meet the plane, and for the Major Medicine ER at University Hospital to be informed with all the vital information.

Dave told the first officer they had to land right away because she was septic and had to be treated immediately. The office said the weather had cleared but the tower was landing the planes low on fuel first. Dave responded that her life was in danger, any plane that could go around again had to, and this plane had to take priority. The officer went back to the flight deck, and the captain came back to talk to Dave.

"Just touch her. Her temp must be a hundred and four. We have got to get her to the hospital now."

A love story and social commentary

The captain returned to the flight deck, and after a time, he announced they would be landing shortly but for all passengers to remain seated until a sick passenger could be removed by an ambulance crew. It was another hour before they got to the gate. The ambulance crew took Sharon off the plane and put her in the ambulance with Dave holding her hand the whole time. The ambulance crew forwarded her vitals to the hospital; her temp was a hundred and five, her BP was 90/50, and her pulse was rapid and weak. She was going into gram-negative shock.

By the time they got her off the plane, into the ambulance and drove to the hospital, it was another hour before they ran into the Major Medicine ER. Dave stood back while they started two IVs, one for fluids and one for antibiotics. They put a Foley catheter in, took a urine culture, and drew blood cultures along with a complete lab panel. She was started on oxygen, triple IV antibiotics therapy, and fluids, then rushed to the ICU. The resident told Dave he would admit her to Dr. Sheffield's private service. Dr. Sheffield was a nephrologist.

Dave took Sharon's hand again. The last thing she said was, "Hold on to me, Dave. Please hold on to me and don't let go."

Connie appeared and brought Dave a chair so he could sit at Sharon's bedside. "Don't worry, Dave, she is going to make it. She loves you too much to ever leave you. Her love for you will pull her through." Connie put her hand on Dave's shoulder. "Dr. Sheffield is the best, you know that."

The adrenaline rush to get her to the hospital was over and Dave caved in, collapsing with his head on Sharon's forearm as he held her hand. Her fever was raging, and she was out of it. Dave knew about gram-negative shock because he had treated it, and he was terrified. He refused to let go of her hand or move from her bedside.

Dr. Sheffield came in. "As you know, she has pyelonephritis with sepsis, and she went into shock. We are treating that, but we don't know yet if she suffered any end-organ damage. Her labs are not good. She is very septic with an extremely high white count and a big left shift. I am not going to patronize you by trying to sugar-coat things. You know how serious this, you know what the survival rate is, and you know the next twenty-four to seventy-two hours will determine the outcome. Understand, I will do everything I can for her, I am here for her, and I will stay at the hospital with her."

Dave thanked him as he left, and Connie returned. "I am going to stay with her too. I will stay here and take care of her for as long as it takes." Dave put his head back down on Sharon's forearm as he held her hand.

He sat in the chair feeling a unique emotion that was so painful it was physical in its intensity. He had spent a large portion of his life becoming a doctor to try to save lives, and now the person who meant the most to him, that he loved more than life itself, was lying in a hospital bed next to him dying, and he couldn't do anything about it. All the years of school, training, work, and sacrifice meant nothing because he couldn't use any of it to save Sharon's life.

Dave thought about *A Farewell to Arms* as Frederic Henry waited as Catherine Barkley lay dying. It hit him like a sledgehammer in his chest; the all-encompassing totally consuming love he and Sharon had was just like the love Frederic and Catherine had. The realization that their love could end the same way caused him real physical pain, and he hurt worse than he had ever hurt in his life. The pain was worse than the injuries he had suffered in sports. The pain was worse than he had with his sister's death. The pain was more than he could bear, and he broke down.

Dave prayed, he bargained, he cajoled, he promised, he called on God, and then he called on whatever gods there may be and on the forces that govern the universe to please let her live. He was doubled over in the chair in physical pain with his head on her forearm, holding her hand, begging her not to die. "Please don't leave me," he said over and over.

Dave knew what death was, he had seen too much of it not to realize he could lose Sharon forever. She would be gone, and he would be left alone for the rest of his life. That thought was too much for him; he cried silently in his anguish, just as he had heard others cry in anguish in the ED.

Connie came to his side again and put her hands on his shoulders. "She hears you. She won't leave you." He stopped crying and a type of numbness set in. It felt like he was in a bad dream and couldn't wake up. It had to be a dream; this couldn't be real.

Dave sat there numb and detached from reality holding Sharon's hand with his forehead on her forearm mumbling to her, begging her not to leave him, begging her not to die. He knew he would not be able to bear a life without her. For the rest of that day, that night, another day, and into the night, he sat with his head on her forearm holding her hand, begging her not to die. Connie went without sleep, taking other nurses' shifts so she could stay with Sharon.

Dr. Sheffield was there twice the next day, and told Dave on the second day that there had not been any change in her status. She was critical, still fighting sepsis and septic shock. She had a high fever, and her white count was far out of the normal range. Before dawn of the third day, Dave woke with a start as he realized his forehead was cool because her forearm was cool, and her hand was cold. "Oh God, she is gone!"

He knew a lot of people died in the early morning hours. He had always seen the early morning as a beginning, but he knew for some they were an ending. He was overcome with the pain of losing her. He felt as if his mind and body had been torn in half, and half of him was gone with her.

Connie came running when she heard him and turned on the overhead light. "Her monitor is fine, and she is not setting off any alarms!" Dave looked up to see Sharon's incredibly beautiful otherworldly eyes looking back at him over the oxygen mask. Dave collapsed and Connie held him.

"It's OK. She is not gone. Her fever broke that's all."

Connie checked her vital signs. "Your BP is 100/70, your pulse is 90, and your temp is 99. Sharon, your fever broke and your vitals are good. I am going to call the on-call nurse to come in. I need to go home to get some sleep. You should too, Dave. She is going to be OK."

Sharon took the oxygen mask off. "How long have I been out of it? The last thing I remember, I was in the ambulance."

Connie answered. "A day and two nights. You had us worried, but you are going to be fine."

Sharon sat up a little. "What about work? Did anyone call my mother?"

Connie smiled. "I called Helen and she called your supervisor, so everything is fine at work. Helen had trouble finding your mother's number, but she got in touch with her yesterday and she is flying in today. Helen is going to pick her up at the airport with Audrey so Audrey can get your car." Dave and Sharon had driven to the airport in Sharon's car so they could park in the employee's parking lot and not have to pay parking. "There are a lot of people waiting to see you. When you get to the floor, there is going to be a flood of well-wishers. We will see that the aids have you presentable by then."

"How can I ever thank you, Connie? Did you stay with me the whole time?" Sharon held her arms out to Connie.

Connie hugged her. "Yes. Dave and I were with you the whole time. He never left your side, and he never let go of your hand."

"I know. I could feel him. I wasn't aware of anything else, but I could feel him near me. When I felt like I was sinking, I could feel him pulling me back. I know that sounds crazy, but it is true." Sharon looked at Dave. "I knew he was there, and I fought to get back to him."

Dave was too shattered to do or say anything, he sat beside her holding her hand until she fell asleep, then he stumbled to the call room and slept until seven. Dave got up, showered, changed into scrubs, and went back to the ICU. Sharon was awake eating breakfast.

"I still don't feel too chipper, but God am I hungry. Dave, how long has it been since you ate? Go get something to eat before Dr. Sheffield gets here." She had almost died yet she was concerned about Dave not eating. Sharon was all woman from her rock-solid inner core to the glow of her outer beauty with the heart of a woman who needed to nurture and care for those she loved.

By the time Dave got back, the aids had put her in a fresh gown and helped her with her hair, so she looked much better. Dr. Sheffield arrived shortly after Dave.

"Well, young lady, your fever broke and your white count is down. We will move you to the floor later today. If you stay afebrile for twenty-four hours on the floor, you can go home on oral antibiotics. Do you have anyone to take care of you other than Dr. Cameron? He needs to get back to his Pedi rotation." Sheffield turned to Dave. "Dr. Cameron, I talked to the chief resident in Pedi. He said you can go home with her tomorrow, take a day off to recover, then start back in the Nursery the following day."

Sharon sat up in bed. "My mother is coming today. Dr. Sheffield, I can't thank you enough for taking care of me. I am so grateful."

Dr. Sheffield smiled at Sharon. "That is what we physicians do. We take care of our patients. When you are married to this young doctor, don't forget that when he has to spend nights at the hospital

A love story and social commentary

caring for his patients. I will see you in the morning and discharge you, then I will have you follow up in the clinic as an outpatient."

Sheffield turned to Dave again. "You don't know it, but there are a lot of doctors and nurses who were concerned about her. Many of them spent their free time in the waiting room hoping for news of her condition."

He turned back to Sharon. "Most of them only know you as Baby. I kept hearing, 'How is Baby? Is Baby going to be alright?' They don't even know your name, but they were here for you."

No sooner had Sheffield left then Nurse Jane appeared with an aid from Medicine 3. "You don't think we would let anyone else take care of Baby, do you, Poncho?" she said to Dave as she brushed past him. "Don't worry, we have a nice private room for you. We are going to get you up walking and let you take a shower. Every nurse on our service feels she knows you, so we are going to take extra special care of you."

They bustled around her, getting her on the gurney, covering her with a warm blanket, putting pillows under her head, and tucking her in. Nurse Jane put Sharon's stuff on the bottom of the gurney, and they started for Medicine 3 with Dave following behind still numb and overcome emotionally.

The nurses barely had Sharon in the room and in bed before they began to show up: Henry, Harven, and George first. They fawned over her and told her how glad they were she was going to be OK. Henry choked up as he hugged her and was at a loss for words to express his feelings.

Tom came. "Jesus, Goldilocks, you look like shit. If I didn't know better, I would think you were the one who had septic shock. Sharon, you are as beautiful as the day I met you. Sepsis seems to agree with you. Are you sure you don't want to dump this panty-waist hippie for a real man like me? I am still available." Then Tom got serious. "I can't tell you how happy I am you pulled through. The world would be a lesser place if you two weren't together in it."

Richard came. "My wife and I prayed for you, and we got our whole church to pray for you. You don't know them, but you had the power of their prayers supporting you. Dave, Tom is right, you look terrible. You need to go home and get some sleep. There are plenty of people here to take care of her. Tom and I will look in on her from time to time. You need to take care of yourself."

Jay came. "I have never met you, but I feel like I know you, and I wanted you to know I was here for you to add my support to your recovery."

Jason came with a blond student nurse. "We came by every day to check on you. I am so glad you are doing better. Lisa and I are together because of you, and I want you to meet her. Sharon, you did a lot to boost my confidence. I would have never been able to be with someone like her without your example. Lisa, this is Sharon."

The pretty student nurse took Sharon's hand. "I feel like I know you because Jason told me so much about you and Dave. He thinks a lot of Dave, and you are just as beautiful as he said you were. I am so glad you are doing better."

Jason had gone through a metamorphosis that had not only transformed him mentally but physically. He no longer slumped but stood up straight with good posture, he was well groomed, and it was obvious he was taking pride in his appearance. He had a confident, open, friendly manner. There was something else Dave noticed—Jason and Lisa both had small strands of matching love beads at their throats.

Several nurses from the ED and wards filed in during, before, or after their shifts to say how happy they were she was doing better. The black RN and the little ward clerk came. "I'm Ella and this is Sherika. I know you don't know us, but we know who you are. I am so glad my white sister is going to be OK." She had an LP with her. "This is for you. I hope it brings you the joy of the blues to help you recover. It's a John Lee Hooker album."

She tried to hand Sharon the record. "I can't take that. Your father left it to you. I would love to have it but please, you keep it. It is part of your legacy."

Ella smiled. "No, his real legacy to me was my love of music. Why do you think I am named Ella? I just wish I had her voice. Please, take the John Lee album. Dave said you love John Lee as much as he does."

Sharon looked into Ella's eyes. "Thank you, you are too kind." Ella looked back directly into Sharon's eyes. "My white sister is welcome." The understanding between them was palpable.

In the afternoon, her mother arrived with Audrey, Jake, and Helen. "Your car is safe, and your bag is in your room. Dave, we have your bag." Helen turned to an attractive well-dressed woman. "Mrs. Kelly, this is Dr. David Cameron; he is Sharon's fiancé."

But the woman ignored Dave and rushed to Sharon's bedside. "Are you Ok? I have been so worried since Helen called me. She said you were in critical condition."

Sharon hugged her. "I was, but I am better now thanks to Dr. Sheffield, the head of the Department of Medicine here and Connie, an ICU nurse who is my friend."

"How did this happen? How did you get so sick? Were you not taking care of yourself?" Sharon's mother was frantic.

Sharon pulled back from her mother and held her by the shoulders. "It's a long story, but I need to tell you some other things first. I am sorry I haven't told you before. I was going to call you before we left, then I was going to call you or come home when we got back. I know what I am going to tell you will come as a shock, but you have to know. The man you were just introduced to and I are getting married, then we are moving to LA for him to do his residency at UCLA Medical Center, and for me to attend UCLA's Graduate School of Business to get an MBA. Remember, I told you I was dating a doctor at Christmas. Well, that's him, and we are getting married and moving to California."

Sharon's mother was mortified. "California! You are getting married and moving to California!"

Sharon looked her mother in the eyes. "I know it is a lot to take in. I should have called or come home to tell you. Dave and I have been together for almost a year. We were in LA finding a place to live. I got sick on the plane coming back, and it got so bad because the flight was delayed by weather. I would have called or come home to tell you if I hadn't gotten so sick. I realize now I should have told you sooner. I am going to stop flying and get my MBA while Dave is doing his Medicine residence, then we are going to live permanently in California. We have our future together planned. Frankly, I didn't tell you sooner because I didn't want to go through this kind of reaction from you."

Sharon's mother pulled away from her. "You are going to quit your job and move to LA with some man on a whim?"

Sharon answered, "It is not a whim. We have been making our plans for some time, and we planned our wedding in the fort on Tom Sawyer's Island at Disneyland before we flew home."

Helen laughed. "Of course, you did. Where else would you two have planned your wedding? Mrs. Kelly, they have been pretty much living together since they met almost a year ago. They are devoted to each other, and the only time they are apart is when Dave is at the hospital or when Sharon is flying."

"We are going to have the ceremony when Connie and Harven get back from Europe. Helen, I want you to be my maid of honor. Audrey, can you and Jake be there?" Sharon asked.

Audrey responded, "Of course, Sharon. Don't worry, we will all be there. I am dying for a Coke. How about you, Helen, wouldn't you like a Coke? Jake, come on; I need a Coke. Dave, can you show us where we can get a Coke? Mrs. Kelly, can we bring you anything?" Audrey herded Dave, Jake, and Helen out of the room with her, leaving Sharon and her mother alone. "Don't worry, Dave, let Sharon handle her. She knows how to deal with her mother; we just need to give them some time and space."

The last thing they heard as they walked out was, "You are living with him, sleeping with him, and you are not married? You planned your wedding without me?"

They met Nurse Jane in the hall. "Sharon is in with her mother, and they need some time alone, so can you keep everyone else out for a while?" Dave asked her.

"Trouble in paradise, Poncho?" Jane responded.

"I don't think my future mother-in-law likes me very much," Dave replied.

"Don't take it personally, Dave. She doesn't like men period, and I can assure you she doesn't like the idea of her daughter sleeping with one, especially one she is not married to," Helen added.

Jane smiled at Dave. "Leave it to Nurse Jane. What did you and Cisco call me?"

"Nurse Jane Fuzzy Wuzzy." Dave laughed.

"Leave it to Nurse Jane Fuzzy Wuzzy." Jane walked away.

Jane went to Sharon's room with an aide. "It is time for your walk, then a shower. I will entertain your mother while you do your turns in the hall." She turned to Mrs. Kelly. "Hi, I am Jane, one of Sharon's nurses."

Sharon left with the aide, and Jane sat down with Sharon's mother. "She is such a beautiful, wonderful girl. We are all so happy for them.

They are the perfect couple. Do you know he calls her every night when he has to stay at the hospital, to check on her, tell her he loves her, and say good night to her? That is why everyone in the hospital knows her as Baby. He calls her Baby when he calls. Let me tell you a little about him, but don't tell Sharon what I tell you, because he protects her from the things he deals with here. He is a good doctor, but he is a better person, and he not only takes care of his patients, but he also takes care of anyone who needs him. He spent the better part of a day finding the ex-husband of a woman dying of cancer so the ex could take their children and the children would not end up in foster care. He finally found him in the oil fields of California and got him to come get his children so the mother could die in peace knowing her children were safe. There is a young nurse who works nights on this station. I am sure you will meet her tonight; he spent time talking to her at night when he was on call instead of sleeping. Her fiancé was in Vietnam; he helped her get through her fears and anxiety about the danger her fiancé was in. He faced down a policeman for beating a prisoner in the ED, and he faced down another policeman for the way he was treating a rape victim. He stood up to a drunk, drugged biker using a broken bottle as a weapon to protect a nurse and other staff in the ED. He is just a good guy. I have been doing this for a long time, I have seen a lot of young doctors come through this station, and he is one of my favorites, not because he is a great doctor, but because he is a good person. You could not ask for a better man for your daughter to marry." Jane stood up. "I have to get back to work now. It was nice to meet you, and I enjoyed talking to you."

Sharon's mother sat alone in the room until Sharon and the aide returned. "That nurse seems to think a lot of…"

"Dave, Mother, his name is David Cameron." Sharon said, feeling exasperated.

Sharon's mother continued, "She seems to think a lot of Dave. I can't say I am not disappointed. I wanted you to marry well. I wanted you to marry someone with social standing and wealth, someone from a prestigious family with influence. With your looks, you could be the wife of a governor or senator. You could marry someone who could make you a socialite or even a celebrity. I wanted to plan a big wedding for you to someone significant."

Sharon responded, "I am sorry you are disappointed. If I married well, it would be for you, not for me. I don't want any of those things, but you do, not for me but for yourself. I would have never married if I had not met Dave. We have a deep connection. It is more than love. When I was critical, I almost died, but one reason I didn't was because I could feel him. I could feel him with me even though I was out of it and not aware of anything else. I was aware of him with me, fighting for my life with me, and holding on to me to keep me from slipping away."

Sharon's mother took Sharon in her arms. "I love you, and I want you to be happy. If he makes you happy, that's all that counts. I would have liked to have planned your wedding with you, though."

Sharon hugged her back. "He makes me happier than I have ever been in my life. I am sorry, but there wasn't much to plan. We did it in a couple of minutes."

"OK, just tell me when and where. I will show up and wear beige." Sharon's mother smiled at her.

On their way back to Sharon's room, Helen told Dave, "Sharon's mother sees herself as some kind of Southern aristocrat. I have seen your charming side; you can be a real Southern gentleman when you turn it on. Charm her, play Ashley for her, but don't let her see your Rhett Butler side. Save that for Sharon. Did you guys really plan your wedding in the fort on Tom Sawyer's Island?"

"Yes," Dave answered.

"Don't lie to me. Did you two do it on Tom Sawyer's Island?" Helen stopped Dave and looked him straight in the eyes.

Dave laughed. "I wanted to, and I knew a good place, but Sharon wouldn't do it, so no, we didn't."

Helen laughed with him. "X rated children. Will you two ever grow up? No, please don't. Don't change or grow up. I like you just the way you are."

Jake looked at Dave in disbelief. "Really, Dave, you were going to do it on Tom Sawyer's Island? I will never think of Disneyland the same way again. I will think about doing it on Tom Sawyer's Island, and I won't be able to get that image out of my head." They all laughed.

They walked into Sharon's room to find Sharon's mother sitting on the bedside talking with Sharon. Sharon's mother stood up and offered Dave her hand. "I am sorry about before, but I was so worried about Sharon, I didn't even hear your name when Helen said it."

Audrey leaned over to Dave. "Nurse Jane Fuzzy Wuzzy was true to her word."

Dave smiled his most charming, "ah shucks, think nothing of it" smile, and took her hand and did a little bow. "When Helen introduced me, I couldn't believe you were Sharon's mother. I thought you were her sister. You are too young and beautiful to be Sharon's mother, Mrs. Kelly."

Helen coughed, Audrey hid a smirk, and Sharon rolled her eyes, but Sharon's mother beamed. "That nurse and Sharon told me a little about you, but they didn't tell me you were so charming and well mannered."

Dave continued to smile as he thought, *here it comes, the same questions the gentry in the South always ask when they meet someone new: Who's your daddy? What parish or county are you from?*

"Where did you develop such lovely manners? Did you go to private school?"

Dave let her hand go. "My family straddles the Texas, Louisiana border. My paternal grandfather is from Louisiana, and my other three grandparents are from East Texas. And yes, I went to a private university."

Sharon added, "His father's family were among the earliest settlers in Louisiana, and his mother's family were in Texas before it was the Republic of Texas, and their roots go back to the colonies." Sharon knew what her mother valued.

Bob and Phil burst into the room and rushed to Sharon's bedside. "Oh, Gorgeous, we have been so worried. You scared the hell out of us. Are you OK?"

Sharon answered, "No, not exactly OK, but better. I am still as weak as a kitten and feel like s—" Sharon stopped and looked at her mother. "Mother, Bob and Phil. Bob and Phil, my mother."

Like Dave, Phil knew how to deal with upscale Southern women. "My God, you are every bit as gorgeous as your daughter. No wonder Sharon is so beautiful." He took her hand.

Then Bob took her hand. "We are Sharon's neighbors, and she is very dear to us. We were devastated when we heard she was in the hospital in critical condition. We are so relieved she is out of the ICU and doing better."

Later in the day, Sigrid, Sam, and Rachael came, so by dinner, Sharon's room was full of people, all of them talking, drinking sodas, and cooing over Sharon. Dave sat on the bed holding Sharon's hand while her mother got to know all their friends. The room was so crowded, the aide couldn't get in to give Sharon her dinner tray, so she returned with a nurse. The nurse forged a path to Sharon's bed and deposited the tray.

"OK, people, she needs to eat, and she needs to rest. It is great she has so many devoted friends, but it is time for everyone who is not family to leave."

The nurse's announcement was followed by hugs, well wishes, and good byes from everyone except Dave, Sharon's mother, and Helen, who was driving Sharon's mother back to the house.

Sharon's mother talked to Sharon while she ate. "That Phil is very nice, but I think he is a little light in the loafers. All your friends are so nice. That Sigrid is so pretty and so tall."

Helen laughed at the comment about Phil and looked at Sharon who said, "He is gay, Mother. He and Bob live together. So are Samantha and Rachael; they live together too."

Sharon's mother looked astonished. "Gay? You mean they are homosexuals?"

"Yes, Mother," Sharon replied.

"Well, I guess he is light in the loafers. But that sweet, pretty girl, Rachael, she is a homosexual too?" Sharon's mother was wide-eyed and shocked.

"Yes, Mother," Sharon answered.

Sharon's mother pursed her lips. "Well, I never. Is everybody in this city gay? Do you have any friends who aren't gay?" Sharon's mother looked horrified. "You're not gay, are you? I mean, I know you sleep with Dave, but you don't sleep with women too, do you?"

Sharon, Dave, and Helen all started laughing. "Don't I wish!" came out of Dave before he could control himself.

"No Mother, I don't sleep with women." She scowled at Dave. "I only sleep with Dave, and we are going to be married, so calm down."

"Thank goodness." But Sharon's mother eyed Dave suspiciously after his comment.

"Mother, he was joking. We love each other. We only sleep with each other. You are overreacting because we have a few gay friends," Sharon reassured her.

"Well, you never know in a city like this where everyone is gay." Sharon's mother looked at them intently.

"We should go and let you get some rest. We have to make up Audrey's room for your mother." Helen and Sharon's mother got ready to leave, then they hugged Sharon and said good night.

When they were gone, Dave lay down on the bed beside Sharon and took her in his arms. They cuddled until a nurse came in, chased him out of the bed, and turned out the lights. "Time to get some sleep."

The next morning, Dave, Henry, Tom, Richard, Harven, Jason, George and Jay were gathered in Sharon's room along with Jane, Carol who stayed after her shift, and several other nurses, when Sheffield appeared at the door. "Don't you doctors have patients to round on, and don't you nurses have things to do?"

A chorus of "Yes, Sir" answered him, but no one left.

Dr. Sheffield made his way to Sharon's bedside. "I guess I need to discharge you, since you seem to be disrupting the operations of the hospital." A little cheer went up from those in the room. Sheffield looked around. "You do know you are in a hospital, don't you?" He looked back at Sharon. "Your labs are normal, your white count is down, you have not had a temperature since you left the ICU, and there is no evidence of any residual effects from your illness. You will be on oral antibiotics for another two weeks, no work until you have your follow-up appointment, and it will be a full two weeks before you feel completely recovered and can return to all your normal activities. Miss Kelly, all my best wishes and congratulations on your upcoming wedding to Dr. Cameron. We will get you out of here sometime after lunch."

Sharon took Sheffield's hand. "Thank you so much. Please forgive me. I am so sorry; I want to apologize for keeping you at the hospital and interrupting your schedule."

Sheffield responded, "Don't be silly, my dear. You don't have to apologize. I told you that's what we doctors do. It was a pleasure to take care of someone like you."

Dr. Sheffield motioned Dave to follow him as he left. When they were out of the room, Sheffield turned to Dave. "David, I would have liked to have had you here for your residency, but the program at UCLA is an excellent one." Dr. Sheffield took Dave's hand. "Dave, you are a good doctor. Learn to trust yourself, control your emotions, rely on your training, and you will be a good physician. Good luck to you at UCLA, and congratulations on your upcoming wedding. I am thankful Sharon survived, and she doesn't seem to have suffered any end-organ damage. The two of you have been given a second chance at a life together, so make sure you take full advantage of it."

Dave waited to go back in the room until everyone had taken their leave of Sharon. She was sitting on the side of the bed. "I called Helen to come get me and take you back to your apartment. My mother is going to stay at the house to take care of me. Oh Dave, I can't believe all this happened. I was so scared."

Dave sat down beside her and hugged her. "I want you with me, I need you with me, but my mother will never tolerate you staying with me with her in the house. She is just too old fashioned and Victorian. God, I don't want to be without you. I know I won't be able to sleep, but she is too difficult to deal with, and I don't have the energy to stand up to her." She hugged him back.

That afternoon, Helen dropped Sharon and her mother at the house, then drove Dave to his apartment. "You know she will never accept you. You did a good job with the Miss Scarlet stuff, and she was impressed with who your family is, but she will never accept that you are fucking her little girl. She went through too much with Sharon's father, and she hates men. Maybe if you were Bar and your family had a lot of money and influence, it might be different, but then you would be an asshole. You are a good guy, but I can tell you, a lot of men aren't."

She left Dave and his bag in the parking lot and drove away. Dave got the impression from what she said that something had happened with Jackson, and that is why she had been with Linda at the match party. Dave wondered if there was more to it than just breaking up with Jackson.

Dave knew there were people who were born gay, it was something in their physiology, it was all nature. He also knew some people were driven gay by their experiences; it was nurture. Both nature and nurture played a part in others. Men were often driven gay by domineering, controlling mothers. Some men and women were driven gay by their experiences with the opposite sex, so they gave up on the other gender and gravitated to their own. He wondered if that was happening with Helen or if she was discovering who she really was with Linda, or

A love story and social commentary

both. Helen seemed to have never liked men. Maybe it had taken someone like Linda to show her why.

Dave unpacked, did his laundry, slept for a while, then got up, showered, shaved, dressed, and drove to Sharon's house in the afternoon. Sharon's mother answered the door. "She is sleeping."

She left Dave standing at the door without asking him in. "Good, I can be there for her when she wakes up. I promised I would stay with her when I was not at the hospital." Dave walked past her into the house and started up the stairs.

"Don't wake her up, she needs her rest." Sharon's mother followed after him.

Dave ignored her and went to Sharon's room where he found her sitting up in bed reading. Sharon got out of bed to hug Dave, and then they sat on the side of the bed. "I am still not too chipper, and I feel so weak, but it is good to be out of the hospital. I fall asleep from time to time, and I don't have any energy, but I am better."

They talked for a while, and then they lay down together in each other's arms and fell asleep. Dave had dinner with Sharon and her mother, then drove to his apartment to go to bed early because he was starting back in the Nursery the next morning.

The David Cameron who walked into the Nursery the next morning was not the man he had been. He had been to the brink and he had suffered more than he thought it was possible to suffer, but he had also matured into a person who was capable of preforming his duties as a doctor without hesitation in a professional and caring manner. The pain of thinking Sharon was dead, followed by the joy of realizing she was alive, had galvanized his transition from an immature, naive, idealistic young medical graduate into a physician. He had become a grown-up, better version of himself capable of dealing with his life and his profession with a much deeper understanding. It had taken the better part of a year of sleep deprivation, long hours, stress, and grueling horrendous work plus the near death of the woman he loved to complete the process. But as he stepped into the Nursery that morning, he was not looking back; he was looking forward to marrying Sharon, moving to California, completing his residency in Medicine, and then living the full, well-lived life he liked to talk about. His step was light, and his heart was full.

Sharon's mother stayed for a week and took care of Sharon until her follow-up appointment. Dave fell into a pattern during that time. He worked for twenty-four hours in the Nursery, slept about four interrupted hours, went home to his apartment to sleep for a few more hours, went to the pool to swim laps, showered, dressed, and drove to Sharon's house. They spent the evenings listening to music in her room, sitting downstairs watching TV, or sitting in the park. Sharon's mother fixed dinner for them and after dinner, Dave would cuddle with Sharon in the front room or in her bedroom before going home to go to bed early before another twenty-four-hour shift the next morning.

He continued to see the same types of cases, mainly happy, healthy newborns with no problems and a scattering of jaundiced babies who had to stay in the hospital for phototherapy. If he had a baby who had serious problems, he would have lunch with the Psych resident to talk out his feelings and he swam more laps the next day before going to Sharon's.

The week slipped by quickly, and Sharon was released to return to work in another week when she was two weeks post-hospitalization. Sharon's mother flew home, so Dave and Sharon had sex for the first time in almost three weeks. Sharon teased Dave about having the worst reltney she had ever seen. Sharon told Dave the chief resident felt her problem was due to dehydration. She had spent two days running around Disneyland in the heat and sun, after a day at the pool in the heat and sun, followed by two days at the beach in the heat and sun, without taking in enough fluids.

They missed Audrey's wedding because Sharon was still recovering. Dave finished the Nursery and started the Pedi ED at the same time Sharon went back to work at the airline. He entered the last rotation of his internship and his last month at University Hospital with his life back to normal. It would be a busy month with Connie and Harven's wedding, their own wedding, and the move, all while Dave was in the Pedi ED doing twenty-four hours on and twenty-four hours off and Sharon was flying. The Pediatrics Department had been great during Sharon's illness, letting Dave miss two shifts in the Nursery, and they also gave him one shift off for his wedding and two off to travel to LA, so he had three days off for the wedding and five days to drive to California.

19
The ED

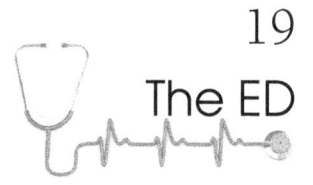

The Pedi ER in June was considerably less busy than it was during the cold and flu season, but there were still the usual sick kids, anxious mothers, injuries, and serious illnesses. Dave was busy, but he had time to get some intermittent sleep at night. There were no teams, just supervising residents that rotated on their own schedules, like the interns and students.

Dave continued the regimen he had started: complete his shift, sleep for a few hours before Sharon arrived, go to the pool and swim, listen to music and smoke some weed, eat dinner, go to bed, make love, go to sleep, and then get up and do it again.

Sharon made all the arrangements for the wedding. She moved the furniture and moved all the chairs to the front room for the ceremony, set up the table in the dining room for the caterer, and had the house professionally cleaned. She found a Justice of the Peace willing to come to the house for the ceremony and hired a caterer. She did the invitations, mailed them, and contacted everyone personally since it was such short notice. She made reservations at the hotel and asked for the same room they had on New Year's Eve. She made reservations for her mother with the airline and got Audrey's old room ready for her. Dave called his parents and brother to tell them he was getting married, but Sharon called his parents too, and made reservations for them along with his brother at a nearby hotel. Dave's brother was in baseball season and would be flying in between games just for the ceremony. She called Mother's Blues, reserved two tables, convinced them to have the house band announce the wedding party and play Fleetwood Mac's "Sentimental Lady" for their first dance, followed by "Warm Ways." By Connie's and Harven's wedding, Sharon had everything in place for her wedding.

She gave her notice to the airline, then she began to dismantle Dave's apartment and her room, packing and preparing everything for the movers. The movers would load Sharon's and Dave's stuff with another couple's things, leave before the wedding, carry their stuff to the new apartment, and deposit it in the appropriate rooms. They would move into Sharon's room with the clothes and other things they needed for the week after the wedding, then carry that stuff with them in their cars on the drive to LA. Sharon did all of it while she was still flying, and Dave continued to do his shifts in the Pedi ER.

Many of the children Dave saw in the ER were there because their mothers were anxious or overly protective, usually because it was their first child, but some were very sick or had major problems. Then there were the children who were there because they had been abused or harmed by an adult.

Dave no longer asked why, lamented about the pathos of the human condition, questioned the presence of a benevolent God, or sought some reason for everything. He accepted life for what it was and dug in to try to improve it in his sphere of influence. He had come to the conclusion there were three types of people who existed in the pile of humanity. There were those who simply sat on the pile riding it along; those who tried to pull the pile back or retard it; and those who tried to push the pile forward and improve it. He resolved to be one of the latter. He would push the pile forward, be a force for good, and exert a positive influence on the pile. He would try to do the right thing, because it was illogical not to do the right thing. He would try to help, but he would always make sure to do no harm.

Dave knew he lived in a consumer-driven society, much like the one Huxley predicted in *Brave New World*, but he vowed he would never succumb to the doctrines of nihilism and existentialism. He would especially oppose Ann Rand's doctrine of libertarianism, social Darwinism, and her dehumanized amoral capitalistic society based on profit and gain. He would value the individual but support the collective efforts to improve the lot of all. He would be a physician and conduct himself in a manner befitting the title.

His compassion for the plight of the abused children he saw in the ED knew no bounds, and his outright hatred of their abusers was even more profound. Dave dealt with abused women in the Surgery ER, but the stories were always plausible, plus the women were never left alone with him or the nurse by the abuser, and if they were, they were afraid to say what really happened. He also knew many abused women never made it to the ED. Several women a day, about a thousand a year, were murdered by their abuser, usually their spouse or boyfriend.

With children, it was harder to come up with a plausible story for the injuries the abuse caused.

Men who beat and abused their wives usually beat and abused their children. Dave saw a child in the Pedi ER with a dislocated elbow, a typical nurse maid's elbow caused by jerking the child up by one arm. The story the parents told was the child fell on his elbow, which was an obvious lie. Dave recognized the mother as a woman he had treated in the Surgery ER for a large scalp laceration she told Dave had been caused by the garage door coming down on her head. Dave had wondered if the laceration was caused by the woman being hit with something. Now he knew he was right. Dave contacted Child Protective Services, and they sent an investigator to the ER to evaluate the child. When the investigator arrived, the father lost his temper, and he had to be restrained by the security guards. The woman became frightened and asked for protection from him for herself and her child.

It amazed Dave there were still men who thought they had a right to beat their wives. In reality, nothing had changed since the days of the "rule of thumb," which stated it was legal to beat your wife as long as you did not use a rod bigger than your thumb. God help the poor woman whose husband had big hands. Today, the beatings usually took place with the fist or open hand, and it was unusual for the abuser to use an object like the man had used on the woman's head.

Dave had no tolerance for the physical abuse of a woman or a child, but to him, sexual abuse was far worse. He had a revulsion for rapists who forced sex on a woman, but his disdain for men who forced themselves on children—pedophiles who prayed on innocent children—was unmeasurable. He saw pedophiles as the embodiment of evil, the most despicable, deplorable, and vile of human creatures.

Dave thought he had seen the worst of what his gender was capable of with the rape cases in the GYN ER. Then he saw a child brought to the Pedi ER by a young mother for a rash on her bottom. The mother told Dave her daughter had a rash that would not go away. When Dave took the diaper off, he saw the girl's vulva was covered with venereal warts—condyloma, a sexually transmitted virus. Dave excused himself, went to the doctors' station, and lost it. He threw the chart against the wall and cursed whoever had sexually molested this child to a fiery hell for eternity. The resident was appalled and asked him what was wrong with him. Dave told her, but she could not believe it. "You must be mistaken."

Dave responded that he was not mistaken, he had seen venereal warts over and over again in GYN Clinic and ER. He led the resident to the exam area, and she gasped, putting her hand over her mouth when she saw the venereal warts. Dave and the resident carefully and gently explained to the mother that her daughter had been sexually assaulted by someone with an STD. The poor woman collapsed into Dave's arms crying uncontrollably. The resident called the police.

The woman was devastated. She told the police her husband was in Vietnam, and she worked but could not afford child care, so she left her daughter with her sister during the day. Her sister was married, but her husband worked and was not there when the baby was at her house, but his younger brother was staying with them because he had lost his job. The police obtained a warrant, picked him up, and brought him in to be examined. He had extensive venereal warts on this penis, so he was arrested and charged.

On his GYN rotations, Dave had seen women with small scars on their arms, their breasts, and even their vulvas. He had no idea what caused them, until he saw a child with the same scars and small round burns. Dave knew right away that they were cigarette burns because he had seen the same burns on rape victims. He realized the scars he had seen on the women were healed cigarette burns the women had suffered repeatedly. This child had the same scars and burns. The mother told Dave she left her child at a day care center while she worked. Again, the police were called, and the owner of the day care was arrested. Dave did not ask what the hell was wrong with these people, because he knew. He just had lunch with the Psych resident and swam more laps than usual.

Most of the horrendous cases Dave was involved with were the results of the abject poverty and the hopelessness of the indigent population he dealt with. The horrid conditions he slogged through were a manifestation of the lack of education, lack of opportunity, lack of basic living conditions, lack of decent food, and lack of any way out or forward for the underprivileged population of the country. There was nothing he could do about it. To eliminate the horror, the conditions that produced the horror had to be eliminated, and Dave came to the conclusion that would never happen.

Those who benefited from privilege would never jeopardize their place on the socioeconomic ladder to benefit those below them who lived in poverty and ignorance. Poor whites were left to struggle in dire circumstances along with poor people of color. Of course, white privilege played a part where racism was involved, but it wasn't all about race; it was about privilege. White groups faced the same bigotry and discrimination. Catholics, Jews, and white ethnic groups also struggled with the issue of privilege.

Dave was aware of white male Protestant privilege before Phil talked about it at lunch the day of the Santana concert. He knew that even though he would never knowingly use it or think about abusing it, he benefited from it. White privilege was tied to the socioeconomic divisions that contributed to the poverty and ignorance plaguing the people of color in the country. Hitler and Germany had taken white privilege to an extreme that destroyed most of Europe, and Dave knew there were still people in this country who harbored those same beliefs. They did everything they could to nurture and foster white male privilege to make sure it was there for them to use and even abuse to perpetuate the current conditions that kept the people of color in poverty and ignorance.

He also knew nothing could be done to change those people. Socialism, a redistribution of wealth, and a decrease in the influence of privilege would never be accepted by a portion of the population.

A lack of understanding added fuel to the fire. Capitalism, socialism, and communism were economic systems, not political systems, but most people confused them with forms of government. The major countries of Europe were parliamentary republics with economic systems that were a blend of capitalism and socialism. The communistic economic systems in Europe and Asia had totalitarian or at best oligarchic forms of government. There were no true forms of democracy in the world. The United States was a capitalistic democratic republic with several socialistic economic programs, like Social Security.

People equated socialism with communism and thought it was a form of government to be shunned in favor of democracy, yet it was really an economic system, not a form of government. Politicians pushed this misconception for nefarious reasons to further their own agenda and to convince the public to vote against their own self-interest. The voting public just did not understand a democracy was a form of government where everyone participated in the decision-making process like ancient Athens. A republic was a representative form of government in which the decisions were made by those representing the general public. An oligarchy was a form of government where the privileged few made the decisions, and in a totalitarian government, only one person made the decisions. A dictatorship could have a capitalistic economic system and a republic could have socialism as its economic system. Most people in the general public simply did not understand.

Dave's view of socialism was straightforward. National defense, education, police, fire protection, health care, mental health care, communication, transportation, work programs that improve and maintained the infrastructure to provide food and shelter to those in need should all be socialized. The collective good should be provided for collectively. The private sector of business should be a regulated capitalistic system where the individual's income and corporate profits are taxed in a graduated fashion to pay for the social programs. This hybrid of capitalism and socialism is present in many social democratic parliamentary countries of Europe, and their populations are the happiest in the world.

Dave was better able to cope with the problems he encountered because he handled his approach to them differently. He called on his competitive spirit. He began to relish tough cases he could manage to a beneficial outcome, then he reveled in the victory of making someone's life better, curing their disease, or relieving their pain and suffering. It was like he had been walking through a long dark tunnel for the last year, but he was now emerging into the bright sunlight again.

He felt good about himself. He felt good about his work. He was confident and enjoyed taking on bigger and more complex challenges, pitting himself against them and exalting in overcoming them. He was hungry for more knowledge and better clinical skills that would propel him to better performance and better results for his patients. He began to have the same feelings he got from sports—going into a game knowing he was well prepared, conditioned, good at the sport and looking forward to the completion, confident he could win.

20
It's Over

Caroline's wedding was a very nice affair with about two hundred guests. Audrey's wedding was a small-town occasion with friends, family, and about one hundred guests. Connie's wedding was the social event of the season. It was covered by the press with Connie's picture in the paper in her haute couture wedding gown from Paris that cost thousands, pictures of the church full of people and the ceremony, then a picture of Connie and Harven leaving the church with a caption about their honeymoon in France.

Harven's mother and father took center stage at the reception. Dave and Sharon ate and drank with their friends but hardly had any contact with Connie and Harven because they were being used by Harven's parents to impress all the important guests. Audrey, Jake, Caroline, Ron, Sharon, Dave, Helen and Helen's plus one, who was Linda, were at one table. Bob, Phil, Sigrid, Henry, Sam, Rachael, George, and the grad student were at another table. At one point, Connie managed to break away long enough to get in a circle with all the girls to jump up and down as the guys looked on laughing.

There were women at the reception who had unlimited time and money to spend on themselves—on their hair, their makeup, and their clothes. They had stylists, cosmeticians, and even plastic surgeons at their beck and call, yet in the midst of all the glitz and glitter, Sharon stood out. Her looks exceeded those of the other women and girls regardless of the amount of money, time, and effort they had expended to look their best. Many of the titans of business, movers and shakers, and politicians chatted her up as she stood drinking Champagne before they were seated for dinner. The men introduced themselves, asked if she would like more champagne, and ignored Dave as they talked to her. Sharon was a well brought-up lady, so she was polite as she listened to them talk about themselves, who they were, their accomplishments, and how wonderful their lives were. When they tried to press her about where she lived and blatantly asked how to get in touch with her, it was too much, so she maneuvered back to Dave's side, took his arm, and looked at him in a way that let them know she wasn't interested in them, regardless of how much money or power they had. But as soon as one left, others swooped in.

Sigrid also attracted a lot of attention. In her four-inch heels she was over six four, so she could literally look straight over the top of the heads of most of the men who tried to chat her up, few of whom were less than twenty-five years her senior. She had nothing but disdain for them, their wealth, and their power. She ignored them, talking to Henry and her friends as if they weren't there. Yet the hauntingly beautiful, tall, pale woman was like a magnet for the powerful men in the room who collected around her, vying for her attention. At one point, after several had asked how to get in touch with her, Sigrid asked the circle of men around her, "Where are your wives? Are they oblivious? Do they not care?"

After dinner, when the dancing started, younger men, the nepotistic sons of the titans, approached Sharon to asked her to dance. She politely told them she was only dancing with her fiancé. Sigrid simply refused when they asked her if she would like to dance.

It was a beautiful ceremony and a great dinner with excellent Champagne and wine, followed by a lively party. Except for the unwanted attention the two women attracted, they had a wonderfully perfect evening. They danced, drank Champagne, laughed and talked. Henry and Dave pulled the two tables together after dinner so they could all sit together. When it was over Connie and Harven left in a cab for the airport to fly to Paris. George hugged everyone and took his leave of each of them since he was leaving for Duke in a week. Caroline and Ron told Sharon they would be back in two weeks for her wedding, and they all vowed to meet at Henry's family's ski lodge in Colorado in January. None of them were in Connie's wedding party because Connie's maid of honor was her sister, and the rest of the attendants had been chosen by Harven's parents for their social status and connections.

As they stood outside the hotel saying goodbye, after sending Connie and Harven off to Paris, Sigrid took Henry to task in a way that gave everyone the impression she and Henry were close to a commitment of their own. "Harven's family is wealthy like yours, yes Henry?"

Henry answered, "I thought you knew that from our conversation in the Zoom room."

Sigrid continued, "Will your family demand you have a wedding like that when you get married?"

Henry became very interested in what Sigrid was saying. "No. My family keeps a low profile; besides, I have my own money. I make my own decisions about what I do and how I do it."

Sigrid's intelligent pale blue eyes flashed. "I would never have a wedding like that. I would never marry a man who wanted a wedding like that. When I get married, I will have a traditional Danish wedding in Denmark with my family and friends, and the family and friends of the man I marry."

Henry put his arm around her. "When I marry, the woman I marry can have any type of wedding she wants, anywhere she wants it." He hugged her and she smiled at him.

The next morning, Dave went back to the Pedi ER, and Sharon flew off to Buffalo. She was going to fly officially until the end of the month but use accumulated time off to cover the last two weeks. She was going to use the week before the wedding to finish the packing and to get with the movers.

Dave still had three hits of LSD from Cousin Jane. He met Henry for breakfast one morning to give them back to him. Henry took two, said he would give one to Harven when they got back, and left one with Dave.

Henry told Dave he had discussed marriage with Sigrid at length the night of Connie and Harven's wedding. She told him she did not want to live like the people at the wedding. She wanted to live the simple life of an academic, like her parents, and all she wanted to do was teach and do research. She didn't want to be rich, and she was worried about Henry's family, especially after what she had seen at Connie and Harven's wedding. She was afraid Henry's ties to his family and to Granny, who controlled the purse strings, would drag her into a lifestyle she did not want and would not be happy in. She hated the people at the wedding and their exploitation of others, but most of all, she hated their disengaged, narcissistic, superior attitude that mimicked the attitude of the aristocrats and royals of Europe. She wanted nothing to do with them, which meant she wanted nothing to do with Henry's family, so that meant she wanted nothing to do with Henry in a long-term relationship like a marriage.

Henry was beside himself because he loved her and could not picture his life without her, but he also loved his mother and father, and he was used to the influence his family's money exerted in his life. Sigrid told him she would not put him in the position of having to choose between her and his family, so there was no reason to talk about marriage. They would continue to live together and to enjoy life together for now.

Dave spoke to his friend from his heart. "Henry, your parents are some of the nicest people I have ever met. Sigrid will love them, they will love her, and they are the only part of your family she will ever have to deal with. The way you have handled your assets and trust proceeds, you have your own money. Plus, you won't be here; you will be living in Europe. Sharon did not want to get married either, but after we were together, her fears dissipated, then went away, and now we are going to be married, and it was her idea. Introduce Sigrid to your parents, let her see what kind of people they are, and do exactly what she said—live together and enjoy your life together. She will come around. But, Henry, even if she doesn't want to get married, don't lose her. Spend your life with her, married or not. That is what Sharon and I were going to do before she decided to marry me."

The days passed quickly for Sharon and Dave. Dave stayed focus on the last days of his internship and let Sharon handle all the other details. Dave was having lunch in the cafeteria before the wedding when Mike approached him. "I ran into Henry in the ER, and he told me you and Sharon were getting married at her house. Are we just supposed to show up?"

Mike sat down at the table with Dave. Dave said, "Sharon doesn't want you at our wedding. You called her a slut to our friends. You called her a slut to me, several times. I knew you did it because you were jealous, so I let it go. If I thought you meant it, I would have beat you to a bloody pulp."

Mike's face turned red and little beads of sweat broke out on his forehead. "But you want me there, don't you? We are friends, aren't we?"

Dave's eyes hardened as he looked at Mike. "Where were you when she was in critical condition? You haven't done anything like bad mouth me to other house officers, have you?" More sweat appeared on Mike's forehead. "Don't show up at the wedding. I would have to throw you out, and I don't want anything negative like that to happen on my wedding day."

Mike's face was red, and his forehead was covered with sweat. "I didn't show up when Sharon was in the hospital because I knew she didn't like me. None of those women like me."

Dave stood up. "You called Sharon a slut to everyone, including me. You walked in on Sigrid every time she was getting out of the shower when Henry was living at the Park house, and you stare at Connie's boobs when you are around her. They are friends, and they talk to each other. Your problem with them is of your own making, not theirs. Mike, don't think I don't know what you have been saying about me to the other house staff. I understand it is because of jealousy; otherwise, like I said, I would beat you to a bloody pulp." Dave walked away feeling good because he had expressed himself appropriately rather than planting his fist squarely in Mike's face.

Mike wiped his sweaty forehead with a shaking hand as he watched Dave walk away. He knew Dave was more than capable of beating him to a bloody pulp, so he was worried about what Dave said, but he was also angry. It never occurred to him he had lost a loyal friend because of his jealousy and envy.

Sharon spent the week before the wedding going back and forth between Dave's apartment and her house getting everything ready for the movers. She and Dave spent their last night at Dave's apartment, then she stayed there the next morning to meet the movers and get everything loaded, first from his apartment, then from her house. It was a bittersweet moment as Sharon watched the truck drive off from her house. She had lived there for five years. She had enjoyed being a flight attendant and living with her three friends, plus the last year had been something special. As she watched the truck disappear down the road, she realized that time of her life was over. Not for the first time, she thought how wonderful it would be if it all could just stay the same. The last year had been the happiest, fullest year of her life.

She walked back to the house to spend a sad, emotional night alone. Dave was at the hospital, both Helen and Linda were on layovers, so she was alone in the big empty house. She knew Dave would call to say good night, but she needed him to help her deal with her emotions and to quell her loneliness. In a way, she was mourning the passing of her previous life, and she needed him to comfort her in her grief, but tonight he was a doctor with obligations. She remembered what Dr. Sheffield said and wondered how many more lonely, unhappy nights she would spend in the coming years because she was a doctor's wife. It was a long, hard night of transition for Sharon, and she had no one to help her through the metamorphosis, so when Dave came in the next morning, sliding into bed next to her, she clung to him, crying softly on his shoulder as he cuddled her.

Dave didn't have to ask what was wrong, because he was dealing with similar feelings. It had all gone so fast, and now things were moving even more quickly. As Dave lay next to Sharon, holding her and feeling her tears on his shoulder, he reflected on his journey. He wondered if he had been so fixed on completing the journey, he had failed to fully appreciate the trip itself. He had been so focused on becoming a doctor that it may have prevented him from becoming fully engaged in the process. He felt as if he had skipped over his life like a stone skipping across the surface of the water, never diving down to see what was beneath.

Dave thought about the ants in the book *The Once and Future King*. Merlin turned Arthur into different animals to teach him how to be a good king and to rule well. For the ants, it was done or not done; done was good, not done was bad. Dave wondered if he had been too much of an ant, living only for the done and missing out on the doing. Not that Dave hadn't taken a big a bite out of life; he had taken full advantage of the activities he enjoyed, the trips he took, and the events he attended. But even his approach to that had been goal-oriented and end-point driven, not an in-depth plunge that immersed him in the doing. He was mourning the loss of things but also grieving for the things he had missed along the way because his journey had been too frantic and phrenetic.

He turned Sharon's face up to his to kiss her tears away. She responded by kissing him passionately, pressing her body against his. This was what she had needed—for Dave to hold her and comfort her. It was what Dave needed—her love and their oneness. They made love with tenderness and care, letting their grief and loss pour out of them in their passion. Then they snuggled until they fell asleep in each other's arms for the rest of the morning. As Dave was falling asleep, his last thought was that his previous approach was over; from now on, he was going to experience life to the fullest with the beautiful, wonderful woman lying beside him. He would pick up his certificate of completion for his internship in a week and apply for a license to practice medicine in California. He would no longer be a skipping stone or ant; he would be a physician, and he would drink fully from the cup of life, delving into its depths before he swallowed.

Dave woke up to find Sharon on her side propped up on her elbow looking at him. "Who the hell are you? What gave you the right to come into my life and turn it upside down?" She put her head down on his chest with her arm over him. "Where were you born? How did you make it? With an engine or a steel wheel? Really, I didn't even know you existed a year ago, and now I can't make it through a night without you next to me. What the fuck? You are the one who is always asking what the fuck about everything. Well, what the fuck about you? I have quit my job, and I am about to move thousands of miles from my home with you." She sat up and looked at him. "I am in love with you, and my heart is full for you. How can you make me that way? Who the hell are you? What the fuck?"

Dave sat up and put his arms around her. "You are the most beautiful, incredible woman I have ever met, and tomorrow you are going to be my wife, which makes me the luckiest man in the world. That's who I am—I am the luckiest man in the world."

They kissed and fell back in the bed together, holding each other. "Wow, that's hard to believe, and then we are off to LA for two years, and who knows what next." Sharon wiggled against him. "I bought something for tomorrow night in New York. Wait until you see it, or more accurately, wait until you see me through it." She laughed and rolled on top of him. "I love you, David Cameron, and tomorrow night, I am going to show you just how much I love you."

Dave pulled her down and kissed her. "Ditto."

They got up, showered together, dressed, and ate lunch then left for the airport for Sharon to pick up her mother and for Dave to meet his parents. Dave's parents had a rental car, but Dave met them, followed them to their hotel, and had them follow him to the house to meet Sharon and her mother. Sharon met her mother at the airport and took her back to the house to wait for Dave and his parents. Dave's brother was flying in the day of the wedding, and Dave's parents were going to pick him up. They all were flying out the day after the wedding, so Dave's parents were going to take Sharon's mother and Dave's brother back to the airport with them.

Dave made reservations at the French restaurant for the five of them, plus Helen, Henry, and Sigrid, for a kind of rehearsal dinner, even though there was no rehearsal. They planned to meet at the house for drinks, then walk to the restaurant, but first, Sharon had to meet Dave's parents, they had to meet Sharon's mother, and all of them would spend the afternoon together. Sharon was so nervous, she changed clothes three times while she and her mother waited for Dave and his parents.

Dave was nervous too, talking incessantly to his parents about Sharon. Finally, Dave's mother interrupted him. "David, I am sure we will love her. You know how much I have always wanted a daughter. Well, now I am going to have one."

Dave's dad added, "She got you to cut your hair, so I like her already."

When Dave and his parents arrived, Sharon and her mother were waiting for them in kitchen. Dave did the introductions and Sharon offered everyone some wine after they sat down. Dave's mother didn't drink, so Sharon got her a Coke.

"I want all my grandchildren to look like Sharon." Dave's dad was beaming with pride over his son marrying someone as stunning as Sharon.

Dave's mother looked at Sharon. "Dave told us you were beautiful and a part-time model, but I had no idea you would be so striking."

Sharon accepted the comments graciously, but was determined Dave's parents would see there was more to her than her looks before the afternoon was over.

Dave's parents and Sharon's mother talked for a while, getting to know each other, and they all three talked to Dave and Sharon about their future plans. They spent the rest of the afternoon with the three parents telling stories about Dave's and Sharon's childhood and school days.

When Dave's parents left, Dave's mother had tears in her eyes as she hugged Sharon and said, "If I had a daughter, I would want her to be just like you. I can't tell you how happy I am you are going to marry my son." Dave's mother did not say if she had a daughter, she would want her to look just like Sharon, but that she would want her to be just like Sharon. That comment was what Sharon wanted to hear.

Sharon smiled at her. "You do have a daughter just like me—it's me. I am your daughter now."

A love story and social commentary

That caused the tears to flow, and Dave's mother hurried out the door with his dad so they wouldn't see her cry.

After Dave and Sharon watched them walk to their car, Sharon turned to Dave. "I don't know how your mother had the courage to try again for a daughter after your sister died. I don't know how she was able to face another pregnancy after what she went through."

Dave looked at his mother getting in the car. "She wanted to try again after my brother was born. She still wanted a daughter so bad she was going have another child, but my dad said, no. He was too afraid something would go wrong and that my mother wouldn't be able to survive a second disaster like my sister. He was worried that something might happen to her too. Pregnancy is not without its risk. You have no idea what you mean to her, even if you are only her daughter-in-law." Dave put his arm around Sharon. Sharon could not imagine what it would be like to lose a child, much less what it would be like to have a child with major disabilities and watch her die a slow, painful death.

Sharon's mother went upstairs to get ready for dinner while Sharon and Dave were saying goodbye to his parents, so Sharon and Dave were alone when they came back in the house. "I see where you get your looks and your BS. Your father is a very nice-looking man, and he is so charming. You obviously learned that smooth Southern gentleman act from him. Was he a good athlete too?"

"No. It was my mother who was the athlete. She was an All-State basketball player in high school. You asked about her courage; I can tell you she is lot tougher than she looks. She raised two wild boys with an iron hand. If we didn't behave or failed to exhibit proper manners, she would put a major hurt on us in a way no one could see, and if we did not respond or we let anyone know she was putting it to us, she cracked down on us more, smiling the whole time. She is just as sweet and nice as she appears. She loved us unconditionally, protected us like a mother lion, encouraging and supporting us in everything we did, but we were raised to be gentlemen and God help us if we failed to meet her expectations in that department." Dave put his arms around Sharon and looked into her eyes. "I am a mama's boy, in case you didn't know. I owe any success I have had in my life to my mother."

Sharon kissed him. "I am glad you love your mother. So many men have a problem with women because they have a problem with their mother. I love my mother too; she is difficult at times, but she did everything for me, loved me, supported me, and has always been there for me. It's a shame my father turned into such an asshole, because she was a lot different before he left us. The whole divorce thing made her bitter, and I know my daddy issues caused my problem with men and marriage." They held hands as they walked upstairs to get ready for dinner.

The small restaurant had pushed two tables together to make a table for eight, and once they were seated, Henry had the waiter open the Champagne and told him to put everything on one check for him. When their glasses were full, Henry stood up and looked at Sharon and Dave. "You are lucky if you have one true friend in your lifetime. Well, I must be lucky, because I have a true friend in Dave. You are fortunate if you meet someone exceptional as you go through life. So I must be fortunate too, because I met Sharon, who is an exceptional person. Words are inadequate to describe how happy I am that my best friend and this exceptional woman are marrying. I knew when I introduced them, they were meant for each other, but I was not prepared, and I don't think they were prepared, for what followed. The terms *love at first sight, sparks flew*, and *the earth moved*, hardly describe what happened. It wasn't simply love at first sight; it was all-consuming, unconditional love at first sight. It wasn't sparks that flew; it was lightning. The earth didn't just move; it trembled and quaked. As I stand here tonight, I am still in awe of the love I wrought the night I brought them together. To my best friend and his exceptional bride to be. I give you Sharon and Dave." Henry raised his glass and they all drank, even Dave's mother.

Helen stood up next. "Sharon is my best friend. We went through training together, have lived together and have flown together for five years. Henry is right, when Sharon and Dave met, it produced shock waves we all felt." Helen looked at Sharon. "Their meeting is now the stuff of legend, known far and wide." Sharon blushed. "But I have seen a different side of their love. I have seen the innocent, childlike devotion they have for each other, the tender caring way they interact, the way they play with each other and make each other happy. I have seen the passion too, make no mistake about that. You have to be careful not to stand too close to them or you might get burned by the heat they generate, but there is so much more to their love than passion. To Sharon and Dave, to their love."

Dave's dad stood up. "First, I want to say how proud I am of my son. Then, I want to welcome Sharon to our family as the daughter we have always wanted. I want to clarify why I am proud of my son; it is not because he became a doctor or any of his other accomplishments; it is because he is marrying Sharon." He looked at Sharon. "What a beautiful, warm, intelligent woman she is. Of all his accomplishments, making her his wife is the one I am most proud of. To my future daughter-in-law, Sharon."

Sharon's mother stood up and looked at her daughter. "I am proud of my daughter, too. I am proud of her courage. She quit her job to get married, to move thousands of miles away, to go back to school, and to start a new life. I must admit, at first, I couldn't understand why. A nurse took me aside at the hospital and told me about Dave. But it wasn't until all nurses and doctors were there for Sharon when she was sick that I began to understand. They didn't know my daughter, some didn't even know her name, but they were there for her because of him. They wanted to support her, in order to support him. When she was sick, I saw how much he loved her, never leaving her side when she was in the hospital and spending every minute he could with her while she recovered at home. I understand now why she is doing what she is doing; it is because of Dave. She loves him, and he makes her happy. To Dave. To the man I know will take care of my daughter." They drank to Dave.

Dave's mother stood up last. "I hope there is enough Champagne for one last toast. I want to drink to the future, to their future, and to the future of our two families. I want to drink to Sharon and Dave's family, to their children, our future grandchildren. To our children's family and our grandchildren." Dave looked at Sharon as they drank. She was smiling at his mother. Dave knew his mother was the quintessential mother, and that all she had ever wanted to be was a mother. She defined herself as a mother, so he was not surprised by her toast, but he was surprised by Sharon's response to it.

Dave felt a little fear grow in the pit of his stomach as he watched his mother and Sharon interact over the toast. Dave knew he could never put Sharon at risk for anything, including a pregnancy, plus he could still see the sadness in his mother's eyes when the word daughter came up. Words are powerful. His mother's toast had a powerful effect on him.

When the toasts were over, they ordered dinner and began to talk. Sigrid leaned over to Henry. "This is the way a wedding should be—family and friends eating, drinking, and having a good time. A simple family affair about love, children, and bring two families together to start a new family. Dave's mother is right, a marriage is about family and children. Do you agree?"

Henry took her hand under the table. "If you marry me, you can have any kind of wedding you want, anywhere you want. And yes, I agree." That was not what Henry had intended to say, but he could not help himself.

Sigrid drew back from Henry. "You are asking me to marry you after what I told you about how I feel?"

Henry responded. "Yes. Please marry me, Sigrid. I love you and I want to spend the rest of my life with you."

"I need a little more time, but yes in time, when I am—no, when we are both ready, yes. There is no reason to rush it. We can take our time to be comfortable with it and to make sure it is what we both want. But yes, Henry, I will marry you, but first we go on like we are for a while, like we agreed. Be patient with me. But yes, I will marry you." She leaned in and kissed him.

"That is good enough for me," Henry responded. Sharon was talking to Dave's mother, Dave's father was talking to Sharon's mother, so only Dave and Helen saw and heard what happened between Henry and Sigrid.

After a bottle of Champagne and six bottles of wine between them, they were a very happy group as they walked back to the house. As they said their good nights, Dave's mother took Sharon's hands and looked straight into her eyes. "Oh, my dear, I am so happy. I am happier than I have been for a long time. Thank you so much." Then she hugged Sharon goodbye and whispered in her ear, "Please have a little girl for me. That is all I ask. Have a sweet little baby girl for me." She stepped back and Sharon saw tears overflow from her eyes as she left.

Sharon's mother said good night and went upstairs, thinking Dave was going back to his apartment, so she was surprised when both Dave and Sharon followed her upstairs to go to Sharon's room, and the look she gave them at the top of the stairs was definitely not one of approval.

A love story and social commentary

When they were in Sharon's room, Dave asked, "Do you have one of those little numbers you can put on so I can take it off?"

Sharon smiled at him. "I have to undress first, and I have a feeling once I have my clothes off, we will never get around to me putting on one of my little numbers." They both undressed, and she was right, Dave couldn't wait for her to put a negligee on.

She frowned. "Dave I can't do it with my mother in the house. I am sorry but after the look she gave us, I feel like she is watching me. I'll make it up to you tomorrow night, I promise."

The day of the wedding was a beautiful warm sunny June day, not too hot and calm without a cloud in the sky. Dave and Sharon slept late and stayed in bed enjoying the peaceful early summer morning. "This is the first day of the rest of our lives. Today everything changes."

Sharon nibbled Dave's ear. "Until the end of time," she whispered.

"Until the end of time," he repeated.

Then there was a knock on the door. "It's late, and you have a wedding at four. You need to get up and get something to eat."

"Mother." Sharon sat up and looked at Dave. "OK, Mom, we are up. We will be down in a minute." Sharon tried to get out of bed, but Dave caught her and pulled her back. "I told you no last night, not with her in the house, and now you want to do it with her right outside the door? Behave." She fell back in his arms and kissed him. "You'll get yours tonight when we are legal. Now, get up and put your robe on."

They put their robes on and went downstairs where, Helen, Caroline, and Audrey were waiting with Sharon's mother. "Hurry and get dressed. We are off to the spa for a steam, sauna, hot tub, hair, nails, and makeup. We can have lunch at the pool. If you hurry, we will be back in time for your wedding." Helen looked at Dave. "Slept late, did we?"

"Dave, can I make you a sandwich or a late breakfast? Say goodbye to Sharon; you won't see her again until the wedding." Sharon's mother looked at Dave.

Dave kissed Sharon goodbye, then she and her friends ran upstairs to get her ready for her spa day. "I am sorry I knocked on the door, but the girls were anxious to go, and it was getting late."

"No problem, we were just enjoying the morning. A sandwich will be fine. Thank you." Dave sat down and waited. It wasn't long before Sharon and her friends rushed out the door giggling, laughing, and shouting bye as they went.

Sharon's mother sat a ham sandwich, chips, and a Coke in front of Dave. "Sharon told me that is what you eat when you are not at the hospital." She sat down and looked at Dave. "Dave, I am sorry I am having trouble adjusting to things. I am a traditionalist, and your Bohemian lifestyle is foreign to me. It is counter to my values and the way I think people should live. I know there is a generation gap, both of you are immersed in the counterculture young people are swept up in today, but the way you live and what you believe goes against my Christian upbringing and flies in the face of everything I was taught to believe. Don't get me wrong, I am not attacking or blaming you. I know Sharon is as much a part of it as you are. I only want you to understand why I am uncomfortable with the situation. I know you love my daughter, I know you will take care of her, and I know you make her happier than she has been since her father left us, but I am still adjusting to a lot of things, so forgive me."

Dave listened to Sharon's mother as he ate his sandwich. "I understand. I have heard some of the same things from my parents. All I can say is, trust your daughter. Sharon is smart. Because of her beauty, her intelligence is often overlooked, and she is not given credit for her overall value. Henry was right last night when he said she is an exceptional person."

Sharon's mother got up and cleared Dave's plate and the Coke bottle. "I know you are right. I put too much value on her looks and forget how smart she is. But it is hard for a mother to let go of her daughter."

Dave stood up. "You are not going to be alone. It's not just you and Sharon any longer; you have me, my parents, and even my brother." Dave gave her a gentle hug. He went upstairs to get dressed to go pick up the rings and flowers.

Dave returned and went straight to Sharon's room to get ready for the wedding. Sharon and the girls were going to get ready in Helen's room. He had two simple matching bands of gold, along with Sharon's bouquet of six white roses with white baby's breath in a sealed plastic bag with the stems in a water vile at the bottom. He sat on the bed and looked at the two bands of gold in one hand and the bouquet in the other. He walked through the bathroom and left the larger ring with the bouquet on Helen's bedside table, went back to the bathroom, stripped off his clothes, and took a nice, long, hot soak in the tub.

As he soaked, he experienced a flashback of the past year, followed by a condensed replay of his life up until the time he met Sharon. He thought about Dickens' *David Copperfield*. "Whether I shall turn out to be the hero of my own life or……I am born." *The day I met Sharon, I was born*, Dave thought as he toweled off. He went back to Sharon's room and lay on the bed looking up at the ceiling.

He smelled Sharon in the bedding, the Chanel and Ambush, her essence, her clean freshness, and he rolled over and buried his face in her pillow inhaling her and remembering smelling Ambush in his bedding after she left his apartment after the first night they spent there. "God, I love her so much, please never let anything happen to her again. Please let everything be OK now," he asked out loud, and then Dave got up and dressed for his wedding.

As he walked downstairs in his new suit, he knew he would never put Sharon in physical danger or at emotional risk, no matter how much he wanted a son to carry on his name, to teach how to ski, sail, and play sports, no matter how much his mother, who had done everything for him, wanted a granddaughter. He would never risk losing her again or having her end up like his mother. That was decided; he was not going to worry about it anymore. He put the whole thing behind him as he walked into the front room.

True to her word, Sharon's mother wore beige and greeted people as they arrived. Bob, Phil, Sam, Rachael, Connie, Harven, Jake, Ron, and Linda, who was Helen's plus one, were already in the front room. Caroline, Helen, and Audrey were upstairs in Helen's room helping Sharon get ready. Henry and Sigrid arrived with Henry in a new custom-tailored suit and Sigrid in a dress Henry bought for her for the occasion, and then Dave's mother, father, and brother were at the front door. The last to arrive were the Justice of the Peace and the caterer.

The girls filed down from Helen's room one at a time with Helen last. She nodded to everyone and took her place beside the judge at the front of the room. Dave gave Henry the ring and went to the bottom of the stairs to wait for Sharon as everyone found a seat, and Henry took his place beside the judge facing Helen. Everything was ready for Sharon.

Sharon sat on the side of Helen's bed, took some deep breaths, stood up and looked at herself in the mirror one last time, then mentally said goodbye to her old life, opened the door, and walked down the stairs into her new one.

Many times, over the course of the last year, Sharon had taken Dave's breath away and made his knees buckle when he saw her, but her appearance on those occasions paled in comparison to the way she looked standing at the top of the stairs on her wedding day. The Rodeo Drive dress displayed her physical assets perfectly. Her makeup had been done by a professional who accentuated her beauty without using an excess of product. The hair stylist had highlighted the gold accents in her hair and produced small ringlets that framed her face. Around her head was a halo of baby's breath that matched the baby's breath in her bouquet and gave her a look of innocence and purity. Her shoes were satin pumps that matched her dress and accentuated her long slender legs.

Dave's heart was pounding as he walked to the foot of the stairs and put his hand out to her. "There are no words to describe how you look. Please, just stand there and let me look at you. I never want to forget how you look today." Sharon smiled and stood in front of him on the stairs holding his hand. She took his arm to walk to the front room. They stopped and stood in the opening between the front room and the hall for a moment so everyone could see them.

Sharon's appearance produced murmurs, and Dave's brother blurted out, "Damn!" He leaned over to his mother. "You told me she was pretty, but damn!"

The civil ceremony went quickly and ended with Dave and Sharon kissing passionately, as everyone crowded around them. Helen laughed. "There will be time for that later."

Dave and Sharon broke the kiss and looked at each other. "We did it." "Yes, we did it."

Helen hugged Sharon. "I am going to miss you."

Henry hugged Dave. "Hey, Poncho, it won't be the same here without you."

Sharon's mother hugged her and then hugged Dave, doing her best to look happy, yet she was disappointed because her dream wedding for Sharon would have been more like Connie's wedding. Dave's mother hugged them, telling them how happy she was. Dave's father just kept smiling as he congratulated the couple, telling Sharon she was the most beautiful bride he had ever seen.

When Sharon met Dave's brother, she did a double take, looking at him and then looking at Dave, because he was simply a bigger version of Dave.

He hugged her, then stepped back looking at her. "I only want to know one thing. Do you have a sister?" Sharon told him no, she was an only child. "Damn!" he said again, then turned to his brother. "Wow, big brother, I am impressed." He laughed and hugged his brother. He turned back to Sharon. "Welcome to our family. I just wish you had a sister who looked like you." He hugged Sharon again then looked at Dave. "How many times do I get to hug her before I get in trouble?"

Sharon looked at Dave. "He looks just like you, only bigger."

Dave laughed. "Yes, but we are different in many ways. He is all jock."

Bob and Phil interrupted. "My God, Gorgeous, I have to find a new name for you. You are more than gorgeous today." Phil hugged Sharon then Bob hugged Sharon as Phil took Dave's hand. "I know I don't have to tell you how lucky you are."

Bob took Dave's hand. "She is special, but you know that."

One by one their friends hugged them, congratulated them, and wished them well. When everyone had their time with Sharon and Dave, Henry put one arm around each of them and pulled them to him in a three-person bear hug. "No matter where we are, no matter what happens, no matter how much time passes, I will always hold you two in my heart. I consider introducing the two of you the finest thing I have done or ever will do in my life." He choked up a bit as he kissed Sharon on the cheek.

Rachael was a photographer, so she took pictures of the ceremony, then of Sharon alone, then of Sharon with Dave, then the parents alone, then the parents with Sharon and Dave, then of Henry with Helen, and finally all of them together.

The girls all clustered together. "Don't!" Jake said. "It's time to grow up. You are all married now."

Sigrid looked at Jake. "I'm not married, and who said we have to grow up? Do we want to grow up?"

There was a chorus of, "No!'

"Do we want to squeal?" Sigrid asked.

There was a second chorus of, "Yes!"

She looked at Jake. "Let's do it!"

Just as Henry came in with the Champagne, the women formed a circle with their arms around each other, jumped up and down, and squealed.

"Oh, Jesus."

"I tried to stop them," Jake said.

"We refuse to grow up."

"We are sisters."

"We will never stop."

"We refuse male dominance."

"And this is our way of showing it."

"Our way of showing solidarity."

"Sisters in solidarity against male dominance."

They jumped up and down again and yelled, "Solidarity." Then they all fell about laughing.

Henry punctuated the whole thing by popping a Champagne cork and yelling, "Come and get it. The glasses are on the dining room table."

Sharon's mother turned to Dave's parents. "It looks like things are about to get wild."

Dave's father answered, "It looks like Sharon and Dave have a close-knit group of good friends who about to celebrate their wedding." Dave's father shouted, "My father, Dave's grandfather, is from Louisiana, and when it is party time in New Orleans, they say *bons temps rouler*, let good times roll. So, *bon temps rouler*. Give me some of that Champagne."

The caterer announced dinner about an hour and a half after the ceremony was over. They sat in groups to have dinner and talk. Once the caterer's helpers had cleared the plates, Henry called for everyone's attention. "I want to be the first to introduce you all to Dr. and Mrs. Cameron." When the applause ended, he raised his glass. "To Sharon and Dave, all my best as they start their new life in California." Everyone drank to Sharon and Dave. "Next to us, the gang. This is probably the last time all of us will be together. George has already left for Duke, Caroline and Ron live in New York now. Audrey and Jake will be moving soon, and Connie, Harven, Sharon, and Dave are off to California. It has been one hell of a year, so one last time, to us." This triggered a series of toasts.

"To the parties."

"To Halloween, the greatest party the Park District has ever seen."

"To Sharon in that cat suit at the Halloween Party."

Followed by, "I told you to forget about that cat."

A love story and social commentary

"To Sharon in the zoom room at the Bar party."

Followed by, "I refuse to drink to that, and I don't want to hear any more about it. My mother is here."

"To Sharon dancing at the 4th of July party."

"To Sharon dancing at any of the parties."

Followed by, "Why is this all about Sharon? What about me?"

Followed by, "Are you serious?" "Have you seen your wife?" "Have you seen your wife dance?" "I know you saw your wife dance at the Halloween party." "I know you saw your wife in the zoom room at the Bar party." "I told you I don't want to hear any more about the zoom room."

"To the Bar party, where it all started."

"Really?"

"To the 4th of July party."

"To the manly game of Frisbee, to beer and barbecue."

"To female power and to the power of squealing."

"To the past year."

"To today, Sharon and Dave's wedding, the last party."

"To the future."

By the time all the toasts were finished, the wine and Champagne were also finished. Those not going dancing began to say their good byes. Bob, Phil, Sam, and Rachael took their leave with Phil asking Sharon when they were going to leave for LA so they could be there to see them off, and then he slipped Dave a baggy of buds. "For later tonight so you start married life off right."

Dave's brother hugged Sharon and said goodbye. "I thought you were doing an internship. It sounds like you were doing post-graduate work in partying." Then he hugged Sharon again and said, "Damn!"

Sharon's mother was teary-eyed as she hugged Sharon and Dave. "I have so many questions now, but I am afraid of the answers." Then she went upstairs to Audrey's room still trying to absorb what had just happened and to reconcile it with the hopes, dreams, and aspirations she had for Sharon before she married Dave.

Dave's dad was riding high on "that's my boy" pride and the joy of his son's marriage. "You have it all now, son. You are a doctor, you have a beautiful wife, a great circle of friends, and an incredibly bright future. I could not be happier for you or prouder of you." He hugged Dave.

But Dave's mother was having trouble saying goodbye. She and Sharon had one arm around each other's waist. "I wish I could spend more time with you, and I wish you were not going to be so far away. Do you think you will ever come back from California?"

Sharon smiled at her. "We are planning to live there permanently, but you can come visit anytime, and we can spend as much time together as you wish."

Dave's mother teared up. She did not want to let Sharon go or say goodbye. "Well, goodbye then. Oh Sharon, I am so glad you married my son. I couldn't ask for a better daughter-in-law." She hugged Sharon and left with Dave's dad and brother.

Henry called for two cabs to take them to the club because they all had been drinking a lot and would be drinking more before the night was over. There were twelve of them, so they squeezed into the two cabs and rode to Mother's Blues.

The band immediately recognized the group, and the front man stepped to the microphone. "We are going to take a short break for a special event." The dance floor cleared. "I want everyone to welcome Dr. and Mrs. Cameron, who just got married, and we are going to let them have their first dance together as husband and wife alone. Dr. and Mrs. Cameron." Dave walked Sharon to the middle of the dance floor as the band began a bluesy version of Fleetwood Mac's "Sentimental Lady."

There was a smattering of applause as the song finished and "Warm Ways" began with their friends joining them on the dance floor led by Connie and Harven, with Harven waving everyone on to the dance floor. The white boy with glasses and the hot blond got some of the black couples' attention, but it was when they saw Sigrid that the black men began to lead their partners on to the dance floor to get a closer look at her. Sigrid had on four-inch heels, she was dressed exquisitely, and she was like a beautiful apparition, in her pale, haunting way.

"That is the whitest white woman I have ever seen," one black man said as he watched her dance.

"That is tallest white woman I have ever seen," his friend added.

"I thought the first one was tall and white, but that one is taller and whiter," another black man said as he led his partner to the dance floor. His partner responded, "I'll bet they are Scandinavian. Those people are tall and white like that."

As the song ended, Harven went to the band stand and got the front man's attention. As he walked away smiling, the band launched into Chuck Berry's "Promised Land" with a guitar riff that split the air. That got everyone out on the dance floor as Harven put his head back and shouted, "We are bound for the Promised Land!"

"Amen!" A black man next to him shouted and they slapped up and down. From that time on, any barriers that may have existed between the two racial groups were broken down, disappearing in the music and dancing. The band started rocking, the music got hotter, and the dancing got more lively as the dance floor became crowded with almost everyone in the club. Sharon found her groove and let the music take control of her as she and Dave danced the night away, celebrating their wedding.

By midnight, Dave informed their friends that he and Sharon were going to the hotel. "We have a marriage to consummate."

Connie responded, "I don't think your marriage can get any more consummated. You two have been steadily consummating since the night you met."

"That was before we were married. But now that we are married, we have to start all over again with the consummating." Dave stood up with Sharon, they hugged their friends, said good night and in some cases goodbye. As they walked across the dance floor to leave, there were cat calls, lewd comments, encouragements to feats of sexual prowess, and cheers with the whole club giving them a loud boisterous send-off. Dave got the bartender to call a cab to take them back to Sharon's house to pick up his car and their overnight bags, and then they drove to the hotel.

The clerk greeted them. "Dr. Cameron, your room has been paid for, and you have been upgraded to a penthouse suite. Here is a card. You will also find a bottle of Champagne and a fruit basket in your room. A group of women, here are their names, ordered that and paid for a wedding breakfast in bed for you in the morning. Simply call room service when you are ready for it. It is a pleasure to have you with us and congratulations. Here are your keys. Oh, one more thing, several packages were delivered for you this afternoon. They are in your room. They came with this card." The first card was from Henry and Harven, the women were Audrey, Caroline, and Helen, and the card with the packages was from Bob and Phil.

The penthouse suite had a living room with a balcony, a bedroom with a king-sized bed, and a large bathroom with an oversized Jacuzzi tub. All the rooms had floor-to-ceiling windows that overlooked the city. The Champagne and fruit basket were in the living room, a stack of boxes from Bob and Phil's were in the bedroom, and the bed was turned down with two robes laid out on the bed with two dark chocolate truffles.

Sharon went to the bathroom with her travel bag while Dave opened the Champagne and rolled a number from the weed Phil had given him. He took his suit off, put on a robe, and turned on the music system. Sharon emerged in a long white negligee that reached the floor and was so shear, it looked like a thin white transparent film covering what it did cover of her body. It had small ruffles at the ends of the long sleeves, around the bottom and the V openings above and below her waist where it fastened with a single hook and eye. She was in her heels and the baby's breath was still in her hair. She stood silhouetted in the door before walking to one of the large windows in the living room that overlooked the city and looked out, just as she had six months before on New Year's Eve. Dave lit the J, took a hit, and walked up behind her with two glasses of Champagne in one hand and the joint in the other. He handed a glass of the Champagne and the joint to her, then stood behind her cupping her breast.

They understood this was their first night as husband and wife, so they took their time to savor every moment of it. They finished their Champagne and ate the chocolate truffles standing in the window looking out over the city. They put their glasses down and Sharon turned to put her arms around Dave's neck as she jumped up, locked her legs around his waist, and kissed him. He carried her to the bedroom and laid her gently on the bed.

Dave hovered over her on his hands and knees, kissed her, and moved to her ear, down her neck, and to her breasts, before he moved lower as she held his head and moaned. He took her to the brink, then moved up over her, and she drew a sharp breath as their bodies merged. Dave wanted them to finish together. He buried himself in her as she locked her legs around him and they rocked together in ecstasy until she moaned louder, squeezed him with her legs, clutched him as tight as she could with her arms and screamed as they both jerked uncontrollably, merged together as one with their passion flowing into each other. When it was finally over, they lay still and quiet for a while, holding each other as they returned from the magical place their lovemaking had taken them.

"Was it us or was it the weed?" Dave fondled her breast.

"I don't know, but every time we really get going, I think it can't get any better, but then it does. Maybe it is because we are married now and it's legal." Sharon raised up on her elbow. "It's funny, I never felt guilty when we did it before, but tonight for some reason, I felt completely relaxed and uninhibited. Maybe there was a hidden element of guilt I didn't even know about that is gone now. I wouldn't doubt it, knowing my mother and what she drilled into me."

"Let's try out the Jacuzzi." They went to the living room, Dave poured two more glasses of Champagne, and lit the number. They both took a hit while sipping their Champagne. They were really high now on all the Champagne, wine, and weed. There were a lot of products in the bathroom, so they added fragrances, bubbles, and bath salts to the Jacuzzi, turned it on, and got in. The tub was big enough for them to float side by side in the bubbles as the jets stirred the water. They were still very high when they got into bed, so they made love one more time before they fell asleep in each other's arms.

The morning sun came streaming in the next day. They got up, and Dave called room service for their breakfast to be served on the balcony. It was a perfect day for breakfast on the balcony overlooking the city. They had eggs Benedict, hash browns, muffins, coffee, and orange juice. They added the leftover Champagne to the orange juice to make mimosas. There were little chocolates for dessert. After breakfast, they were back in the Jacuzzi, which led to morning sex, followed by another round in the Jacuzzi, then they got dressed, gathered up and packed their things and checked out.

When they returned to her house, Sharon helped Dave carry their stuff inside. The dining room table was covered with gifts from their friends. Her mother was gone, Helen and Linda were gone, so they had the house to themselves. "I want to spend the afternoon in the park. We can fly my kite and have a picnic with the fruit basket. I can open the presents from Bob and Phil, then there is something I want to discuss with you." They changed into shorts, T-shirts, and sandals, and Sharon bustled around putting things together to go to the park: her kite, a blanket, the fruit basket, some waters, a bottle of wine, and the boxes from Bob and Phil.

"Let's go. I don't want to waste our first day of married life." She skipped out the door leading Dave by the hand.

Sharon was happy and as carefree as any little girl excited to go to the park and fly her kite. She was a beautiful, hot woman—a stone-cold fox men could not resist, yet she was as innocent as a child who liked to play and enjoy things in an uncomplicated simple way. As he helped her get the kite up, it was hard for him to believe she was the same sensual, sexual woman who carried him to the heights of carnal pleasure.

Once the kite was up, Dave staked it out. They spread the blanket out and lay down on their sides propped up on their elbows facing each other with the fruit basket between them. They nibbled fruit, sipped wine, watched the kite, and basked in the warm soft sunshine until Sharon sat up to open the boxes.

Bob and Phil had given her a small wedding trousseau with a nighty, panties, a casual outfit, and a nice dress. Then she lay down with Dave and snuggled into his arms. "Dave, we agreed to never get married, and now we are married." She sat up and looked across the park at the houses. "So much has changed in the last year." Her mood saddened as she looked at the houses that had once been so full of people and life, hosting great parties and the events that had changed her life. George was at Duke with the grad student; Connie and Harven left for the Bay Area that morning; Henry was living downtown with Sigrid; Mike was the only one left in the Park house, and she didn't care what happened to him; Caroline and Ron lived in New York; Audrey and Jake were living in Jake's old apartment waiting to see where he would be based with his promotion; Helen and Linda were moving to an apartment together near the airport; in a few days, she and Dave would be on the road for LA. In her heart, she wanted to see Bob and Phil coming across from the houses with some wine to join them, but she knew they were at their store.

She lay back down. "Something else has changed. I told you I didn't want to have children, and I know we agreed on that, but now I want to have a child." A small knot of fear appeared in Dave's chest. "In two years, you will finish your residency, and I will have my MBA. It will take another year for you to establish your practice and for us to buy a house, and then I want to have a child. I don't want to be any older than that when I get pregnant." She leaned up on her elbow and

A love story and social commentary

looked at Dave. "Dave, I had a lot of time to think when I was sick. Knowing I almost died changed a lot of things for me. I realized if I died, there would be nothing left of me, no part of me left in this world. It would be like I never existed. If we have a child, there will be some part of us left when we are gone." She lay back down and put her head on his chest. "You said it. We have a biological obligation to propagate. That is the only real reason we are here. Our lives would be forever unfulfilled if we failed in that obligation. That is why the sex drive is so strong, why sex feels so good, and why it is so much fun." She laughed. "We have to do this, we have no choice, and we will be a family, a real family, a family of our own." She sat up. "Something deep inside me wants to be a mother, and I cannot deny that drive and desire. I have to do it, or I will never truly be happy and fulfilled."

Dave sat up beside her and put his arms around her. He was terrified. He knew she was right, yet he knew he would continue to be terrified until she and the child were safe. Putting her at risk and the risk having a child with a problem galvanized him with fear, but the thought of having his own family filled him with a sense of joy. "Jesus Christ, Sharon, it scares the hell out of me, but if that is what you want, I want it too, but God, you have to be alright and the child has to be alright." The risk was more than he could take, but the reward was more than they could forego.

They spent the rest of the afternoon enjoying the warm day, talking, cuddling, and watching the kite in the clear blue cloudless sky as they snacked on the fruit and drank the wine. When they went in, the house felt empty and lonely. Sharon knew she could not be happy now until she was in her own place—their home in Santa Monica. The time of her time had come and gone, she needed to move on to her future—a future where the gang was not her family anymore because she and Dave would have their own family. The gang would simply be a circle of close friends. For Sharon, the day had been an ending and a new beginning.

Dave went back for his last few shifts in the Pedi ER, marking time, already having moved on in his mind, ready for what came next. Then on his last shift, a child was admitted to the ER with exactly the same defects and deformities his sister had, only they weren't as severe, so not only had the child survived, but she could walk, albeit with difficulty, and talk again with impairment, but she was functional, and her cognitive abilities were normal. Dave had always suspected that mentally, his sister had been normal, and that was one of the things that made it so bad, knowing she could feel and perceive.

The child had gotten into poison oak and had the typical irritated rash on one of her legs. It was not the fact she had poison oak and needed a prescription for a topical steroid that affected Dave; it was the fact that she was a happy, normal acting child, interacting with her mother and others as if there was nothing wrong with her. What struck Dave was her relationship with her mother. It was obvious her mother loved her, and that love overcame any physical issues she had and gave her the emotional support she needed to deal with others as if she were totally normal. It was as if her mother's love had emotionally healed her physical defects. This child's behavior let Dave see the power of love in healing.

His whole interaction with the child and her mother was very powerful. The encounter made him understand the realities of human existence. The search for understanding was a mental exercise he needed to carry on, because through that search, he would learn how to make things better. But in the practical day-to-day management of his life and the practice of medicine, it did not matter; the only thing that mattered was an analytic, thoughtful, careful, data-driven approach that led to a solution to the problem in an unemotional results-driven manner—work the problem, solve it, and make it better. Figure out the right thing to do, then do it, and never give up hope or underestimate the power of love.

As Dave drove to Sharon's house the next morning, he felt a sense of relief, not only because his internship was over, but because he finally felt he understood things. Like iron is forged, hardened, and hammered into steel, a tougher product that could better perform tasks and withstand usage, he had been hardened and hammered into a better version of himself in order to become a physician. As it had many times in the past year, Invictus came to him again. "I thank whatever gods may be for my unconquerable soul…. My head is bloody but unbowed….. I am master of my fate: I am captain of my soul."

Dave knew at the bottom of it all, the only things mankind had were love and hope. You had to have hope in order to carry on in face of the pathos of the human condition, and love gave you that hope. He could not wait to see Sharon; he could not wait to get on the road to LA and to their future together—a future filled with love and hope.

Epilogue

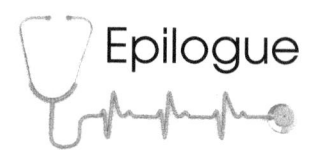

We've arranged a society on science and technology in which nobody understands anything about science and technology, and this combustible mixture of ignorance and power sooner or later is going to blow up in our faces. I mean, who is running the science and technology in a democracy if the people don't know anything about it? Science is more than a body of knowledge, it's a way of thinking. If we are not able to ask skeptical questions to interrogate those who tell us something is true, to be skeptical of those in authority, then we're up for grabs for the next charlatan political or religious leader who comes ambling along. It's a thing that Jefferson lay great stress on. It wasn't enough, he said, to enshrine some rights in the Constitution and the Bill of Rights, the people had to be educated and they have to practice their skepticism and their education. Otherwise, we don't run the government, the government runs us.

—Carl Sagan

The US ranks twenty seventh in the world in education, and medical education falls somewhere in that dismal ranking. Traditional postgraduate medical training started with an internship. The term "intern" was derived from the fact that the doctor was interred in the hospital for a period of one year. By being present in the hospital constantly, the intern was exposed to the maximum number of cases and training experiences possible. If a physician specialized, then a residency was done in that specialty. The term "residency" was derived from the fact that the physician lived in the hospital or was a resident of the hospital during the training period.

By the time of this story, things had already changed. The intern was no longer interred in the hospital, and the resident no longer lived in the hospital, although both spent the majority of their time there. Straight internships were leading directly to residencies because the number of cases necessary to become proficient in a field had increased to the point where another year of training was needed. The internship year was appropriated by the specialties and broad-based rotating internships were phased out.

Reforms were instituted to protect doctors in training. These reforms reversed the trend toward increased physician training and markedly decreased the number of cases and training experiences doctors were exposed to during internship and residency. This resulted in interns and residents not seeing the number of cases or doing the number of procedures necessary to become well trained and competent in their field.

The problem was further exacerbated by medical schools becoming businesses in order to stay financially viable. Their focus shifted away from producing well-trained, competent physicians toward being successful health care plans with good patient retention and earnings.

Next, the advent of technology changed medical training. Order the right test and imaging studies to get the correct diagnosis then use the best practice guidelines to institute the proper treatment. The role of the physician was diminished to that of a provider. But what about critical thinking and judgment? They are not in the computer program; they have to come from the physician. Healing is and always has been an art as well as a science. The human factor, the art of healing, has been lost in the technology. If this cookbook method of one-shoe-fits-all and the current training methods worked, why is the US ranked eleventh in the world in health care?

Where is the outcry, where is the anger, where is the outrage? The richest country in the world is twenty-seventh in education and eleventh in health care! The most important thing a human being has is their life. Why are people not up in arms about the state of health care in this country? Our foundation is life, liberty, and the pursuit of happiness—good health care prolongs life; there is no liberty without the good health to enjoy it, or any happiness in the face of poor health. Health care should be the number one priority of our society. Good health care depends on education to produce adequately trained physicians.

Today, our medical schools are not training institutions; they are businesses like Harvard Medical and Stanford Medical. Their goals have shifted from medical education to patient retention and earnings. They are not producing physicians; they are producing Dr. Feel Good, a provider concerned about patient retention and profit who will do whatever it takes to meet those goals, including over-prescribing opioids. The prescribing behavior of doctors led to the opioid epidemic.

Adding to the problems with medical education and training, drug companies now fund the drug trials for their new drugs at medical schools and training institutions. The trials are no longer funded by impartial government grants. Medical schools need the funds from these trials, so Big Pharma has leverage over them and the outcome. Profit drives a drug company's behavior, not concerns for humanity. They have co-opted medical schools and training institutions into their business model.

This country needs to wake up to the fact that money and material goods are not the most important things in life; one's life and health are the most valuable things one possesses. You can't take money and material things with you if you die due to poor health care.

> "*I have never seen a hearse with a luggage rack on it.*"
> —Don Henley

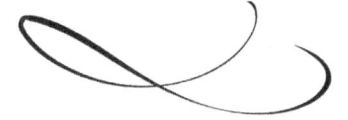

Essay on Health Care in the U.S.

A doctor refuses to refer a patient to a specialist, even though the patient asked to be referred. This "gate keeping" is meant to hold costs down.

Tests are withheld by the doctor, decreasing overhead for the health plan by doing a minimum work-up.

The doctor is on the computer, treating the chart and not the patient, failing to listen to the patient and missing important information.

The patient gets a poor outcome because too much cost would be incurred to treat the patient properly, or what is needed is not covered by insurance and the patient cannot afford the out-of-pocket costs necessary for the proper treatment.

The case is botched because the doctor is poorly trained, incompetent, or disengaged with the patient because postgraduate training hospitals and medical schools have become businesses instead of institutes of higher learning.

Lives are lost because decisions are made by business people rather than medical personnel. Physicians are simply employees in a business model.

The list of problems is endless. The business of health care is failing because health care should not be a business.

Health care in the United States was assassinated by the country's politicians. The hit was carried out by presidents, the Senate, and the House of Representatives, but it was ordered by the powerful, wealthy, oligarchical elite who control this country. Once the contract on health care was ordered, the politicians were facilitated in their murderous act by corporate greed and business interests eager to add fuel to the funeral pyre and fan the flames.

Those in power, the movers and shakers, the titans of business, the corporate oligarchs, the decision-makers, came to the conclusion that too much of the gross domestic product was being spent on health care and the cost of health care was rising too quickly. The American people were spending too much of their output on taking care of themselves and prolonging their lives. Money spent on health care did not benefit consumerism, businesses, and the military industrial complex. There was no limit to the amount of money the U.S. was willing to spend on endless wars, being fought for no valid reason, with no achievable end point because it supported American industry and its industrialists. The sky was the limit where killing people was concerned, but spending to relieve suffering, to prevent disability, and to prolong life needed to be curtailed. Health care's escalating costs were impinging on corporate America's profits. After all, the business of America is business.

Harvard MBAs examined the situation and came to this conclusion: the doctors were the problem. The greedy doctors were charging too much and making too much money. Humans beings see things through their own paradigm, and they evaluate everything based on their own experiences. An honest person thinks everyone is honest; a liar believes everyone lies. The Harvard MBAs thought doctors were being greedy because the markets they worked in were driven by greed. They decided the solution was simple: apply the basic principle of supply and demand. There were too few doctors demanding too much money. Make more doctors to increase the supply, and that would drive down the demand, decreasing what doctors could charge, and consequently controlling the escalating cost of health care.

There were two fallacies in their thinking. Doctors are a large part of health care costs, but whether there are too few doctors charging too much or more doctors charging less, the overall cost remains the same because it is driven by patients' needs. The continuing escalation of health care costs weren't being caused by doctors. Technology and science were the main factors in the equation. CT scanners, MRI scanners, the ever-evolving advances in medical equipment, new methodology demanding new technical devices, new testing, new drugs, and the advancements in the science of medicine in general were causing the increasing costs. Drugs are twenty percent of health care costs, more than the cost of maintaining the bricks and mortar of the hospitals and clinics used to administer patient care. Big pharma was one of the problems, but big pharma is part of the business community, and the business community had to be protected. The advancement in the ability to better relieve suffering, to prevent disability, and to prolong life was costing more. But Harvard MBAs missed the point and focused on doctors.

The idea was that making more doctors would solve the problem, so the number of medical schools and the size of their classes were increased. Increasing the number of medical schools resulted in decreasing the quality of the schools and their facility. Increasing the size of medical school classes decreased the quality of the applicants the school accepted. Both resulted in a decrease in the quality of graduates the schools produced. The outcome of this approach was that the costs of health care kept escalating at an accelerated rate, but the quality of those administering it decreased.

Because the costs continued to spiral out of control, the door was open for more Draconian measures. Health care was turned over to the private sector and became a business. So now Americans pay more for health care and get less than any other country in the world. Plus, the quality of health care in this country has fallen below almost all other industrialized nations. The final blow came when drug companies were allowed to advertise and market directly to patients. Drug companies can advertise chemotherapy drugs directly to cancer patients desperate for a cure encouraging those patients to try their drug. But the most outrageous action of the drug companies is their marketing to the mentally ill. Schizophrenia is a psychosis and is defined as a loss of contact with reality, yet drug companies are marketing directly to schizophrenics. The illness is very difficult to treat and patients constantly stop taking their meds, but the drug companies are marketing directly to them in order to get them to change their medication to increase profits regardless of the outcome that produces. Bipolar disorder is another mental illness drug companies are making harder to treat to increase their profits. Bipolar patients also constantly stop taking their meds. By marketing directly to them, drug companies are giving bipolar patients a reason to get off their meds to try a new drug. Prescription medications should be prescribed by doctors, not patients, and they should be marketed to doctors, not patients.

Yet big pharma has gone even further. Drug companies were found guilty of paying unethical doctors to prescribe addicting narcotics to patients to get them hooked on their meds to increase the drug's usage in order to increase their profits. The doctors were nothing more than drug pushers, and the drug companies were no better than drug cartels. They combined to produce the opioid epidemic that has ravaged our country, destroying families and taking lives. All this has been done in the name of business in order to make more money for corporate executives and wealthy shareholders.

This entire process has been orchestrated by the country's self-serving politicians in an unending attempt to force health care into a corporate entity that serves business interests and not the populous. The end result of their frankly evil effort is the disaster we face today in health care. Costs are still escalating at an even more alarming rate because corporate executives and shareholders must make as much as possible out of the business of health care. Quality is sinking at an astonishing pace because of the failure of medical education and training in a corporate atmosphere at the teaching hospitals coupled with the diminished number of cases in the humane training programs of today. The population of the country is receiving overpriced substandard care or no care at all.

Health care should not be a business, and it had never been a business until it became one in this country. Even our medical schools are businesses now. Medical school is not only about education and training; it is a rite of passage. It is a trial to weed out the unworthy and a baptismal for those who make the grade. It is the foundation a doctor stands on for their entire career. That foundation must be solid for a society to have good physicians, and good health care in any society depends on good physicians. The population is growing, and as it grows, more doctors are needed to serve it, but those doctors need to be properly educated and trained in order to serve society well. It is not only a numbers game; it must also be a quality game.

There are solutions to the problems with health care in the US, but politicians and the medical profession have to have the political will to address the problems and to solve them for those they serve and not for the special interests vested in the health care industry, corporate or business interest, political party ideation, or their own self-serving need to stay in office. The failure of the health care system in this country is primarily due to the failure of the political system and its politicians. Until the voters stop voting against their own self-interest and in favor of dogma or emotional issues that do not affect them directly, the critical changes that need to be made will be left unaddressed.

Two simple changes to medical education and training could solve the problem of physician quality. The medical school curriculum could be changed to eliminate the majority of courses in the basic science years by pushing those courses down to the college level and making them prerequisites for medical school. That would free up time for the senior year of medical school to replace the internship year in training. The number of cases the doctor in training would be exposed to could be increased without the time constraints that forced the untenable approach of the old system. The specialties could be further subdivided to narrower fields requiring fewer cases to become adequately trained and competent. Internal Medicine could become Hospital Care, Elder Care, and Clinical Care. The same could be done for the other specialties. Medical school could be standardized to teach the same courses, and tests could be developed to be given to all students to determine if they are ready to advance. A baseline for physician quality could be established, maintained, and monitored.

The health care system could be modified to mimic the best of the systems in other countries. The US doesn't need to reinvent the wheel. It can pick and choose the best parts of other countries' wheels. A hybrid tiered system seems to work best. The lowest income levels would be covered by a national insurance reimbursement system. As income levels rise the part covered by this national insurance would decrease and the part covered by the individual and/or employer through private or privatized socialized programs would rise. The employer's part of that cost would decrease as the employee's income rose. Doctors and hospitalized would be free to operate as doctors and hospitals, not as businesses or corporate entities.

Certainly, there are other solutions to the problems, but those solutions must be based on what is best for the country's citizens, not what is best for corporate America, business, political parties, or individual politicians. The citizens of the richest country in the world deserve the best health care in the world. To have the best health care in the world, those citizens must be willing to pay for it, and the politicians must be willing to give it to them.

A love story and social commentary

Modern Hippocratic Oath

"I swear to fulfill, to the best of my ability and judgment, this covenant:

I will respect the hard-won scientific gains of those physicians in whose steps I walk, and gladly share such knowledge as is mine with those who are to follow.

I will apply, for the benefit of the sick, all measures that are required, avoiding those twin traps of overtreatment and therapeutic nihilism.

I will remember that there is art to medicine as well as science, and that warmth, sympathy, and understanding may outweigh the surgeon's knife or the chemist's drug.

I will not be ashamed to say "I know not," nor will I fail to call in my colleagues when the skills of another are needed for a patient's recovery.

I will respect the privacy of my patients, for their problems are not disclosed to me that the world may know.

Most especially must I tread with care in matters of life and death. If it is given me to save a life, all thanks. But it may also be within my power to take a life; this awesome responsibility must be faced with great humbleness and awareness of my own frailty.

Above all, I must not play at God.

I will remember that I do not treat a fever chart, a cancerous growth, but a sick human being, whose illness may affect the person's family and economic stability. My responsibility includes these related problems, if I am to care adequately for the sick.

I will prevent disease whenever I can, for prevention is preferable to cure.

I will remember that I remain a member of society, with special obligations to all my fellow human beings, those sound of mind and body as well as the infirm.

If I do not violate this oath, may I enjoy life and art, respected while I live and remembered with affection thereafter.

May I always act so as to preserve the finest traditions of my calling and may I long experience the joy of healing those who seek my help."

Ancient Oath Translation by W.H.S. Jones
(originally written by Hippocrates).

I swear by Apollo the Healer, by Asclepius, by Hygieia, by Panacea, and by all the gods and goddesses, making them my witnesses, that I will carry out, according to my ability and judgment, this oath and this indenture.

To hold my teacher in this art equal to my own parents; to make him partner in my livelihood; when he is in need of money to share mine with him; to consider his family as my own brothers, and to teach them this art, if they want to learn it, without fee or indenture; to impart precept, oral instruction, and all other instruction to my own sons, the sons of my teacher, and to indentured pupils who have taken the Healer's oath, but to nobody else.

I will use those dietary regimens which will benefit my patients according to my greatest ability and judgment, and I will do no harm or injustice to them. Neither will I administer a poison to anybody when asked to do so, nor will I suggest such a course. Similarly, I will not give to a woman a pessary to cause abortion. But I will keep pure and holy both my life and my art. I will not use the knife, not even, verily, on sufferers from stone, but I will give place to such as are craftsmen therein.

Into whatsoever houses I enter, I will enter to help the sick, and I will abstain from all intentional wrong-doing and harm, especially from abusing the bodies of man or woman, bond or free. And whatsoever I shall see or hear in the course of my profession, as well as outside my profession in my intercourse with men, if it be what should not be published abroad, I will never divulge, holding such things to be holy secrets.

Now if I carry out this oath, and break it not, may I gain for ever reputation among all men for my life and for my art; but if I break it and forswear myself, may the opposite befall me.

Let me remind you, "Ask not for whom the bell tolls, it tolls for thee."

About the Author

The author has a B.S. in biology, an M.D. degree, and three years of postgraduate training – Internship and Residency. He is Board Certified and practiced medicine for thirty-two years, serving as a hospital Chief of Staff, Vice Chief of Staff, and on multiple hospital committees, including appointments as the project leader for programs analyzing old systems and developing new systems to improve quality, decrease cost, and improve efficiency for a large medical group. He was a volunteer facility member for two medical schools and trained both medical students and residents, as well as nurse practitioners.

He has served his community as a high school team physician, was elected to four county boards, and was on the board of directors for two nonprofits; one for hospice care and one for environmental preservation.

He is married and has two adult children with his wife of almost fifty years and one grandchild. He is retired and lives in Northern California.

CPSIA information can be obtained
at www.ICGtesting.com
Printed in the USA
FSHW020051140521
81272FS